Lecture Notes:
General Surgery

Companion website

The book is supported by a website containing a free bank of interactive questions and answers. These can be found at:

www.testgeneralsurgery.com

The website includes:
- Interactive Multiple-Choice Questions for each chapter
- Interactive Short Answer Questions for each chapter

Lecture Notes:
General Surgery

Harold Ellis

CBE DM MCh FRCS
Emeritus Professor of Surgery, Guy's Hospital, London

Sir Roy Calne

MS FRCS FRS
Emeritus Professor of Surgery, Addenbrooke's Hospital, Cambridge

Christopher Watson

MD BChir FRCS
Reader in Surgery and Honorary Consultant, Addenbrooke's Hospital,
Cambridge

Twelfth Edition

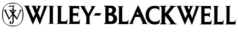

A John Wiley & Sons, Ltd., Publication

This edition first published 2011© 1965, 1968, 1970, 1972, 1977, 1983, 1987, 1993, 1998, 2002, 2006, 2011 © 2011 Harold Ellis, Sir Roy Y. Calne, Christopher J. E. Watson

Blackwell Publishing was acquired by John Wiley & Sons in February 2007. Blackwell's publishing program has been merged with Wiley's global Scientific, Technical and Medical business to form Wiley-Blackwell.

Registered office: John Wiley & Sons Ltd, The Atrium, Southern Gate, Chichester, West Sussex, PO19 8SQ, UK

Editorial offices: 9600 Garsington Road, Oxford, OX4 2DQ, UK
              The Atrium, Southern Gate, Chichester, West Sussex, PO19 8SQ, UK
              111 River Street, Hoboken, NJ 07030-5774, USA

For details of our global editorial offices, for customer services and for information about how to apply for permission to reuse the copyright material in this book please see our website at www.wiley.com/wiley-blackwell

The right of the author to be identified as the author of this work has been asserted in accordance with the UK Copyright, Designs and Patents Act 1988.

First published 1965   Fifth edition 1977   Ninth edition 1998
Revised edition 1966   Sixth edition 1983   Reprinted 1999, 2000
Second edition 1968   Reprinted 1984, 1985, 1986   Tenth edition 2002
Third edition 1970   Seventh edition 1987   Reprinted 2003, 2004, 2005
Fourth edition 1972   Reprinted 1989 (twice)   Eleventh edition 2006
Reprinted 1974   Eighth edition 1993   Twelfth Edition 2010
Revised reprint 1976   Reprinted 1994, 1996

Greek edition 1968
Portuguese edition 1979
Indonesian edition 1990
Turkish edition 2005

Wiley also publishes its books in a variety of electronic formats. Some content that appears in print may not be available in electronic books.

Designations used by companies to distinguish their products are often claimed as trademarks. All brand names and product names used in this book are trade names, service marks, trademarks or registered trademarks of their respective owners. The publisher is not associated with any product or vendor mentioned in this book. This publication is designed to provide accurate and authoritative information in regard to the subject matter covered. It is sold on the understanding that the publisher is not engaged in rendering professional services. If professional advice or other expert assistance is required, the services of a competent professional should be sought.

Library of Congress Cataloging-in-Publication Data

Ellis, Harold, 1926–
      Lecture notes. General surgery / Harold Ellis, Sir Roy Calne, Christopher Watson. – 12th ed.
         p. ; cm.
      General surgery
      Includes bibliographical references and index.
      ISBN 978-1-4443-3440-1 (pbk. : alk. paper)
   1. Surgery. I. Calne, Roy Yorke. II. Watson, Christopher J. E. (Christopher John Edward) III. Title. IV. Title: General surgery.
      [DNLM: 1. Surgical Procedures, Operative. WO 100]
      RD31.E4 2011
      617–dc22
                                                        2010036446

A catalogue record for this book is available from the British Library.

Set in 8.5/11pt Utopia by Toppan Best-set Premedia Limited
Printed and bound in Malaysia by Vivar Printing Sdn Bhd

03 2013

Contents

Companion website

The book is supported by a website containing a free bank of interactive questions and answers. These can be found at:

www.testgeneralsurgery.com

The website includes:
- Interactive Multiple-Choice Questions for each chapter
- Interactive Short Answer Questions for each chapter

Introduction

The ideal medical student at the end of the clinical course will have written his or her own textbook – a digest of the lectures and tutorials assiduously attended and of the textbooks meticulously read. Unfortunately, few students are perfect, and most approach the qualifying examinations depressed by the thought of the thousands of pages of excellent and exhaustive textbooks wherein lies the wisdom required of them by the examiners.

We believe that there is a serious need in these days of widening knowledge and expanding syllabus for a book that will set out briefly the important facts in general surgery that are classified, analysed and as far as possible rationalized for the revision student. These lecture notes represent our own final-year teaching; they are in no way a substitute for the standard textbooks but are our attempts to draw together in some sort of logical way the fundamentals of general surgery.

Because this book is written at student level, principles of treatment only are presented, not details of surgical technique.

The need after only 4 years for a new, 12th, edition reflects the rapid changes which are taking place in surgical practice. We are confident that our constant updating will ensure that this volume will continue to serve the requirements of our medical students. We advise you to read this book in conjunction with *Clinical Cases Uncovered – Surgery*, which provides illustrated case studies, MCQs, EMQs and SAQs, cases that correspond to the chapters in this volume.

H.E.
R.Y.C.
C.J.E.W.

Acknowledgements

We are grateful to our colleagues – registrars, housemen and students – who have read and criticized this text during its production, and to many readers and reviewers for their constructive criticisms. In particular, we are indebted to Simon Dwerryhouse (Chapters 20 and 21); Justin Davies (Chapters 22, 23 and 25); Gordon Wishart (Chapters 35, 37 and 38); Neville Jamieson (Chapters 30–33 and 40); Kathryn Nash (Chapters 21 and 30); and Andrew Doble (Chapters 41–46).

Finally, we would like to acknowledge the continued help given by the staff at Wiley Blackwell, in particular to Jane Fallows, who has created some new diagrams and brought colour to others, Rebecca Huxley, who oversaw the production, and Lindsey Williams, who has meticulously steered this edition from text to finished product.

Abbreviations

ABPI	ankle brachial pressure index	HHT	hereditary haemorrhagic telangiectasia
ACE	angiotensin-converting enzyme	HHV	human herpes virus
ACTH	adrenocorticotrophic hormone	HIV	human immunodeficiency virus
ADH	antidiuretic hormone	HLA	human leucocyte antigen
AFP	α-fetoprotein	HPOA	hypertrophic pulmonary osteoarthropathy
AIDS	acquired immune deficiency syndrome	HPV	human papilloma virus
ALP	alkaline phosphatase	HRT	hormone replacement therapy
ALT	alanine transaminase	HTIG	human tetanus immunoglobulin
APACHE	Acute Physiology And Chronic Health Evaluation	ICP	intracranial pressure
		ICSI	intracytoplasmic sperm injection
APUD	amine precursor uptake and decarboxylation	IFN-γ	interferon γ
		IPMN	intraductal papillary mucinous tumour
ASA	American Society of Anesthesiologists	IVC	inferior vena cava
AST	aspartate transaminase	IVF	in vitro fertilization
ATN	acute tubular necrosis	IVU	intravenous urogram
BCG	bacille Calmette–Guérin	JVP	jugular venous pressure
CABG	coronary artery bypass graft	KSHV	Kaposi sarcoma herpes virus
CEA	carcinoembryonic antigen	'KUB'	kidneys, ureters and bladder
CNS	central nervous system	LAD	left anterior descending artery
CRP	C-reactive protein	LCIS	lobular carcinoma in situ
CSF	cerebrospinal fluid	LHRH	luteinizing hormone-releasing hormone
CT	computed tomography	MAG3	mercapto-acetyl triglycine
DCIS	ductal carcinoma in situ	MCN	mucinous cystic neoplasm
DIC	disseminated intravascular coagulopathy	MEN	multiple endocrine neoplasia
DMSA	dimercaptosuccinic acid	MHC	major histocompatibility complex
DOPA	dihydroxyphenyl alanine	MIBG	meta-iodobenzylguanidine
DTC	differentiated thyroid cancer	MIBI	methoxyisobutylisonitrile
DTPA	diethylene triamine pentaacetic acid	MR	magnetic resonance
ECG	electrocardiograph	MRCP	magnetic resonance cholangiopancreatography
EMG	electromyography		
ER	oestrogen receptor	MRSA	meticillin-resistant Staphylococcus aureus
ERCP	endoscopic retrograde cholangiopancreatography	NAFLD	non-alcoholic fatty liver disease
		NPI	Nottingham Prognostic Index
ESBL	extended spectrum beta-lactamase	NSAIDs	non-steroidal anti-inflammatory drugs
ESR	erythrocyte sedimentation rate	NSGCT	non-seminomatous germ cell tumour
ESWL	extracorporeal shock wave lithotripsy	NST	'no special type'
EUS	endoscopic ultrasound	OCP	oral contraceptive pill
FAP	familial adenomatous polyposis	OPG	orthopantomogram
FEV$_1$	forced expiratory volume in 1 second	PET	positron emission tomography
GCS	Glasgow coma scale	PNET	primitive neuroectodermal tumour
GFR	glomerular filtration rate	POSSUM	Physiological and Operative Severity Score for the enUmeration of Mortality and morbidity
GGT	gamma glutamyl transferase		
GLA	gamma linolenic acid		
GTN	glyceryl trinitrate	PSA	prostate-specific antigen
HAART	highly active anti-retroviral treatment	PTA	percutaneous transluminal angioplasty
HbA1c	glycosylated haemoglobin	PTC	percutaneous transhepatic cholangiography
HCC	hepatocellular carcinoma		
HER2	human epidermal growth factor receptor 2	PTCA	percutaneous transluminal coronary angioplasty

PTFE	polytetrafluoroethylene	TIA	transient ischaemic attack
PTH	parathormone	TIPS	transjugular intrahepatic portosystemic
SGOT	serum glutamic oxaloacetic transaminase		shunt
	(synonymous with AST)	TNF	tumour necrosis factor
SGPT	serum glutamic pyruvic transaminase	TOE	transoesophageal echocardiography
	(synonymous with ALT)	TPA	tissue plasminogen activator
SIADH	syndrome of inappropriate antidiuretic	TPN	total parenteral nutrition
	hormone	TSH	thyroid-stimulating hormone
SLE	systemic lupus erythematosus	TUR	transurethral resection
SLN	sentinel lymph node	UW	University of Wisconsin
T3	tri-iodothyronine	VAC	vacuum-assisted closure
T4	tetra-iodothyronine, thyroxine	VATS	video-assisted thoracoscopic surgery
TACE	transarterial chemoembolization	VIP	vasoactive intestinal polypeptide
TCC	transitional cell carcinoma	VRE	vancomycin-resistant *Enterococcus*
TED	thromboembolism deterrent	β-HCG	β-human chorionic gonadotrophin

Surgical strategy

Learning objectives
✓ To understand the principles of taking a clear history, performing an appropriate examination, presenting the findings and formulating a management plan for surgical diagnosis.

✓ To understand the common nomenclature used in surgery.

Students on the surgical team, in dealing with their patients, should recognize the following steps in their patients' management.

1 *History taking.* Listen carefully to the patient's story.
2 *Examination of the patient.*
3 *Writing notes.*
4 *Constructing a differential diagnosis.* Ask the question 'What diagnosis would best explain this clinical picture?'
5 *Special investigations.* Which laboratory and imaging tests are required to confirm or refute the clinical diagnosis?
6 *Management.* Decide on the management of the patient. Remember that this will include reassurance, relief of pain and, as far as possible, allaying the patient's anxiety.

History and examination

The importance of developing clinical skills cannot be overemphasized. Excessive reliance on special investigations and extensive modern imaging (some of which may be quite painful and carry with them their own risks and complications) is to turn your back on the skills necessary

Lecture Notes: General Surgery, 12th edition. © Harold Ellis, Sir Roy Y. Calne and Christopher J. E. Watson. Published 2011 by Blackwell Publishing Ltd.

to become a good clinician. Remember that the patient will be apprehensive and often will be in pain and discomfort. Attending to these is the first task of a good doctor.

The history

The history should be an accurate reflection of what the patient said, not your interpretation of it. Ask open questions such as 'When were you last well?' and 'What happened next?', rather than closed questions such as 'Do you have chest pain?'. If you have a positive finding, do not leave the subject until you know everything there is to know about it. For example, 'When did it start?'; 'What makes it better and what makes it worse?'; 'Where did it start and where did it go?'; 'Did it come and go or was it constant?'. If the symptom is one characterized by bleeding, ask about what sort of blood, when, how much, were there clots, was it mixed in with food/faeces, was it associated with pain? Remember that most patients come to see a surgeon because of pain or bleeding (Table 1.1). You need to be able to find out as much as you can about these presentations.

Keep in mind that the patient has no knowledge of anatomy. He might say 'my stomach hurts', but this may be due to lower chest or periumbilical pain – ask him to point to the site of the pain. Bear in mind that he may be pointing to a site of referred pain, and similarly do not accept 'back pain' without clarifying where in the back – the

Table 1.1 Example of important facts to determine in patients with pain and rectal bleeding

Pain	Rectal bleeding
Exact site	Estimation of amount (often inaccurate)
Radiation	Timing of bleeding
Length of history	Colour – bright red, dark red, black
Periodicity	Accompanying symptoms – pain, vomiting (haematemesis)
Nature – constant/colicky	Associated shock – faintness, etc.
Severity	Blood mixed in stool, lying on surface, on paper, in toilet pan
Relieving and aggravating factors	
Accompanying features (e.g. jaundice, vomiting, haematuria)	

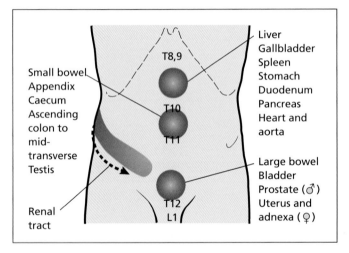

Figure 1.1 Location of referred pain for the abdominal organs.

sacrum, or lumbar, thoracic or cervical spine, or possibly loin or subscapular regions. When referring to the shoulder tip, clarify whether the patient means the acromion; when referring to the shoulder blade, clarify whether this is the angle of the scapula. Such sites of pain may suggest referred pain from the diaphragm and gallbladder, respectively.

It is often useful to consider the viscera in terms of their embryology. Thus, epigastric pain is generally from foregut structures such as stomach, duodenum, liver, gallbladder, spleen and pancreas; periumbilical pain is midgut pain from small bowel and ascending colon, and includes the appendix; suprapubic pain is hindgut pain, originating in the colon, rectum and other struc-

tures of the cloaca such as the bladder, uterus and fallopian tubes (Figure 1.1). Testicular pain may also be periumbilical, reflecting the intra-abdominal origin of these organs before their descent into the scrotum – never be fooled by the child with testicular torsion who complains of pain in the centre of his abdomen.

The examination

Remember the classical quartet in this order:

1 inspection;
2 palpation;
3 percussion;
4 auscultation.

Learn the art of careful inspection, and keep your hands off the patient until you have done so. Inspect the patient generally, as to how he lies and how he breathes. Is he tachypnoeic because of a chest infection or in response to a metabolic acidosis? Look at the patient's hands and feel his pulse.

Only after careful inspection, proceed to palpation. If you are examining the abdomen, ask the patient to cough. This is a surrogate test of rebound tenderness and indicates where the site of inflammation is within the peritoneal cavity. Remember to examine the 'normal' side first, the side that is not symptomatic, be it abdomen, hand, leg or breast. Look at the patient while you palpate. If there is a lump, decide which anatomical plane it lies in. Is it in the skin, in the subcutaneous tissue, in the muscle layer or, in the case of the abdomen, in the underlying cavity? Is the lump pulsatile, expansile or mobile?

Writing your notes

Always write up your findings completely and accurately. Start by recording the date and the time of the interview. Write all the negative as well as positive findings. Avoid abbreviations since they may mean different things to different people; for instance, PID – you may mean pelvic inflammatory disease but the next person might interpret it as a prolapsed intervertebral disc. Use the correct surgical terminology (Table 1.2).

Illustrate your examination unambiguously with drawings – use anatomical reference points and measure the diameter of lumps accurately. When drawing abdominal findings use a hexagonal representation (Figure 1.2). A continuous line implies an edge; shading can represent an area of tenderness or the site where pain is experienced. If you can feel all around a lump, draw a line to indicate this; if you can feel only the upper margin, show only this. Annotate the drawings with your findings (Figure 1.2). At the end of your notes, write a single paragraph summary, and make a diagnosis, or write down a differential diagnosis. Outline a management plan and state what investigations should be done, indicating which you have already arranged. Sign your notes and print your name, position and the time and date legibly underneath.

Case presentation

The purpose of presenting a case is to convey to your colleagues the salient clinical features, diagnosis or differential diagnosis, management and investigations of your patient. The presentation

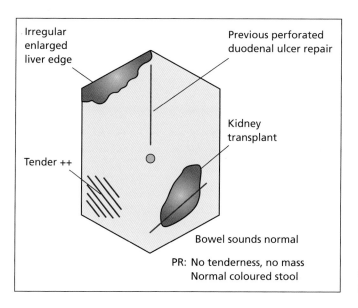

Irregular enlarged liver edge

Previous perforated duodenal ulcer repair

Kidney transplant

Tender ++

Bowel sounds normal

PR: No tenderness, no mass
Normal coloured stool

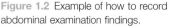

Figure 1.2 Example of how to record abdominal examination findings.

Table 1.2 Common prefixes and suffixes used in surgery

Prefix	Related organ/structure
angio-	blood vessels
arthro-	a joint
cardio-	heart
coelio-	peritoneal cavity
cholecysto-	gallbladder
colo- and colon-	colon
colpo-	vagina
cysto-	urinary bladder
gastro-	stomach
hepato-	liver
hystero-	uterus
laparo-	peritoneal cavity
mammo- and masto-	breast
nephro-	kidney
oophoro-	ovary
orchid-	testicle
rhino-	nose
thoraco-	chest

Suffix	Procedure
-centesis	surgical puncture, often accompanied by drainage, e.g. thoracocentesis
-desis	fusion, e.g. arthrodesis
-ectomy	surgical removal, e.g. colectomy
-oscopy	visual examination, usually through an endoscope, e.g. laparoscopy
-ostomy	creating a new opening (mouth) on the surface, e.g. colostomy
-otomy	surgical incision, e.g. laparotomy
-pexy	surgical fixation, e.g. orchidopexy
-plasty	to mould or reshape, e.g. angioplasty; also to replace with prosthesis, e.g. arthoplasty
-rrhapy	surgically repair or reinforce, e.g. herniorrhaphy

should not be merely a reading of the case notes, but should be succinct and to the point, containing important positive and negative findings. Do not use words such as 'basically', 'essentially' or 'unremarkable', which are padding and meaningless. Avoid saying that things are 'just' palpable – either you can feel it or you cannot. Make up your mind. At the end of a good presentation, the listener should have an excellent word picture of the patient and his/her problems, what needs to be watched and what plans you have for management.

Fluid and electrolyte management

Learning objective
✓ To understand the distribution and composition of body fluids, and how these may change following surgery.

The management of a patient's fluid status is vital to a successful outcome in surgery. This requires preoperative assessment, with resuscitation if required, and postoperative replacement of normal and abnormal losses until the patient can resume a normal diet. This chapter will review the normal state and the mechanisms that maintain homeostasis, and will then discuss the aberrations and their management.

Body fluid compartments (Figure 2.1)

In the 'average' person, water contributes 60% to the total body weight: 42 L for a 70 kg man. Forty per cent of the body weight is intracellular fluid, while the remaining 20% is extracellular. This extracellular fluid can be subdivided into intravascular (5%) and extravascular, or interstitial (15%). Fluid may cross from compartment to compartment by osmosis, which depends on a solute gradient, and filtration, which is the result of a hydrostatic pressure gradient.

The electrolyte composition of each compartment differs. Intracellular fluid has a low sodium and a high potassium concentration. In contrast, extracellular fluid (intravascular and interstitial) has a high sodium and low potassium concentra-

Lecture Notes: General Surgery, 12th edition. © Harold Ellis, Sir Roy Y. Calne and Christopher J. E. Watson. Published 2011 by Blackwell Publishing Ltd.

tion. Only 2% of the total body potassium is in the extracellular fluid. There is also a difference in protein concentration within the extracellular compartment, with the interstitial fluid having a very low concentration compared with the high protein concentration of the intravascular compartment.

Knowledge of fluid compartments and their composition becomes very important when considering fluid replacement. In order to fill the intravascular compartment rapidly, a plasma substitute or blood is the fluid of choice. Such fluids, with high colloid osmotic potential, remain within the intravascular space, in contrast to a saline solution, which rapidly distributes over the entire extravascular compartment, which is four times as large as the intravascular compartment. Thus, of the original 1 L of saline, only 250 mL would remain in the intravascular compartment. Five per cent dextrose, which is water with a small amount of dextrose added to render it isotonic, will redistribute across both intracellular and extracellular spaces.

Fluid and electrolyte losses

In order to calculate daily fluid and electrolyte requirements, the daily losses should be measured or estimated. Fluid is lost from four routes: the kidney, the gastrointestinal tract, the skin and

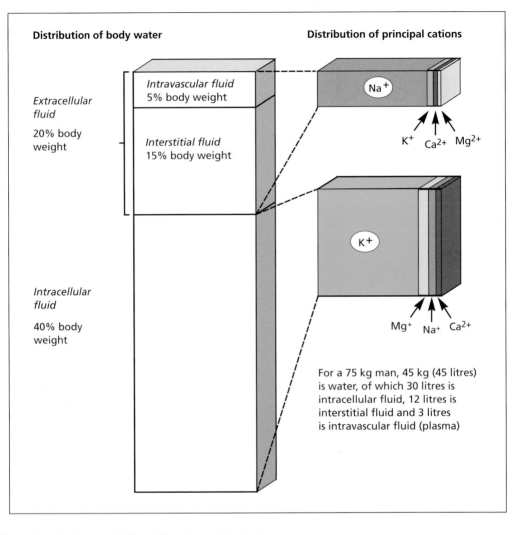

Distribution of body water

Distribution of principal cations

Extracellular fluid

20% body weight

Intravascular fluid
5% body weight

Interstitial fluid
15% body weight

Na$^+$

K$^+$ Ca^{2+} Mg^{2+}

Intracellular fluid

40% body weight

K$^+$

Mg$^+$ Na$^+$ Ca^{2+}

For a 75 kg man, 45 kg (45 litres) is water, of which 30 litres is intracellular fluid, 12 litres is interstitial fluid and 3 litres is intravascular fluid (plasma)

Figure 2.1 Distribution of fluid and electrolytes within the body.

the respiratory tract. Losses from the last two routes are termed insensible losses.

Normal fluid losses (Table 2.1)

The kidney

In the absence of intrinsic renal disease, fluid losses from the kidney are regulated by aldosterone and antidiuretic hormone (ADH). These two hormone systems regulate the circulating volume

Table 2.1 Normal daily fluid losses

Fluid loss	Volume (mL)	Na$^+$ (mmol)	K$^+$ (mmol)
Urine	2000	80–130	60
Faeces	300		
Insensible	400		
Total	2700		

and its osmolarity, and are thus crucial to homeostasis. Aldosterone responds to a fall in glomerular perfusion by salt retention. ADH responds to the increased solute concentration by retaining water in the renal tubules. Normal urinary losses are around 1500–2000 mL/day. The kidneys control water and electrolyte balance closely, and can function in spite of extensive renal disease, and abuse from doctors prescribing intravenous fluids. However, damaged kidneys leave the patient exquisitely vulnerable to inappropriate water and electrolyte administration.

The gastrointestinal tract

The stomach, liver and pancreas secrete a large volume (see Table 2.3) of electrolyte-rich fluid into the gut. After digestion and absorption, the waste material enters the colon, where the remaining water is reabsorbed. Approximately 300 mL is lost into the faeces each day.

Insensible losses

Inspired air is humidified in its passage to the alveoli, and much of this water is lost with expiration. Fluid is also lost from the skin, and the total of these insensible losses is around 700 mL/day. This may be balanced by insensible production of fluid, with around 300 mL of 'metabolic' water being produced endogenously.

Abnormal fluid losses

The kidney

Most of the water filtered by the glomeruli is reabsorbed in the renal tubules so impaired tubular function will result in increased water loss. Resolving acute tubular necrosis (Chapter 41, p. 349), diabetes insipidus and head injury may result in loss of several litres of dilute urine. In contrast, production of ADH by tumours (the syndrome of inappropriate ADH, or SIADH) causes water retention and haemodilution.

The gastrointestinal tract

Loss of water by the gastrointestinal tract is increased in diarrhoea and in the presence of an ileostomy, where colonic water reabsorption is absent.

Vomiting, nasogastric aspiration and fistulous losses result in loss of electrolyte-rich fluid. Disturbance of the acid–base balance may also occur if predominantly acid or alkaline fluid is lost, as occurs with pyloric stenosis and with a pancreatic fistula, respectively.

Large occult losses occur in paralytic ileus and intestinal obstruction. Several litres of fluid may be sequestered in the gut, contributing to the hypovolaemia. Resolution of an ileus is marked by absorption of the fluid and the resultant hypervolaemia produces a diuresis.

Insensible losses

Hyperventilation, as may happen with pain or chest infection, increases respiratory losses. Losses from the skin are increased by pyrexia and sweating, with up to 1 L of sweat per hour in extreme cases. Sweat contains a large amount of salt.

Effects of surgery

ADH is released in response to surgery, conserving water. Hypovolaemia will cause aldosterone secretion and salt retention by the kidney. Potassium is released by damaged tissues, and the potassium level may be further increased by blood transfusion, each unit containing in excess of 20 mmol/L. If renal perfusion is poor, and urine output sparse, this potassium will not be excreted and instead accumulates, the resultant hyperkalaemia causing life-threatening arrhythmias. This is the basis of the recommendation that supplementary potassium may not be necessary in the first 48 hours following surgery or trauma.

Prescribing fluids for the surgical patient

The majority of patients require fluid replacement for only a brief period postoperatively until they resume a normal diet. Some require resuscitation preoperatively, and others require replacement of specific losses such as those from a fistula. In severely ill patients, and those with impaired gastrointestinal function, long-term nutritional support is necessary.

Replacement of normal losses

Table 2.1 shows the normal daily fluid losses. Replacement of this lost fluid in a typical adult is

Table 2.2 Electrolyte content of intravenous fluids

Intravenous infusion	Na$^+$ (mmol/L)	Cl$^-$ (mmol/L)	K$^+$ (mmol/L)	HCO$_3^-$ (mmol/L)	Ca^{2+} (mmol/L)
Normal saline (0.9% saline)	150	150	–	–	–
4% dextrose/ 0.18% saline	30	30	–	–	–
Hartmann's (compound sodium lactate)	131	111	5	29	2
Normal plasma values	134–144	95–105	3.4–5.0	22–30	2.2–2.6

Table 2.3 Daily volume and composition of gastrointestinal fluids

Fluid	Volume (mL)	Na$^+$ (mmol/L)	K$^+$ (mmol/L)	Cl$^-$ (mmol/L)	H$^+$/HCO$_3^-$ (mmol/L)	
Gastric	2500	30–80	5–20	100–150	H$^+$	40–60
Bile	500	130	10	100	HCO$_3^-$	30–50
Pancreatic	1000	130	10	75	HCO$_3^-$	70–110
Small bowel	5000	130	10	90–130	HCO$_3^-$	20–40

achieved by the administration of 3 L of fluid, which may comprise 1 L of normal saline (150 mmol NaCl) together with 2 L of water (as 5% dextrose) (Table 2.2). Potassium may be added to each 1 L bag (20 mmol/L). Alternatively, compound sodium lactate (Hartmann's solution) has been advocated as the more effective fluid replacement in the postoperative period since it is similar in composition to plasma (Table 2.2). Adjustments to this regimen should be based on regular clinical examination, measurement of losses (e.g. urine output), daily weights (to assess fluid changes) and regular blood samples for electrolyte determination. For example, if the patient is anuric, 1 L/day of hypertonic dextrose without potassium may suffice, which has the added advantage of reducing catabolism with the breakdown of protein and accumulation of urea.

Replacement of special losses

Special losses include nasogastric aspirates, losses from fistulae, diarrhoea and stomas and covert losses such as occur with an ileus. Loss of plasma in burns is considered elsewhere (Chapter 8). All fluid losses should be measured carefully when possible, and this volume added to the normal daily requirements. The composition of these special losses varies (Table 2.3) but, as a rough guide, replacement with an equal volume of normal saline should suffice. Extra potassium supplements may be required when losses are high, such as in diarrhoea. Biochemical analysis of the electrolyte content of fistula drainage may be useful.

Resuscitation

Estimation of the fluid deficit in patients is important in order to enable accurate replacement. Thirst, dry mucous membranes, loss of skin turgor, tachycardia and postural hypotension, together with a low jugular venous pressure, suggest a loss of between 5% and 15% of total body water. Fluid losses of under 5% body water are difficult to detect clinically; over 15%, there is marked circulatory collapse.

As an example, consider a 70 kg man presenting with a perforated peptic ulcer. On examination he is noted to have dry mucous membranes, a tachycardia and slight postural fall in arterial blood pressure. If the loss is estimated at 10% of the total body water, itself 60% of body weight, the volume deficit is 10% × 60% of 70 kg, or 10% of 42 L = 4.2 L.

As this loss is largely isotonic (gastric juices and the peritoneal inflammatory response), infusion of a balanced crystalloid solution (e.g. Hartmann's solution) is appropriate. A general rule of thumb is to replace half of the estimated loss quickly, and then reassess before replacement of the rest. The best guide to the success of resuscitation is the resumption of normal urine output; therefore, hourly urine output should be measured. Central venous pressure monitoring will help in the adjustment of the rate of infusion.

Nutrition

Many patients undergoing elective and emergency surgery are reasonably well nourished and do not require special supplementation pre- or postoperatively. Recovery from surgery is usually swift, and the patient resumes a normal diet before he/she has become seriously malnourished. There are, however, certain categories of patients in whom nutrition prior to surgery is poor, and this may be a critical factor in determining the outcome of an operation by lowering their resistance to infection and impairing wound healing. Such patients include those with chronic intestinal fistulae, malabsorption, chronic liver disease, neoplasia and starvation, and those who have undergone chemo- and radiotherapy. Wherever possible in such patients, nutritional support should be instituted before surgery, as postoperative recovery will be much quicker.

Enteral feeding

If the gastrointestinal tract is functioning satisfactorily, oral intake can be supplemented by a basic diet introduced through a fine nasogastric tube directly into the stomach. The constituents of the diet are designed to be readily absorbable protein, fat and carbohydrate. Such a diet can provide 8400 kJ with 70 g protein in a volume of 2 L. The commonest complication is diarrhoea, which is usually self-limiting.

If a prolonged postoperative recovery is anticipated, or a large preoperative nutritional deficit needs to be corrected, consideration should be given to insertion of a feeding jejunostomy at the time of surgery. This has the advantage of avoiding a nasogastric tube.

Parenteral feeding

For patients with intestinal fistulae, prolonged ileus or malabsorption, nutrition cannot be supplemented through the gastrointestinal tract, and therefore parenteral feeding is necessary. This is usually administered via a catheter in a central vein because of the high osmolarity of the solutions used; there is a high risk of phlebitis in smaller veins with lower blood flow. However, peripheral parenteral nutrition with less hyperosmolar solutions can be used for short-term feeding. The principle is to provide the patient with protein in the form of amino acids, carbohydrate in the form of glucose, and fat emulsions such as Intralipid. Energy is derived from the carbohydrate and fat (30–50% fat), which must be given when amino acids are given, usually in a ratio of 1000 kJ/g protein nitrogen. Trace elements, such as zinc, magnesium and copper, as well as vitamins such as vitamin B_{12} and ascorbic acid, and the lipid-soluble vitamins A, D, E and K, are usually added to the fluid, which is infused as a 2.5 L volume over 24 hours. Daily weights as well as biochemical estimations of electrolytes and albumin are useful guides to continued requirements.

The ability of a patient to benefit from intravenous feeding depends on the general state of metabolism and residual liver function. Nutritional support should be continued in the postoperative period until gastrointestinal function returns and the patient is restored to positive nitrogen balance from the perioperative catabolic state. Restoration of a positive nitrogen balance is often apparent to the nurses and doctors as a sudden occurrence, when the patient starts smiling and asks for food. Occasionally, in chronic malnutrition with intestinal fistulae or in patients who have lost most of the small bowel, parenteral feeding may be necessary on a long-term basis.

Complications of total parenteral nutrition (TPN) include sepsis, thrombosis, hyponatraemia, hyperglycaemia and liver damage. To minimize sepsis, the central venous catheter is tunnelled with a subcutaneous Dacron cuff at the exit site to reduce the risk of line infection. Thrombosis may occur on any indwelling venous catheter, and, in patients requiring long-term TPN, this is a major cause of morbidity. Hyperglycaemia is common, particularly following pancreatitis, and may necessitate infusion of insulin.

3

Preoperative assessment

Learning objectives

✓ To be aware of the principles of preoperative assessment.
✓ To be able to identify and manage likely complicating factors prior to surgery.

The preoperative assessment involves an overall analysis of the patient's condition and preparation of the patient for the proposed procedure. This involves taking a careful history, confirming that the indication for surgery still exists (e.g. that the enlarged lymph node that was to be removed for biopsy has not spontaneously regressed), and that the patient is as fit as possible for the procedure. Do not accept someone else's diagnosis – it might be wrong. In particular, verify the proposed side of surgery and mark the side; write the operation name next to the arrow.

Fitness for a procedure needs to be balanced against urgency – there is no point contemplating a referral to a diabetologist for better diabetic control for someone with a ruptured aortic aneurysm in need of urgent repair. The assessment process can be considered in terms of factors specific to the patient and to the operation.

Patient assessment

In assessing a patient's fitness for surgery, it is worth going through the clerking process with this in mind.

History of presenting complaint

An emergency presentation may warrant an emergency procedure, so the assessment aims to iden-

Lecture Notes: General Surgery, 12th edition. © Harold Ellis, Sir Roy Y. Calne and Christopher J. E. Watson. Published 2011 by Blackwell Publishing Ltd.

tify factors that may be a problem during or following surgery. Some problems may be readily identifiable and treated in advance; for example, a history of vomiting or intestinal obstruction would indicate that fluid volume replacement is necessary, and this can be done swiftly prior to surgery. A long history of a condition that is scheduled for elective surgical treatment may afford time in which the patient's comorbid conditions can be improved before surgery.

Past medical history

- *Diabetes* – whether controlled by insulin, oral hypoglycaemics or diet. Severe diabetes may be complicated by gastroparesis with a risk of aspiration on induction of anaesthesia.
- *Respiratory disease* – what is the nature of the chest problem, and is the breathing as good as it can be or is the patient in the middle of an acute exacerbation?
- *Cardiac disease* – has the patient had a recent myocardial infarct, or does he/she have mild stable angina? What is his exercise tolerance?
- *Rheumatoid arthritis* – may be associated with an unstable cervical spine so a cervical spine X-ray is indicated.
- *Rheumatic fever or valve disease* or presence of a prosthesis – necessitating prophylactic antibiotics.
- *Sickle cell disease* – a haemoglobin electrophoresis should be checked in all patients of African–Caribbean descent. Homozygotes are prone to sickle crises under general anaesthetic, and postoperatively if they become hypoxic.

Past surgical history

- *Nature of previous operations* – what has been done before? What is the current anatomy? What problems were encountered last time? Ensure a copy of the previous operation note is available.
- *Complications of previous surgery*, e.g. deep vein thrombosis, MRSA wound infection or wound dehiscence.

Past anaesthetic history

- *Difficult intubation* – usually recorded in the previous anaesthetic note, but the patient may also have been warned of previous problems.
- *Aspiration during anaesthesia* – may suggest delayed gastric emptying (e.g. owing to diabetes), suggesting that a prolonged fast and airway protection (cricoid pressure) are indicated prior to induction.
- *Scoline apnoea* – deficiency of pseudocholinesterase resulting in sustained paralysis following the 'short-acting' muscle relaxant suxamethonium (Scoline). It is usually inherited (autosomal dominant) and so there may be a family history.
- *Malignant hyperpyrexia* – a rapid excessive rise in temperature following exposure to anaesthetic drugs due to an uncontrolled increase in skeletal muscle oxidative metabolism and associated with muscular contractions and rigidity, sometimes progressing to rhabdomyolysis; it carries a high mortality (at least 10%). Most of the cases are due to a mutation in the ryanodine receptor on the sarcoplasmic reticulum, and susceptibility is inherited in an autosomal dominant pattern, so a family history should be sought.

'Social' habits

- *Smoking* – ideally patients should stop smoking before any general anaesthetic to improve their respiratory function and reduce their thrombogenic potential.
- *Alcohol* – a history suggestive of dependency should be sought, and management of the perioperative period instituted using chlordiazepoxide to avoid acute alcohol withdrawal syndrome.
- *Substance abuse* – in particular a history of intravenous drug usage should be sought and

appropriate precautions taken; such patients are a high risk for transmission of hepatitis B, hepatitis C and human immunodeficiency virus (HIV).

Drugs

Most drugs should be continued on admission. In particular, drugs acting on the cardiovascular system should usually be continued and given on the day of surgery. The following are examples of drugs that should give cause for concern and prompt discussion with the surgeon and anaesthetist:

- *Warfarin* – when possible it should be stopped before surgery. If continued anticoagulation is required, then convert to a heparin infusion.
- *Aspirin and clopidogrel* cause increased bleeding and should also be stopped whenever possible at least 10 days before surgery.
- *Oral contraceptive pill* is associated with an increased risk of deep vein thrombosis and pulmonary embolism; it should be stopped at least 6 weeks preoperatively. The patient should be counselled on appropriate alternative contraception since an early pregnancy might be damaged by teratogenic effects of some of the drugs used in the perioperative period.
- *Steroids* – patients who are steroid dependent will need extra glucocorticoid in the form of hydrocortisone injections to tide them over the perioperative stress.
- *Immunosuppression* – patients are more prone to postoperative infection.
- *Diuretics* – both thiazide and loop diuretics cause hypokalaemia. It is important to measure the serum potassium in such patients and restore it to the normal range prior to surgery.
- *Monoamine oxidase inhibitors* are not widely used nowadays, but do have important side-effects such as hypotension when combined with general anaesthesia.

Allergies

It is important to determine clearly the nature of any allergy before condemning a potentially useful drug to the list of allergies. For example, diarrhoea following erythromycin usually reflects its action on the motilin receptor rather than a true allergy, but a skin rash does suggest an allergy such that its use should be avoided. In particular, consider allergies to the following:

- *anaesthetic agents*;
- *antimicrobial drugs*;
- *skin preparation substances*, e.g. iodine;
- *wound dressings*, e.g. Elastoplast.

Management of pre-existing medical conditions

Diabetes

Patients with diet-controlled diabetes require no special preoperative treatment. Patients on oral hypoglycaemics or on subcutaneous insulin should stop therapy the night before, and be commenced on a glucose and insulin infusion. In particular, long-acting insulin preparations should be avoided the night before surgery in order to prevent unexpected intraoperative hypoglycaemia. Patients with diabetes should be placed first on the operating list.

Respiratory disease

Asthma

The degree of respiratory compromise can be readily assessed with a peak flow meter. In addition, patients will know whether their chest is as good as it can be, or whether they are currently having an exacerbation. Some patients with allergic asthma have poor peak flows in summer owing to pollen allergies, but have no problems in winter months. Elective surgery should be planned to avoid the summer in such patients.

Obstructive pulmonary disease

This is often more of a problem, since there is less reversibility and, even at the patient's best, respiratory reserve might be poor. Consider whether the patient will require postoperative ventilation on an intensive care unit, or whether epidural analgesia would be sensible to avoid opiates early postoperatively.

Cardiac disease

Angina is not a contraindication to general anaesthesia provided it is stable. An indication of the severity of angina can be gauged by the frequency with which the patient uses glyceryl trinitrate preparations for acute attacks. High usage is an indication to refer to a cardiologist for improved management. Similarly if the patient has a good exercise tolerance, regularly walking his or her dogs half a mile, for example, it suggests that the cardiac disease is not limiting.

Coronary artery bypass graft (CABG) surgery

Patients who have had successful CABG surgery should have better cardiac function than they had prior to surgery; the same applies following balloon angioplasty and stenting. If CABG surgery was done some time previously, ascertain whether the patient's symptoms have changed, particularly whether there was any recurrence of angina or breathlessness, suggesting that the graft(s) may have thrombosed or the disease progressed.

Routine electrocardiogram (ECG) may detect abnormalities at rest. To rule out significant cardiac disease, consider stressing the heart, such as with an exercise ECG, stress-echocardiogram or radionuclide myocardial perfusion scan. Local anaesthesia should be considered in all patients with a history of cardiac or respiratory disease.

Other problems

Bleeding disorders or anticoagulation

Patients should be managed in close collaboration with the haematology department. Patients with haemophilia A or B should be given the specific clotting factor replacement. Patients on warfarin should be converted to heparin preoperatively. When patients are anticoagulated on account of previous thromboembolic disease, additional prophylaxis should be given, including measures such as thromboembolism deterrent (TED) stockings, intermittent compression boots while on the operating table and early mobilization (when possible with local anaesthesia to facilitate this). Rapid reversal of warfarin may be achieved with clotting factor replacement (human prothrombin complex, e.g. Beriplex) or pooled fresh frozen plasma.

Obstructive jaundice

Patients with obstructive jaundice often have a prolonged prothrombin time and require vitamin K and either human prothrombin complex (e.g. Beriplex) or fresh frozen plasma prior to surgery to correct the abnormality. They are also more prone to infection and poor wound healing. Intraoperatively, it is important to maintain a diuresis with judicious fluid replacement and diuretics (such as mannitol) to prevent acute renal failure (hepatorenal syndrome) to which these patients are susceptible. In the presence of liver impairment, metabolism of some commonly used drugs may be reduced.

Chronic renal failure

Chronic renal failure carries many additional perioperative problems. Electrolyte disturbances, particularly hyperkalaemia, are common and, in the absence of adequate renal function, fluid balance is difficult to achieve. Uraemia impairs platelet function, but the effect can be reversed using desmopressin (DDAVP). Clearance of narcotics is poor and postoperative narcosis should be reversed by the opiate antagonist naloxone, which should be given as a bolus and must be followed by an extended infusion, since the half-life of naloxone is much shorter than that of opiate analgesia. Venous access should be carefully chosen since such patients may have, or may require, arteriovenous dialysis fistulas. In patients with chronic renal failure, avoid using the arm with a fistula *in situ*, and avoid using either cephalic vein. Similarly, central lines should be placed in the internal jugular veins rather than the subclavian veins, since a resultant subclavian vein stenosis could prevent satisfactory fistula function.

Operative factors influencing preoperative management

Nature of the surgery

Some operations require special preparation of the patient, such as bowel preparation prior to colonic surgery or preoperative localization of an impalpable mammographic abnormality prior to breast surgery. Different degrees of fitness are acceptable for different procedures. So, a patient with severe angina might be a candidate for removal of a sebaceous cyst under a local anaesthetic but not for a complex incisional hernia repair under a general anaesthetic. When the surgery will correct the comorbidity, different criteria apply; thus, the same patient with angina would be a candidate for a general anaesthetic if it was given to enable myocardial revascularization with aortocoronary bypass grafts.

Urgency of the surgery

When patients present with life-threatening conditions, the risk–benefit balance often changes in favour of surgical intervention even if there is significant risk attached, but the alternative is probable death; a good example is a patient presenting with a ruptured aortic aneurysm, in whom death is often an immediate alternative to urgent surgery, and there is little time for preoperative preparation.

Objective operative risk assessment

The American Society of Anesthesiologists (ASA) has produced a grading scheme to estimate comorbidity (Table 3.1). Half of all elective surgery will be in patients of grade 1, i.e. normal fit individuals with a minimal risk of death. As the patient's grade increases, reflecting increased comorbidity, the postoperative morbidity and mortality increases. Alternative predictive scoring schemes exist, both in general and tailored for specific operations. The Acute Physiology And Chronic Health Evaluation (APACHE) score looks at different physiological variables (e.g. temperature, blood pressure, heart rate, respiratory rate) to derive a measure of how ill someone is. It is of most use in an ITU setting, and is less useful as a preoperative risk estimation tool. In contrast, the Physiological and Operative Severity Score for the enUmeration of Mortality and morbidity (POSSUM) was developed as a predictive scoring system for surgical mortality and combines information regarding the patient's physiological status and the operative procedure (Table 3.2). A subsequent refinement resulted in P-POSSUM, which is now widely used as an audit tool to compare estimated mortality with actual mortality.

Table 3.1 The ASA grading system

ASA grade	Definition	Typical mortality (%)
I	Normal healthy person, no comorbidity	<0.1
II	Mild systemic disease that does not limit activity	0.3
III	Severe systemic disease that limits activity, but is not incapacitating	2–4
IV	Incapacitating systemic disease which is constantly life-threatening	20–40
V	Not expected to survive 24 hours, with or without surgery	>50

Table 3.2 Factors involved in the estimation of risk using P-POSSUM

Physiological parameters	Operative parameters
Age	Operation severity, e.g. minor, moderate, major
Cardiac disease, e.g. heart failure, angina, cardiomyopathy	Number of procedures
Respiratory disease, e.g. degree of exertional dyspnoea	Operative blood loss
ECG, e.g. presence of arrhythmia	Peritoneal soiling
Systolic blood pressure	Presence of malignancy
Heart rate	Urgency, e.g. elective, urgent, emergency
Leucocyte count	
Haemoglobin concentration	
Urea concentration	
Sodium concentration	
Potassium concentration	
Glasgow coma score	

Postoperative complications

Classification

Any operation carries with it the risk of complications. These can be classified according to the following:

1 Local or general complication.
- *Local* – involving the operation site itself.
- *General* – affecting any of the other systems of the body, e.g. respiratory, urological or cardiovascular complications.
2 Time of occurrence postoperatively.
- *Immediate* – within the first 24 hours.
- *Early* – within the first 30 days.
- *Late* – any subsequent period, often long after the patient has left hospital.
 In addition, when considering the factors contributing to any postoperative complication the following classification should be used:
  - *Preoperative* – factors already existing before the operation is carried out.
  - *Operative* – factors that come into play during the operation itself.

Lecture Notes: General Surgery, 12th edition. © Harold Ellis, Sir Roy Y. Calne and Christopher J. E. Watson. Published 2011 by Blackwell Publishing Ltd.

  - *Postoperative* – factors introduced after the patient's return to the ward.

A useful table of postoperative complications following abdominal surgery is presented in Table 4.1. This scheme can be modified for operations concerning any other system.

Wound infection

The incidence of wound infection after surgical operations is related to the type of operation. The common classification of risk groups is as follows:

1 *Clean* (e.g. hernia repair) – an uninfected operative wound without inflammation and where no viscera are opened. Infection rate is 1% or less.
2 *Clean contaminated* – where a viscus is open but with little or no spillage. Infection rate is less than 10%.
3 *Contaminated* – where there is obvious spillage or obvious inflammatory disease, e.g. a gangrenous appendix. Infection rate is 15–20%.
4 *Dirty or infected* – where there is gross contamination (e.g. a gunshot wound with

Table 4.1 Postoperative complications following abdominal surgery

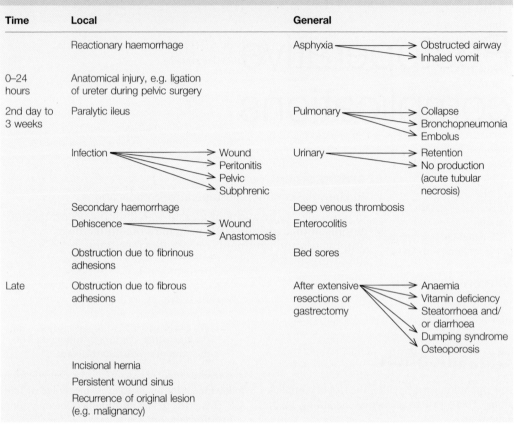

Time	Local	General
	Reactionary haemorrhage	Asphyxia → Obstructed airway / Inhaled vomit
0–24 hours	Anatomical injury, e.g. ligation of ureter during pelvic surgery	
2nd day to 3 weeks	Paralytic ileus	Pulmonary → Collapse / Bronchopneumonia / Embolus
	Infection → Wound / Peritonitis / Pelvic / Subphrenic	Urinary → Retention / No production (acute tubular necrosis)
	Secondary haemorrhage	Deep venous thrombosis
	Dehiscence → Wound / Anastomosis	Enterocolitis
	Obstruction due to fibrinous adhesions	Bed sores
Late	Obstruction due to fibrous adhesions	After extensive resections or gastrectomy → Anaemia / Vitamin deficiency / Steatorrhoea and/or diarrhoea / Dumping syndrome / Osteoporosis
	Incisional hernia	
	Persistent wound sinus	
	Recurrence of original lesion (e.g. malignancy)	

devitalized tissue), or in the presence of frank pus or gross soiling (e.g. a perforated large bowel). Anticipated infection rate up to 40%.

In pre-antibiotic days, the haemolytic *Streptococcus* was feared most, but now, as this is still usually penicillin sensitive, the principal causes of wound infection are the penicillin-resistant *Staphylococcus aureus*, together with *Streptococcus faecalis*, *Pseudomonas*, coliform bacilli and other bowel bacteria including *Bacteroides*. With continued use of antibiotics, more resistant strains of the organisms are appearing, such as the meticillin-resistant *Staphylococcus aureus* (MRSA) and the vancomycin-resistant *Enterococcus* (VRE).

Preoperative factors

1 *Local factors* – pre-existing infection, e.g. a perforated appendix or an infected compound fracture.

2 *General factors* – nasal carriage of staphylococci; concurrent skin infection, e.g. a crop of boils; malnutrition, e.g. gastric carcinoma; immunosuppression.

Operative factors

These are lapses in theatre technique, e.g. failure of adequate sterilization of instruments, the surgeon's hands or dressings. There may be nasal or skin carriers of staphylococci among the nursing and surgical staff. Wound infections are especially common when the alimentary, biliary or urinary tract is opened during surgery, allowing bacterial contamination to occur. Wounds placed in poorly vascularized tissue, such as an amputation stump, are also prone to infection, in particular gas gangrene from anaerobic clostridial contamination, since necrotic tissue is a good medium for bacterial growth.

Postoperative factors

1 *Cross-infection* from elsewhere on the patient's body or from other infected cases in the ward during dressing changes or wound inspection.
2 *New infection* due to contamination of the wound from the nose or hands of the surgical or nursing staff.

The use of basic infection control and hygiene discipline cannot be overstated. Healthcare professionals, be they nurses, doctors, ward clerks or cleaners, have a duty to care for their patients. This includes avoidance of cross-contamination or infection by basic hand washing before touching any patient or whenever entering their bed space, and isolation of any patient infected with a contagious or dangerous organism such as MRSA, VRE, extended spectrum beta-lactamases (ESBL) (see p. 18) or *Clostridium difficile* (see p. 18).

Clinical features

The onset of wound infection is usually a few days after operation; this may be delayed still further, even up to weeks, if antimicrobial chemotherapy has been employed. The patient complains of pain and swelling in the wound and of the general effects of infection (malaise, anorexia, vomiting) and runs a swinging pyrexia. The wound is red, swollen, hot and tender. Removal of sutures or probing of the wound releases the contained pus.

Treatment

Prophylaxis comprises scrupulous theatre and dressing technique, the isolation of infected cases and the elimination of carriers with colds or septic lesions among the medical and nursing staff.

Established infection is treated by drainage; antibiotics are given if there is, in addition, a spreading cellulitis. Open wounds may benefit from use of a negative pressure wound therapy device (vacuum-assisted closure (VAC) system), although direct application onto an open abdomen runs the risk of creating an enteric fistula.

Antimicrobial prophylaxis

Prophylactic antimicrobial chemotherapy ('prophylactic antibiotics') was, in the early days of its use, believed to herald the end of wound infections. Unfortunately, the widespread and prolonged use of antimicrobials resulted in the emergence of resistant strains of bacteria, and side-effects such as diarrhoea and skin rashes.

Principles of antimicrobial prophylaxis

1 *Antimicrobial selection* in order to target the bacterial flora likely to be encountered.
2 *Treatment before contamination* occurs, in order to achieve adequate antimicrobial concentration in the blood at the time of exposure to infection.

Specific examples

- *Valvular heart disease.* In patients with valvular heart disease, commonly rheumatic mitral valve disease, prophylaxis is given against haematogenous bacterial colonization of the valve resulting in infective endocarditis.
- *Implantation or presence of a foreign body.* Where a foreign body such as a prosthetic heart valve or prosthetic joint is implanted, antimicrobials are used to prevent infection of the prosthesis at the time of surgery. The commonest infecting agent is *S. aureus*, therefore the antimicrobial spectrum should cover this organism. The likely presence of MRSA should inform the choice of antimicrobial. Haematogenous spread of an organism during other procedures should also be borne in mind, occurring in a similar manner to infective endocarditis.
- *Vascular surgery.* Used especially where prosthetic material is used and where ischaemia exists.
- *Amputation of an ischaemic limb.* Here the risk of gas gangrene is high, particularly following above-knee amputations where contamination by perineal and faecal organisms may occur: penicillin is the antibiotic of choice.
- *Penetrating wounds and compound fractures.* Penicillin prophylaxis against clostridial infections (metronidazole if penicillin allergic).
- *Organ transplant surgery.* Prophylaxis should be given against wound infection, but also against opportunist viral, fungal and protozoan infections occurring as a consequence of immunosuppression.
- *Where there is a high risk of bacterial contamination.* In operations such as those

that involve opening the biliary or alimentary tract (especially the large bowel), prophylactic systemic broad-spectrum antimicrobials are indicated. In colonic surgery, cover against anaerobic organisms is particularly important and is afforded by metronidazole. Systemic anti-candidal therapy with fluconazole may also be indicated.

Antibiotic-associated enterocolitis: *Clostridium difficile*

Broad-spectrum antibiotics disrupt the normal commensal organisms in the gut, selecting out resistant forms, such as the toxin-producing strains of *C. difficile*. The patient experiences severe watery diarrhoea due to extensive enterocolitis, and the bowel shows mucosal inflammation with pseudomembrane formation – pseudomembranous colitis.

When first described, there was a strong association with preceding lincomycin or clindamycin therapy; today, cephalosporins and co-amoxiclav are the commonest culprits, reflecting their widespread use in clinical practice.

Clinical features

Antibiotic-associated enterocolitis usually occurs in patients who have received broad-spectrum antibiotics. The condition is particularly likely to occur after large-bowel surgery. Mild cases present simply with watery diarrhoea. Severe cases have a cholera-like picture with a sudden onset of profuse, watery diarrhoea with excess mucus, abdominal distension and shock due to the profound fluid loss. Occasionally, *C. difficile* infection may present with a toxic dilatation of the colon.

Sigmoidoscopy reveals a red, friable mucosa with whitish yellow plaques, which may coalesce to form a pseudomembrane. Diagnosis is made by identification of the *C. difficile* toxins (A and B) in the stool.

Recently, a new strain of *C. difficile*, known as type 027, has been detected in the UK, having first been identified in North America. Type 027 produces more toxins and is associated with increased mortality and more relapses.

Treatment

Fluid and electrolyte replacement is essential. Broad-spectrum antibiotics are stopped when possible, and oral metronidazole is prescribed. Oral vancomycin, which is not absorbed from the gut, rapidly eliminates *C. difficile* but is avoided as first-line therapy to prevent the occurrence of vancomycin-resistant enterococci.

C. difficile is highly contagious; so in order to prevent further spread on the ward, scrupulous hand hygiene should be practised and the patient placed in isolation. Spores of *C. difficile* are quite hardy and persist in the environment, resulting in relapse and reinfection unless cleaning practices are thorough.

The best prophylaxis against *C. difficile* infection is the judicious use of antibiotics, avoiding broad-spectrum antibiotics wherever possible.

Meticillin-resistant *Staphylococcus aureus* (MRSA)

Pathology

Most community-acquired species of *S. aureus* are sensitive to flucloxacillin and meticillin (previously called methicillin); increasingly in hospital, the organism is resistant to these and other antibiotics, including cephalosporins and gentamicin. *S. aureus* has a record of developing resistance to antibiotics; for example, most species, whether acquired in hospital or in the community, already possess a beta-lactamase that confers resistance to penicillin. MRSA strains have been increasing in incidence and most remain sensitive to vancomycin, although MRSA species with reduced or no sensitivity to vancomycin (vancomycin-intermediate *S. aureus* (VISA) and vancomycin-resistant *S. aureus* (VRSA)) are now commonly encountered.

Clinical features

MRSA is spread by contact, and scrupulous hand hygiene is a cheap and effective way to reduce infection. Once colonized, it is difficult to clear the organism from patients, particularly if they have a urinary catheter, intravenous cannula or open wound. Typically, the organism causes a local infection in the same way that non-MRSA species do. It is commonly found in sick patients, particularly those on intensive care units who have been on broad-spectrum antibiotics and who are already severely debilitated. MRSA is the cause of 40% of all staphylococcal bacteraemias in the UK, and it is associated with one-fifth of all deaths involving hospital-acquired infection.

One of the reasons for the prevalence of MRSA is the failure of healthcare professionals to follow good infection control practice, such as hand washing. Increased nursing workload has also been shown to correlate with increased infection. Screening of patients and staff for MRSA carriage, with decolonization or isolation of carriers, does reduce infection rates. Such simple practices reduce not only the incidence of MRSA but also infections by other bacteria.

Treatment

Hand hygiene to prevent transmission between patients and intravenous vancomycin to treat those patients with the infection are the principles of management. Infected patients should be isolated, particularly when the organism is in the nose or lungs with the potential for droplet spread.

Colonization of a patient with MRSA is not an indication for treatment, although current or previous history of colonization would alter the choice of antibacterial prophylaxis for surgical procedures to include cover against MRSA. Attempts to eradicate MRSA are worthwhile in patients due to undergo procedures involving implantation of prosthetic material, such as hip replacements and hernia repairs.

Extended spectrum beta-lactamases (ESBL)

While MRSA is one of the most prevalent antibiotic-resistant bacteria, still others exist. One such class of bacteria are the Gram-negative bacteria such as *Klebsiella* and *Escherichia coli* that produce an extended spectrum beta-lactamase, an enzyme that hydrolyses the beta-

lactam ring of beta-lactam antibiotics including second- and third-generation cephalosporins (e.g. cefotaxime) and carbapenems (e.g. meropenem). Most ESBL-producing bacteria are also exceptionally resistant to non-beta-lactam antibiotics such as quinolones and aminoglycosides, the resistance for which is carried and spread to other bacteria by plasmids. As with other resistant organisms, they are commonly found in patients treated with prolonged courses of broad-spectrum antibiotics.

Vancomycin-resistant enterococci (VRE)

Enterococci constitute a significant portion of the normal gut flora. The emergence of resistance of enterococci to vancomycin is an inevitable consequence of the increased usage of vancomycin for prophylaxis and treatment of MRSA, as well as the use of similar drugs in animal foodstuffs to enhance growth. First identified in 1986, VRE is now commonly isolated in patients who have had prolonged admissions with exposure to antibiotics, such as those on intensive care units, transplant units and haematology wards.

At present there are few antibiotics capable of treating VRE, and treatment is best delayed until microbiological sensitivities are known. As with MRSA and ESBL, VRE is best contained by appropriate infection-control measures, such as hand washing and isolation.

Pulmonary collapse and infection

Some degree of pulmonary collapse occurs after almost every abdominal or transthoracic procedure. Mucus is retained in the bronchial tree, blocking the smaller bronchi; the alveolar air is then absorbed, with collapse of the supplied lung segments (usually the basal lobes). The collapsed lung continues to be perfused and acts as a shunt, which reduces oxygenation. The lung segment may become secondarily infected by inhaled or aspirated organisms, and, rarely, abscess formation may occur.

Aetiology

Preoperative factors

- *Pre-existing acute or chronic pulmonary infection* increases the amount of bronchial secretion and adds the extra factor of pathogenic bacteria.
- *Smokers* are at particular risk, with increased secretions and ineffective cilia.
- *Chronic pulmonary disease*, e.g. emphysema.
- *Chest wall disease*, e.g. ankylosing spondylitis, which makes coughing difficult.

Operative factors

- *Anaesthetic drugs* increase mucus secretion and depress the action of the bronchial cilia.
- *Atropine* in addition increases the viscosity of the mucus.

Postoperative factors

- *Pain.* The pain of the thoracic or abdominal incision, which inhibits expectoration of the accumulated bronchial secretions, is the most important cause of mucus retention.

Clinical features

Pulmonary collapse occurs within the first post-operative 48 hours. The patient is dyspnoeic with a rapid pulse and elevated temperature. There may be cyanosis. The patient attempts to cough, but this is painful and, unless encouraged, he or she may fail to expectorate. The sputum is at first frothy and clear, but later may become purulent, diagnostic of secondary infection.

Examination reveals that the patient is distressed, with a typical painful 'fruity cough'. This results from the sound of the bronchial secretions rattling within the chest and a good clinician should be able to make the diagnosis while still several yards away from the patient. The chest movements are diminished, particularly on the affected side; there is basal dullness and air entry is depressed with the addition of coarse crackles.

Pulse oximetry indicates a reduced saturation, and chest X-ray may reveal an opacity of the involved segment (usually basal or mid-zone), together with mediastinal shift to the affected side.

Treatment

- *Preoperatively*, breathing exercises are given, smoking is forbidden and antibiotics prescribed if any chronic respiratory infection is present. Surgery should be postponed when possible until all pre-existing chest infection has resolved.
- *Postoperatively*, the patient is encouraged to cough, and breathing exercises are instituted, usually under the supervision of a physiotherapist. Small repeated doses of opiates diminish the pain of coughing but are insufficient to dull the cough reflex. Epidural anaesthesia and intercostal nerve blocks may help reduce the inhibitory pain of an abdominal or thoracic incision, without affecting the respiratory drive. Antibiotics are prescribed only if the sputum is infected; their selection is based on the sensitivity of the cultured organisms.

Deep vein thrombosis in the lower limb

In the operative and postoperative periods, the patient has an increased predisposition to venous thrombosis in the veins of the calf muscles, the main deep venous channels of the leg and pelvic veins. This predisposition has three main components (Virchow's triad):

1 *Increased thrombotic tendency.* Following blood loss and platelet consumption intraoperatively, more platelets are produced, numbers peaking around day 10. The new platelets have an increased tendency to aggregate. Fibrinogen levels also increase, predisposing to clot formation.
2 *Changes in blood flow.* Increased stagnation within the veins occurs as a result of immobilization on the operating table and postoperatively in bed, and with depression of respiration.
3 *Damage to the vein wall* prompts thrombus formation on the damaged endothelium. The damage may be due to an inflammatory process in the pelvis, or may be produced by pressure of the mattress against the calf or direct damage at operation (particularly the pelvic veins during pelvic procedures) or by disease (e.g. pelvic sepsis).

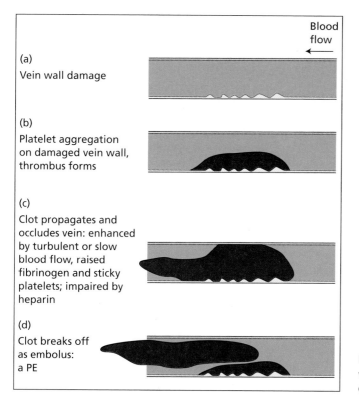

(a)
Vein wall damage

(b)
Platelet aggregation on damaged vein wall, thrombus forms

(c)
Clot propagates and occludes vein: enhanced by turbulent or slow blood flow, raised fibrinogen and sticky platelets; impaired by heparin

(d)
Clot breaks off as embolus: a PE

Blood flow

Figure 4.1 (a–d) Progression of deep vein thrombosis. PE, pulmonary embolus.

Platelets deposit on the damaged endothelium, the vein is occluded by thrombus and a propagated fibrin clot then develops, which may detach and embolize to the lung (a pulmonary embolus, see below; Figure 4.1).

This complication is particularly likely to occur in elderly patients, the obese, those with malignant disease, patients who have a history of previous deep vein thrombosis, those undergoing abdominal, pelvic and particularly hip surgery and women who are taking oestrogen-containing oral contraceptives and hormone replacement tablets. Thrombosis is commonly observed in the deep veins during lower limb amputation for ischaemia, the thrombus resulting from the low flow and immobilization. In addition, some patients may be predisposed to thrombosis because of reduced levels of the endogenous anticoagulants protein C, protein S and antithrombin III, or because they carry the Leiden mutation of coagulation factor V or the prothrombin 20210 mutation.[1]

[1]Factor V Leiden is a G to A substitution at nucleotide 1691 of the factor V gene; the thrombophilic factor II (prothrombin) mutation is G to A at nucleotide 20210.

Clinical features

Deep vein thrombosis can be 'silent', but typically symptoms and signs occur during the second postoperative week, although they may come earlier or later. Studies using radioiodine-labelled fibrinogen, which is deposited as fibrin in the developing thrombus and which can be detected by scanning the leg, suggest that the thrombotic process usually commences during, or soon after, the operation. Earlier thrombosis may occur when a patient has already been immobile in hospital for some time preoperatively.

The patient complains of pain in the calf, and on examination there is tenderness of the calf and swelling of the foot, often with oedema, raised skin temperature and dilatation of the superficial veins of the leg. This is accompanied by a mild pyrexia. If the pelvic veins or the femoral vein are affected, there is massive swelling of the whole lower limb.

Special investigations

- *Duplex scanning*. The course of the iliac and femoral veins can be scanned and filling defects due to thrombi detected. In skilled hands, duplex scanning can detect thrombi in all the major veins at and above the knee, but is less reliable below this. It has the advantage that it is simple and non-invasive.

- *Venography*. This is the definitive investigation but can be neither repeated frequently nor employed for routine screening.
- *^{125}I-labelled fibrinogen*. A highly sensitive test that enables the legs to be scanned at daily intervals. It demonstrates the presence of a deep vein thrombus in approximately one-third of all postoperative patients, with a particularly high incidence in the high-risk groups listed above. Only half of the thrombi picked up on scanning can be detected on careful clinical examination. Owing to scatter from the radioactive iodine excreted in the urine and held in the bladder, the test is unreliable in the pelvic and thigh region and is significant only from the knee downwards.

Management

Prophylaxis

- *Treat avoidable risk factors*. Elective surgery on anyone with a treatable risk factor should be avoided. For example, elective surgery on a patient taking the contraceptive pill should be delayed for 6 weeks (one normal cycle) after stopping the pill.
- *Active mobilization*. Stimulation of blood flow by encouraging early mobilization reduces the risks.
- *Intermittent calf compression* using inflatable cushions wrapped around the lower legs may be used intraoperatively to reduce the incidence of thrombosis.
- *Thromboembolic deterrent (TED) stockings* (graded compression stockings) and elevation of the legs to increase venous return are simple and effective.
- *Subcutaneous low molecular weight heparin injections*, such as enoxaparin, should be started preoperatively and continued while the patient remains at risk. Controlled trials have shown a reduction in the incidence of venous clot formation, with a less certain reduction in pulmonary embolism in the treated groups. These drugs are eliminated by the kidneys and, in the presence of renal failure, factor Xa levels

should be checked to avoid inadvertent over-anticoagulation.

Treatment

In the established case, anticoagulant therapy with an intravenous heparin infusion or subcutaneous low molecular weight heparin is commenced to prevent further propagation of the clot, and to increase fibrinolysis. Once anticoagulated, the patient can be mobilized with the lower limbs supported in elastic stockings to prevent oedema, and initial parenteral anticoagulation can be replaced by oral anticoagulation with warfarin.

The decision to anticoagulate a patient is particularly difficult if thrombosis occurs in the immediate postoperative period, as anticoagulation carries a serious risk of haemorrhage at the operation site. In this setting, a heparin infusion is usually used since the infusion can be immediately discontinued, and its effects reversed with protamine, if bleeding occurs.

If pulmonary embolism occurs in spite of anticoagulation, or when anticoagulation is contraindicated, percutaneous insertion of an umbrella-like filter into the inferior vena cava may be indicated to prevent recurrent episodes of pulmonary embolization. Emboli get caught up in the umbrella rather than in the pulmonary arteries.

Pulmonary embolus

This occurs when a clot from a vein, usually originating in a femoral vein or a pelvic vein (and occasionally in the calf muscles), detaches and travels to the heart to becomes lodged in the pulmonary arterial tree.

Clinical features

The clinical features of pulmonary embolus may vary from dyspnoea or mild pleuritic chest pain to sudden death due to an occlusion of the pulmonary artery trunk. Minor symptoms include pleuritic chest pain, dyspnoea and haemoptysis. Severe dyspnoea may occur with cyanosis and shock, and larger emboli may prompt acute right heart failure and death.

The dyspnoea may be sudden in onset, or progressive as further showers of emboli dislodge. The chest pain is pleuritic, and, when basal lung segments are affected, diaphragmatic irritation may occur and result in shoulder-tip pain. In elderly patients, confusion due to hypoxia may be the presenting symptom. Pulmonary emboli classically occur around the 10th postoperative day. They often occur while straining at stool, as the increased intra-abdominal pressure dislodges a pelvic venous thrombus.

Examination

On examination, the patient is tachypnoeic, often with a spike of fever. There is a tachycardia and a raised jugular venous pressure (JVP) reflecting the pulmonary hypertension. There may be tenderness in the calves at the site of a deep vein thrombosis, but this is not common. Cyanosis may be present if the embolus is large, and a pleural rub may be audible in small and peripherally located emboli.

If the patient survives the embolus, complete clearing of the clot occurs quite rapidly. Infarction of the lung is uncommon because the lungs themselves are perfused via the bronchial arteries. It may occur in those patients with cardiac failure in whom there is pre-existing pulmonary congestion.

Diagnosis of an embolus is often difficult. The main differential diagnosis of a major embolus is a myocardial infarction, while small emboli may be confused with a chest infection.

Special investigations

- *Chest X-ray* in the early stages is often normal, although within a few hours patchy shadowing of the affected segment takes place.
- *Electrocardiogram (ECG)* may help in differentiating pulmonary embolus from myocardial infarction. In the case of an embolus, there may be rhythm changes (atrial fibrillation, heart block) or features of right heart strain (ST segment depression in leads V1 to V3, III and aVF, with right axis deviation), as the heart pumps against the obstructed pulmonary arterial tree. The characteristic 'S1–Q3–T3' pattern (S wave in lead I, with a Q wave and an inverted T wave in lead III) is seldom present.
- *Arterial blood gases* may confirm the hypoxia. Hypocapnia (low CO_2) may also be present secondary to tachypnoea.
- *Ventilation–perfusion scintigraphy (V/Q scan)*. This is a radionuclide technique in which a

radiolabelled inert gas such as krypton-81m is inhaled and its distribution throughout the lung compared with the distribution of intravenously injected technetium-99m-labelled human albumin particles. The albumin particles are trapped in the lung capillaries and their distribution reflects lung perfusion. In a pulmonary embolus, the perfusion scan will show uneven circulation through the lungs, with multiple perfusion defects, but a simultaneous ventilation scan is normal in the absence of pre-existing pulmonary disease (mismatch).
- *Computed tomographic pulmonary angiography (CTPA)* is the definitive diagnostic test used when V/Q scan is unreliable, such as when pulmonary disease is present.

It is important to appreciate that pulmonary embolus may occur without any preceding warning signs of thrombosis in the leg. Indeed, once there are obvious clinical features of deep vein thrombosis, detachment of an organized and adherent clot from this limb is rather unlikely, especially if anticoagulant therapy has been commenced so that fresh clot formation is inhibited. The great majority of fatal pulmonary emboli are unheralded.

Treatment

When the person is in pain, opiate analgesia is given, oxygen is administered and heparin is commenced if the patient is not already on anticoagulants. Lysis of a massive embolus may be effected with an intravenous infusion of streptokinase, especially if delivered via a pulmonary catheter at the time of pulmonary angiography. Recent surgery is a relative contraindication to thrombolysis. In the critically ill patient, pulmonary embolectomy carried out with cardiopulmonary bypass may be successful.

Burst abdomen

Aetiology

Dehiscence of the abdominal wound may result from a number of factors, preoperative, operative and postoperative.

Preoperative

Uraemia, cachexia with protein deficiency, vitamin C deficiency, jaundice, obesity and steroids all impair wound healing.

Operative

Poor technique in closing the abdominal wound or the use of suture material of low tensile strength, which ruptures postoperatively. Badly tied knots may come undone and sutures too near the edge of the incision may cut through the tissues like a wire through cheese, especially if these tissues are weakened by infection.

Postoperative

Cough or abdominal distension, which puts a strain on the suture line; infection or haematoma of the wound, which weakens it.

Clinical features

The abdomen usually dehisces on about the 10th day. There may be a warning of this if pink fluid discharges through the abdominal incision. This represents the serous effusion (which is always present during the first week or two within the abdominal cavity after operation), which is tinged with blood and which seeps through the breaking down wound. If this 'pink fluid sign' is ignored, the patient finds a loop of intestine or the omentum protruding through the wound, usually after a cough or strain – a most alarming finding for both the patient and staff.

Sometimes, the deep layer of the abdominal incision gives way but the skin sutures hold; such cases result in a massive incisional hernia.

Treatment

The patient with a burst abdomen is usually in mortal fear. The patient should be reassured and the reassurance supplemented by an injection of morphine combined with an antiemetic. The abdominal contents should be covered with sterile towels soaked in saline and the patient prepared for operation. The abdominal wound should be resutured under a general anaesthetic using strong nylon stitches passed through all the layers of the abdominal wall including the skin. The prognosis after this procedure is good unless the patient succumbs to the underlying disease.

The wound usually heals rapidly, but there is a high incidence of subsequent incisional hernia.

Postoperative fistula

Definition

A fistula is defined as an abnormal connection between two epithelial surfaces.

Aetiology

The development of a fistula involving the alimentary canal or its biliary or pancreatic adnexae following abdominal surgery is a serious complication. A fistula may be consequent upon general or local factors.

General factors

The patient's general condition may be poor due to uraemia, anaemia, jaundice, protein deficiency or cachexia from malignant disease.

Local factors

- *Poor surgical technique.*
- *Poor blood supply* at the anastomotic line, particularly in operations on the oesophagus and rectum.
- *Sepsis* incurred before or during the operation leading to suture line breakdown. (Sepsis is inevitable once leakage has occurred.)
- *Presence of distal obstruction.* A biliary fistula is likely to occur if stones are left behind in the common bile duct after cholecystectomy.
- *Local malignant or chronic inflammatory disease*, e.g. Crohn's disease.

Clinical features

Diagnosis is usually all too obvious, with the escape of bowel contents or bile through the wound or drainage site. If there is any doubt, methylene blue given by mouth will appear in the effluent of an alimentary fistula, and the fluid can be tested for bile to diagnose a biliary leak, or creatinine for a urinary tract leak, while the fluid from a pancreatic leak is rich in amylase. An injection of radio-opaque fluid will outline the fistulous tract and provide valuable information about its size and whether or not distal obstruction exists.

The enzyme-rich fluid of the upper alimentary tract and of a pancreatic fistula produces rapid excoriation of the surrounding skin. This is much less marked in a faecal fistula, as the contents of the colon are relatively poor in proteolytic enzymes. The patient is toxic and passes into a severe catabolic state compounded by infection and starvation due to loss of intestinal fluid. Rapid wasting occurs from fluid loss and protein depletion.

Treatment

The early management has three aims:

1 *To protect the skin around the fistula from ulceration.* The edges of the wound are covered by Stomahesive (which adheres even to moist surfaces), or aluminium paint or silicone barrier cream. It may be possible to collect the effluent by means of a colostomy appliance and thus reduce skin soiling. If the mouth of the fistula is large, continuous suction may be necessary.
2 *To replace the loss of fluid, electrolytes, nutrients and vitamins.* In a high alimentary fistula, this will require intravenous feeding via a central line (total parenteral nutrition). Calories are given in the form of glucose and fat emulsion and protein depletion is countered by amino acids. Vitamins and electrolytes are also required. Such prolonged intravenous feeding must be carefully monitored by serial biochemical studies. If the fistula is low in the alimentary tract, an elemental diet can be given by mouth. This is rapidly absorbed in the upper intestine and is thus not lost through the fistula.
3 *To reduce sepsis.* This is achieved by judicious drainage of pus collections and by antibiotic therapy.

On this conservative regimen, a side-fistula without distal obstruction may well heal spontaneously. However, if the fistula is large or complete, or if there is a distal obstruction or if the fistula is malignant in origin or at the site of an inflammatory disease such as Crohn's disease, subsequent surgery is required to close the leak and deal with the cause. This can only be successful if carried out at the stage when the patient's condition has improved and when a positive nitrogen balance has been achieved.

Postoperative pyrexia

There are many causes of a pyrexia following surgery, and diagnosis requires a methodical approach. A mild pyrexia is a common postoperative feature immediately following surgery and is a normal response to tissue injury. The following procedure is valuable in elucidating the cause of such a fever.

1 *Inspect the wound*: superficial wound infection or haematoma.
2 *Inspect venous cannula sites*: thrombophlebitis is common when a cannula has remained *in situ* for a few days, or when irritant infusions have passed through it.
3 *Examine the chest clinically* and if necessary order a chest X-ray and ultrasound: exclude pulmonary collapse, infection, infarction and subphrenic abscess.
4 *Examine the legs*: deep vein thrombosis.
5 *Rectal examination*: pelvic abscess.
6 *Urine culture*: urinary infection.
7 *Stool culture*: for *C. difficile* toxin to exclude enterocolitis.
8 Finally, consider the possibility of *drug sensitivity*.

5

Acute infections

Learning objectives

✓ To know the common surgical infections and their management.

✓ To be particularly cognizant of tetanus and gas gangrene, including prophylaxis and treatment.

There is an important general principle in treating acute infection anywhere in the body; antibiotics are invaluable when the infection is spreading through the tissues (e.g. cellulitis, peritonitis, pneumonia), but drainage is essential when abscess formation has occurred.

Diabetics are very prone to infection; in any infection, test the blood or urine for sugar.

Cellulitis

Cellulitis is a spreading inflammation of connective tissues. It is generally subcutaneous, but the term may also be applied to pelvic, perinephric, pharyngeal and other connective tissue infections. The common causative agent is the β-haemolytic *Streptococcus*. The invasiveness of this organism is due to the production of hyaluronidase and streptokinase, which dissolve the intercellular matrix and the fibrin inflammatory barrier respectively.

Characteristically, the skin is dark red with local oedema and heat; it blanches on pressure. There may be vesicles and, in severe cases, cutaneous gangrene. Cellulitis is often accompanied by lym-

phangitis and lymphadenitis, and there may be an associated septicaemia.

Treatment

Immobilization, elevation and antibiotics. If a local abscess forms, this must be drained.

Abscess

An abscess is a localized collection of pus, usually, but not invariably, produced by pyogenic organisms. Occasionally, a sterile abscess results from the injection of irritants into soft tissues (e.g. thiopentone).

An abscess commences as a hard, red, painful swelling, which then softens and becomes fluctuant. If not drained, it may discharge spontaneously onto the surface or into an adjacent viscus or body cavity. There are the associated features of bacterial infection, namely a swinging fever, malaise, anorexia and sweating with a polymorph leucocytosis.

Treatment

An established abscess in any situation requires drainage. Antimicrobial agents cannot diffuse in sufficient quantity to sterilize an abscess

Lecture Notes: General Surgery, 12th edition. © Harold Ellis, Sir Roy Y. Calne and Christopher J. E. Watson. Published 2011 by Blackwell Publishing Ltd.

completely. Pus left undrained continues to act as a source of toxaemia and becomes surrounded by dense, fibrous tissue.

The technique of abscess drainage depends on the site. The classical method, which is applicable to a superficial abscess, is to wait until there is fluctuation and to insert the tip of a scalpel blade at this point. The track is widened by means of sinus forceps, which can be inserted without fear of damaging adjacent structures. If there is room, the surgeon's finger can be used to explore the abscess cavity and break down undrained loculi. Drainage is then maintained until the abscess cavity heals – from below outwards – since otherwise the superficial layers can close over, with recurrence of the abscess. The cavity is therefore kept open by means of a gauze wick, a corrugated drain or a tube; the drain is gradually withdrawn until complete healing is achieved.

Deep abscesses can be localized and drained percutaneously using ultrasound or CT guidance.

Boil

A boil (furuncle) is an abscess, usually due to the pyogenic *Staphylococcus*, which involves a follicle and its associated glands. It is therefore not found on the hairless palm or sole, but is usually encountered where the skin is hairy, injured by friction or is dirty and macerated by sweat; thus, it occurs particularly on the neck, axilla and the perianal region. Occasionally, a furuncle may be the primary source of a staphylococcal septicaemia and may be responsible for osteomyelitis, perinephric abscess or empyema, particularly in debilitated patients. A boil on the face may be complicated by a pyelophlebitis spreading along the facial veins resulting in thrombosis of the cavernous sinus.

Differential diagnosis

- *Hidradenitis suppuritiva*. Multiple infected foci in the axillae or groins due to infection of the apocrine sweat glands of these regions are usually misdiagnosed as boils. They do not respond to antimicrobial therapy and can only be treated effectively by excision of the affected skin; if this is extensive, the defect may require grafting.

Treatment

When pus is visible, the boil should be incised. Recurrent crops of boils should be treated by improving the general hygiene of the patient, and by the use of ultraviolet light and hexachlorophene baths, but systemic antibiotic therapy is seldom indicated.

Carbuncle

A carbuncle is an area of subcutaneous necrosis that discharges onto the surface through multiple sinuses. It is usually staphylococcal in origin. The subcutaneous tissues become honeycombed by small abscesses separated by fibrous strands. The condition is often associated with general debility, and diabetes, in particular, must be considered.

Treatment

Surgery is rarely indicated initially. Antibiotic therapy is given and the carbuncle merely protected with sterile dressings. Occasionally, a large sloughing area eventually requires excision and a skin graft. Diabetes, if present, must be controlled.

Specific infections

Tetanus

Tetanus is now a rare disease in the Western world, thanks to a comprehensive immunization policy. In the developing world, it remains prevalent with a mortality of up to 60%.

Pathology

Tetanus is caused by *Clostridium tetani*, an anaerobic, exotoxin-secreting, Gram-positive bacillus. It is characterized by formation of a terminal spore ('drumstick'), and is a normal inhabitant of soil and faeces. The bacillus remains at the site of inoculation and produces a powerful exotoxin, tetanospasmin. Tetanospasmin principally affects inhibitory neurones that secrete gamma-aminobutyric acid (GABA) and glycine. By blocking the inhibitory effects of these neurones, there is unopposed excitatory activity from motor and autonomic neurones. Motor effects include increase in muscle tone, with rigidity and reflex spasms; autonomic effects include sympathetic overactivity with tachycardia, increased cardiac output and reduced vascular tone.

Tetanus follows the implantation of spores into a deep, devitalized wound where anaerobic conditions occur. Infection is related less to the severity of the wound than to its nature; thus, an extensive injury that has received early and adequate wound toilet is far less risky than a contaminated puncture wound that has been neglected.

Clinical features

The incubation time is 24 hours to 24 days, the initial injury often being trivial and forgotten. Muscle spasm first develops at the site of inoculation and then involves the facial muscles and the muscles of the neck and spine. As a rule, it is the trismus of the facial spasm (producing the typical 'risus sardonicus') that is the first reliable indication of developing tetanus. This may be so severe that it becomes impossible for the patient to open his or her mouth ('lock-jaw'). The period of spasm is followed, except in mild cases, by violent and extremely painful convulsions, which occur within 24–72 hours of the onset of symptoms and may be precipitated by some trivial stimulus, such as a sudden noise. The convulsions, like the muscle spasm, affect the muscles of the neck, face and trunk. Characteristically, the muscles remain in spasm between the convulsions. The temperature is a little elevated but the pulse is rapid and weak.

In favourable cases, the convulsions, if present at all, become less frequent and then cease and the tonic spasm gradually lessens. It may, however, be some weeks before muscle tone returns to normal and the risus sardonicus disappears. In fatal cases, paroxysms become more severe and frequent; death occurs from asphyxia due to involvement of the respiratory muscles or from exhaustion, inhalation of vomit or pneumonia.

Poor prognostic features are a short incubation period from the time of injury to the onset of spasm (under 5 days) and the occurrence of convulsions within 48 hours of the onset of muscle spasm.

Differential diagnosis

- *Hypocalcaemic tetany*: characteristically affects the limbs, producing carpopedal spasm (see p. 324)
- *Strychnine poisoning*: flaccidity occurs between convulsions, whereas in tetanus the spasm persists.
- *Meningitis*: neck stiffness.
- *Epilepsy*.
- *Hysteria*.

Treatment

Prophylaxis

Active immunization
This comprises two initial injections of tetanus toxoid (formalin-treated exotoxin) at an interval of 6 weeks. Booster doses are given at intervals of 10 years, or at the time of any injury. Toxoid should be given to any population at risk of injury, particularly the elderly in whom cover may have lapsed.

Wound toilet
The risk of tetanus can be reduced almost to zero if penetrating and contaminated wounds are adequately excised to remove all dead tissue and a course of prophylactic penicillin (or erythromycin for penicillin-sensitive patients) is given. Antibiotic therapy is no substitute for thorough wound debridement.

Passive immunization
This is done to neutralize the toxin. Patients who have previously received toxoid should be given a booster dose. If toxoid has not been given in the past, human tetanus immunoglobulin (HTIG), prepared from fully immunized subjects, should be given if the wound is heavily contaminated or is a puncture wound, and more than 6 hours have elapsed before treatment is received. HTIG is insufficient to confer long-term immunity, and a course of toxoid should also be given.

Curative treatment

Control of convulsions
The patient is nursed in isolation, quiet and darkness, and is heavily sedated. In severe cases, pharmacological paralysis with tracheostomy and intermittent positive-pressure mechanical ventilation is required and this may have to be continued for several weeks. It is terminated when the spasms and rigidity are absent during a trial period without muscle relaxants.

Control of the local infection
Excision and drainage of any wound is carried out under a general anaesthetic. High-dose penicillin

(or erythromycin if the patient is penicillin sensitive) is administered.

Nutrition
Feed the patient by fine-bore nasogastric tube to maintain the general condition and electrolyte balance.

Gas gangrene

Pathology

Gas gangrene results from infection by *Clostridium perfringens* (*welchii*) and other *Clostridium* species. The organism, a Gram-positive, anaerobic spore-forming bacillus such as *Clostridium tetani*, also produces powerful exotoxins. The toxins have various activities, including phospholipase, collagenase, proteinase and hyaluronidase, which facilitate aggressive local spread of infection along tissue planes, with liberation of CO_2, H_2S and NH_3 by protein destruction. The organisms are found in soil and in faeces.

Gas gangrene is a typical infection of deep penetrating wounds, particularly of war, but sometimes involvement of the abdominal wall or cavity may follow operations upon the alimentary system. Occasionally, gas gangrene complicates amputation of an ischaemic lower limb, or follows abortion or puerperal infection.

Clinical features

The incubation period is about 24 hours. Severe sudden onset of pain is characteristic, together with severe toxaemia with tachycardia, shock and vomiting. The temperature is first elevated and then becomes subnormal. The affected tissues are swollen, and crepitus is palpable due to gas. The skin becomes gangrenous and the infection spreads along the muscle planes, producing at first dark red swollen muscle and then frank gangrene.

Treatment

Prophylaxis

Debridement
Adequate excision of wounds removes both the organisms and the dead tissues which are essential for their anaerobic growth. Seriously contused wounds (such as those produced by a gunshot) or contaminated wounds are left open and lightly packed with gauze. Delayed primary suture can then safely be performed after 5–6 days, by which time the wound is usually healthy and granulating. The dangers of primary closure of contaminated wounds has been learned and forgotten after every war and catastrophe since 1914!

Antimicrobial therapy
Penicillin is given in all heavily contaminated wounds and to patients undergoing amputation of an ischaemic leg.

Curative treatment

In the established case, all involved tissue must be excised. Involvement of all muscle groups in a limb is an indication for amputation, which in the lower limb may mean a disarticulation at the hip. High-dose penicillin is given, and other supportive measures as required. Hyperbaric oxygen therapy, to eliminate the anaerobic environment, has been used with varying degrees of success. The value of antiserum against gas gangrene, as either a prophylactic or curative measure, is not proven.

Synergistic gangrene

Pathology

Synergistic gangrene, also known as progressive bacterial gangrene and Meleney's gangrene[1], is caused by the synergistic action of two or more organisms, commonly aerobic haemolytic *Staphylococcus* and microaerophilic non-haemolytic *Streptococcus*. It is more common in patients with diabetes and is often related to recent trauma or infection. Where it affects the scrotum and perineum, it has been termed Fournier's gangrene.[2]

Clinical features

There may be no precipitating factor, but most follow infections or recent surgery (previously termed progressive postoperative gangrene). Around the wound an area of cellulitis appears, which spreads rapidly. The area is exquisitely tender, and, as gangrene evolves, it liberates an offensive odour. The patient becomes profoundly septic and unwell.

[1]Frank L. Meleney (1889–1963), Professor of Clinical Surgery, Columbia University, OH, USA.
[2]Jean Alfred Fournier (1832–1914), 'Professeur des maladies cutanées et syphilitiques', Hôpital St. Louis, Paris, France.

Treatment

High-dose, broad-spectrum antibiotics should be commenced immediately, but the mainstay of treatment is a radical debridement of all the affected area. Following the initial debridement, the wound should be inspected twice daily at least for evidence of spread, and further debridement performed until all the affected area is cleared.

Surgical infections and bioterrorism

Recent events have focused attention on the potential for bioterrorism, in particular with anthrax. Its inclusion here reflects manifestations that might present to the surgeon.

Anthrax

Anthrax is caused by *Bacillus anthracis*, a Gram-positive aerobic spore-forming bacillus that lives in the soil. It may manifest in one of three ways:

1 *cutaneous anthrax* – infection through a break in the skin;
2 *gastrointestinal anthrax* – spore entry through the gut mucosa;
3 *inhalational anthrax* – inhalation of spores causing pulmonary disease.

It is an occupational disease of people working with wool ('wool sorter's disease') and the hides from infected animals.

- *Cutaneous anthrax.* This is the commonest manifestation and presents as a painless, pruritic papule that develops into a vesicle 1–2 cm in diameter. The vesicle ruptures, undergoes necrosis and enlarges to form a black eschar with surrounding oedema. Associated features include lymphangitis and regional lymphadenopathy as well as general manifestations of sepsis.
- *Gastrointestinal anthrax.* Manifests as nausea, vomiting, fever and abdominal pain, with bloody diarrhoea and features suggestive of an acute abdomen. Symptoms first appear 2–5 days after ingestion of contaminated food. Haemorrhagic mesenteric adenitis and ascites are late features, and mortality is around 50%.

Prophylaxis and treatment of anthrax is with ciprofloxacillin.

Botulism

Botulism is caused by an exotoxin of *Clostridium botulinum*, botulism is associated with ingestion of contaminated food, originally described with contaminated sausages ('botulus' is Latin for sausage). The botulinum toxin is a heat-labile toxin (hence destroyed by cooking) that penetrates cholinergic neurones and prevents neurotransmitter release, thus inhibiting muscular contraction. While botulism is itself a condition more familiar to infectious disease units, the toxin is becoming increasingly used in surgery for conditions as diverse as fissure *in ano*, achalasia, facial wrinkles and hyperhidrosis (excess sweating, especially of the palms). As an aerosol, the toxin has been considered for biological warfare.

6

Shock

Learning objective

✓ To understand what shock is, what causes it, and how it is best managed according to the cause.

Shock is characterized by inadequate perfusion of vital organs, principally the heart and brain.

Aetiology

Tissue perfusion requires an adequate blood pressure, which is dependent upon the systemic vascular resistance and cardiac output; the cardiac output is a function of the heart rate and the stroke volume. These may be expressed in mathematical terms:

$$CO = HR \times SV$$
$$BP = CO \times SVR$$

where CO is cardiac output, SV is stroke volume, HR is heart rate, BP is arterial blood pressure and SVR is systemic vascular resistance.

Normal regulation of tissue perfusion

The autonomic nervous system is able to alter heart rate and peripheral vascular resistance in response to changes in blood pressure detected by the carotid sinus and aortic arch baroreceptors; changes in systemic vascular resistance may alter venous return by changing the amount of fluid circulating in the cutaneous and splanchnic vascular beds. Venous return determines stroke volume; increasing venous return causes an increase in stroke volume, the heart acting as a permissive pump (Starling's law:[1] the output depends on the degree of stretch of the heart muscle at the end of diastole). Volume regulation is achieved by the kidney, in particular by the regulation of sodium loss by the renin–angiotensin–aldosterone system (Chapter 11, p. 77 and antidiuretic hormone (ADH) produced by the posterior pituitary; in addition, a fall in circulating volume prompts the sensation of thirst, stimulating increased fluid intake.

Abnormal regulation of tissue perfusion

Inadequate tissue perfusion (shock) may result from factors related to the pump (the heart) and factors relating to the systemic circulation. The causes of shock may be classified accordingly, as follows:

1 *Cardiogenic shock.* A primary failure of cardiac output in which the heart is unable to maintain adequate stroke volume in spite of satisfactory filling. Compensation involves an increase in heart rate and systemic vascular resistance, manifested clinically by a tachycardia, sweating (due to sympathetic nervous system outflow), pallor and coldness (due to cutaneous vasoconstriction). Causes include the following:

[1]Ernest Henry Starling (1866–1927), Professor of Physiology, University College, London, UK. Described capillary flow dynamics and discovered secretin (with Bayliss).

a massive myocardial infarction;
b pulmonary embolism;
c acute ventriculoseptal defect following myocardial infarction affecting the septum;
d mitral or aortic valve rupture;
e acute cardiac tamponade.

2 *Fluid loss.* Reduction in circulating volume results in a reduction in stroke volume and cardiac output. Blood pressure is initially maintained as in cardiogenic shock, with increased sympathetic activity raising the peripheral vascular resistance leading to the clinical picture of a cold, clammy patient with a tachycardia. As volume losses increase, the blood pressure falls. In severe cases, the patient is confused or semiconscious. Causes include:

a haemorrhage, revealed or internal (e.g. ruptured aneurysm; bleeding into the bowel or around a closed fracture);
b burns, with massive loss of plasma and electrolytes;
c severe diarrhoea or vomiting, with fluid and electrolyte loss, particularly in colitis or pyloric stenosis;
d bowel obstruction, in which large amounts of fluid are sequestered into the gut, in addition to the losses due to vomiting;
e peritonitis, with large fluid losses into the abdomen as a consequence of infection or chemical irritation;
f gastrointestinal fistulae with fluid and electrolyte loss;
g urinary losses, e.g. the osmotic diuresis of diabetic ketoacidosis, or polyuria in resolving acute tubular necrosis (Chapter 41, p. 349).

3 *Reduction in systemic vascular resistance.* Reduction in systemic vascular resistance increases the size of the systemic vascular bed, producing a relative hypovolaemia, reduced diastolic filling, reduced stroke volume and thus a fall in blood pressure. Unlike the previous two causes, vasodilatation occurs as part of the pathogenesis, so the patient appears warm ('hot shock'), not cold and peripherally shut down. The heart compensates with an increase in output. The principal causes are:

a anaphylaxis;
b sepsis;
c spinal shock.

4 *Confounding factors.* Pre-existing medical conditions and medications may confuse the clinical picture. Consider a patient, with hypertension and taking a β-blocker such as atenolol. For that patient, a systolic blood pressure of 110 mmHg may be very low, and the atenolol prevents a compensatory tachycardia in response.

Special causes of shock

Adrenocortical failure

Loss of the hormones produced by the cortex of the suprarenal gland may follow bilateral suprarenal haemorrhage, adrenalectomy, Addison's disease[2] or lack of corticosteroid replacement in patients who have been on long-term glucocorticoids.

Failure of aldosterone secretion results in volume depletion and glucocorticoid deficiency, which impairs autonomic responses. The ability to respond to minor stress is severely compromised and may provoke an Addisonian crisis characterized by bradycardia and postural hypotension, which is responsive to corticosteroid replacement. Adrenocortical failure should be considered and a bolus of hydrocortisone given in all patients with unexplained hypotension.

Sympathetic interruption

This reduces the effective blood volume by widespread vasodilatation. It follows transection of the spinal cord (spinal shock), but may also occur after a high spinal anaesthetic.

The vasovagal syndrome (faint)

The vasovagal syndrome is produced by severe pain or emotional disturbance. It is the result of reflex vasodilatation together with cardiac slowing owing to vagal activity. Hypotension is caused by a fall in cardiac output due to both bradycardia and reduced venous return; the latter the result of peripheral vasodilatation. Clinically, it is recognized by the presence of a bradycardia and responds to the simple measure of laying the patient flat with elevation of the legs.

[2] Thomas Addison (1793–1860), Physician, Guy's Hospital, London, UK. His original specimens may still be seen in the Gordon Museum at Guy's Hospital.

Septic shock

Shock may be produced as the result of severe infection from either Gram-positive or, more commonly, Gram-negative organisms. The latter are seen particularly after colonic, biliary and urological surgery, and with infected severe burns. The principal effect of endotoxins is to cause vasodilatation of the peripheral circulation together with increased capillary permeability. The effects are partly direct and partly due to activation of normal tissue inflammatory responses such as the complement system and release of cytokines such as tumour necrosis factor (TNF).

Disseminated intravascular coagulation (DIC) results from activation of the clotting cascade and may lead to blockage of the arterial microcirculation by microemboli. Fibrin and platelets are consumed excessively, with resultant spontaneous haemorrhages into the skin, the gastrointestinal tract, the lungs, mouth and nose.

Sequelae of shock

A continued low blood pressure produces a series of irreversible changes, so that the patient may die in spite of treatment. The lack of oxygen affects all the vital organs.

- *Cerebral hypoperfusion* results in confusion or coma.
- *Renal hypoperfusion* results in reduced glomerular filtration, with oliguria or anuria. As renal ischaemia progresses, tubular necrosis may occur, and profound ischaemia may lead to cortical necrosis (Chapter 41).
- *The heart* may fail owing to inadequate coronary perfusion.
- *Pulmonary capillaries* may reflect the changes in the systemic circulation with transudation of fluid resulting in pulmonary oedema, hampering oxygen transfer and causing further arterial hypoxaemia and thus tissue hypoxia. Pulmonary capillary function may also be impaired following multiple blood transfusions and contusions resulting from chest trauma, a condition known as acute lung injury (previously termed 'shock lung').
- *DIC*, precipitated by sepsis, may be further aggravated by hypothermia unless active re-warming is undertaken.

Principles in the management of patients in shock

Immediate measures

The immediate treatment of patients in shock varies according to cause. Two causes merit mention for immediate treatment: bleeding and anaphylaxis.

Bleeding

Direct pressure should be applied to a bleeding wound. Immediate surgical exploration is indicated where continued bleeding is likely, such as in peptic ulcer haemorrhage, ruptured spleen, ruptured aortic aneurysm or ruptured ectopic pregnancy. In these cases, resuscitation cannot overcome the losses until the rate of blood loss is curtailed.

Anaphylaxis

In surgical practice, this may arise as an allergic reaction to an antibiotic or radiological contrast medium. In addition to hypotension (due to vasodilatation), bronchospasm and laryngeal oedema may be present and warrant immediate therapy. The immediate treatment for anaphylaxis is the administration of adrenaline (epinephrine; 0.5 mL of 1:1000 concentration) intramuscularly or subcutaneously, repeated every 10–30 minutes as required. Subsequently, hydrocortisone and antihistamine agents may be given (e.g. chlorphenamine).

For milder reactions, aliquots of 1 mL of 1:10 000 adrenaline are given and titrated to effect.

Monitoring and subsequent management

The severely shocked patient should be admitted to an intensive care ward where continuous supervision by specially trained nursing staff is available. As well as careful clinical surveillance, the following need to be monitored:

- Core temperature, pulse, respiration rate and blood pressure.
- Hourly urine output (via a urinary catheter).
- Central venous pressure.

- Pulse oximetry. Oxygen is administered to ensure adequate oxygenation. Mechanical ventilation may be required.
- Electrocardiogram (ECG).
- Serum electrolytes, haemoglobin and white blood cell count.
- Arterial blood gases (Po_2, Pco_2, [H^+]).
- The cardiac output, and left atrial and pulmonary arterial pressures using a Swan–Ganz catheter (see below).

The frequency of these measurements depends on the patient's condition and response to treatment. It is particularly important that doctors remember that, in this environment of recording machinery and scientific nursing, the patient remains a human being, who deserves to be treated with dignity and tenderness. If the patient is conscious, he or she may well be terrified, in pain and acutely aware of all that is going on. Proper explanations and appropriate analgesia must be provided.

Swan–Ganz catheter[3]

The Swan–Ganz catheter is a multiple lumen catheter that is passed via a central vein (internal jugular or subclavian) into the right atrium. At this stage, a small balloon on the end of the catheter is inflated. The inflated balloon then 'floats' with the blood, returning to the heart across the tricuspid and pulmonary valves into the pulmonary artery. Once there, the catheter is advanced until it wedges itself in a small branch of the pulmonary arterial tree. The balloon is then deflated. During insertion, the position of the catheter can be monitored by the changing pressure waveform recorded by a transducer connected to the lumen. The catheter also has a temperature probe near its tip, which facilitates the measurement of cardiac output as well as core temperature.

Cardiac output is calculated by the Fick[4] principle after injecting a bolus of cold saline through the catheter and monitoring the change in temperature. Importantly, the catheter also allows

calculation of the systemic and pulmonary vascular resistances.

When the balloon is inflated, no flow comes past the tip. The catheter is wedged and the pressure that is recorded, referred to as the wedge pressure, is an approximation of the left atrial pressure.

Fluid management

See Chapter 2.

Prevention of hypothermia

Patients may cool down because of neglect, infusion of cold fluids, particularly unwarmed blood, and extracorporeal circulations such as haemodialysis or haemofiltration circuits. Allowing a patient to cool down to subnormal temperatures (35°C and below) impairs the coagulation cascades and platelet aggregation, and promotes fibrinolysis, possibly resulting in DIC. To prevent this, all infusions should be prewarmed, and the patient actively re-warmed using warm air blankets.

Pharmacological agents

The shocked patient may require significant pharmacological support. The principal drugs used are catecholamines or their derivatives, in addition to drugs to treat specific causes such as antimicrobial therapy for septicaemia. Patients in cardiogenic shock benefit from positive inotropic agents, whereas patients with low systemic vascular resistance due to sepsis require agents to increase vascular resistance. The drugs used in this context are sympathomimetics, with differing degrees of α (peripheral vasoconstriction), β_1 (inotropic and chronotropic) and β_2 (peripheral vasodilatation) effects. Examples of such drugs include the following.

Dopamine

Dopamine has three separate actions according to dose:

---

[3]Harold J. C. Swan (1922–2005), Cardiologist, Cedars of Lebanon Hospital, Los Angles, CA, USA. William Ganz (1919–2009), Professor of Medicine, UCLA, and Senior Research Scientist, Cedars of Lebanon Hospital, Los Angeles, CA, USA.
[4]Adolf Eugen Fick (1829–1901), born in Germany, Professor of Physiology, Zurich, Switzerland.

1 At *low doses* (2 µg/kg/min) dopaminergic actions dominate, causing increased renal perfusion. This is the commonest indication for the use of dopamine.
2 At *moderate doses* (5 µg/kg/min), β_1 effects predominate with positive inotropic activity (increasing myocardial contractility and rate).
3 At *higher doses* (over 5 µg/kg/min), α effects predominate with vasoconstriction.

Dopexamine

Dopexamine has predominantly β_2 actions, increasing myocardial contractility; it also acts on peripheral dopamine receptors, increasing renal perfusion.

Dobutamine

Dobutamine has predominantly β_1 actions, increasing myocardial contractility and rate, thus increasing cardiac output. It is used principally in cardiogenic shock.

Noradrenaline (norepinephrine)

Noradrenaline has predominantly α effects, but with modest β activity. It is used to increase systemic vascular resistance through its vasoconstrictor α effects.

Adrenaline (epinephrine)

Adrenaline has strong α and β actions, and may be used to increase peripheral resistance while also increasing cardiac output. The powerful vasoconstrictor actions of both adrenaline and noradrenaline may result in ischaemia and infarction of peripheral tissues, most commonly fingers, toes and the tips of the nose and ears.

7

Tumours

Learning objectives

✓ To know the pathology and clinical features of tumours, as well as the ways in which a tumour might present, the histological features which influence prognosis, and the principles of tumour staging.

✓ To know the treatment options, including the principles of cytotoxic chemotherapy and the broad classes of agents available.

New growths are so common and widespread that their consideration must at least pass through the mind in most clinical situations. It therefore behoves the student, both for examinations and, still more importantly, for his or her future practice of medicine, to have a standard scheme with which to tabulate the pathology, diagnosis, treatment and prognosis of neoplastic disease.

Pathology

When considering the tumours affecting any organ, this simple classification should be used:

1 Benign.
2 Malignant:
   a primary;
   b secondary.

It is surprising how often failure to remember this basic scheme leads one to omit such an elementary fact that common tumours of brain and bone are secondary deposits.

For each particular tumour, the following headings should be used:

- Incidence.
- Age distribution.

Lecture Notes: General Surgery, 12th edition. © Harold Ellis, Sir Roy Y. Calne and Christopher J. E. Watson. Published 2011 by Blackwell Publishing Ltd.

- Sex distribution.
- Geographical distribution (where relevant).
- Predisposing factors.
- Macroscopic appearances.
- Microscopic appearances.
- Pathways of spread of the tumour.
- Prognosis.

Clinical features and diagnosis

A malignant tumour may manifest itself in any or all of four ways.

1 The effects of the *primary tumour* itself.
2 The effects produced by *secondary deposits*.
3 The general effects of *malignant disease*.
4 *Paraneoplastic syndromes*. These are remote effects caused by hormone or other tumour-cell products, which are most common in carcinoma of the lung, particularly small cell tumours. For example, production of ectopic adrenocorticotrophic hormone (ACTH) may present like Cushing's syndrome, and production of ectopic parathormone (PTH) may present with hypercalcaemia and its symptoms.

The only common exceptions to this scheme are primary tumours of the central nervous system (CNS), which seldom produce secondary deposits.

Diagnosis is always made by history, clinical examination and, where necessary, special investigations.

Let us now, as an example, apply this scheme to carcinoma of the lung – the commonest lethal cancer in the UK, accounting for 22% of all deaths from cancer; bowel (10%), breast (8%) and prostate (7%) follow lung cancer in this deadly league table.

History

- *The primary tumour* may present with cough, haemoptysis, dyspnoea and pneumonia (sometimes recurrent pneumonia due to partial bronchial obstruction).
- *Secondary deposits* in bone may produce pathological fracture or bone pains; cerebral metastases may produce headaches or drowsiness; liver deposits may result in jaundice.
- *General effects of malignant disease*: the patient may present with malaise, lassitude or loss of weight.
- *Paraneoplastic syndromes*, such as
  - ectopic hormone production (e.g. PTH, ACTH);
  - myasthenia-like syndrome (Eaton–Lambert syndrome[1]);
  - hypertrophic pulmonary osteoarthropathy (HPOA) and finger clubbing.

Examination

- *The primary tumour* may produce signs in the chest.
- *Secondary deposits* may produce cervical lymph node enlargement, hepatomegaly or obvious bony deposits.
- *The general effects of malignancy* may be suggested by pallor or weight loss.

[1]Lealdes M. Eaton (1905–1958), Professor of Neurology at the Mayo Clinic, Rochester, MN, USA. Edward Lambert (1915–2003), Professor of Physiology and Neurology, Mayo Clinic, Rochester, MN, USA.

Special investigations

- *The primary tumour*: chest X-ray, computed tomography (CT), bronchoscopy, cytology of sputum and needle biopsy.
- *Secondary deposits*: isotope bone scan, bone X-ray and ultrasound of liver.
- *General manifestations of malignancy*: a blood count may reveal anaemia. The erythrocyte sedimentation rate (ESR) may be raised.
- *Paraneoplastic hormone production*: hormone assay.

This simple scheme applied to any of the principal malignant tumours will enable the student to present a very full clinical picture of the disease with little mental effort.

Tumour markers

These are blood chemicals (often fetal proteins) produced by the malignant cells. Some tumours have a characteristic marker associated with them, such as α-fetoprotein (AFP) in hepatoma and teratoma and prostate-specific antigen (PSA) in carcinoma of the prostate (Table 7.1). Tumour markers may indicate malignant change in a benign condition, and are useful in postoperative monitoring. If a marker was raised before treatment, it should fall when the disease is controlled, but will rise again if recurrence occurs. Some tumours produce excess amounts of the appropriate hormone, such as medullary carcinoma of the thyroid and calcitonin, in which case hormone assay may be used to detect tumour activity.

Treatment

The treatment of malignant disease should be considered under two headings:

1 *Curative*: an attempt is made to ablate the disease completely.
2 *Palliative*: although the disease is incurable or has recurred after treatment, measures can still be taken to ease the symptoms of the patient.

In this section, we shall summarize the possible lines of treatment for malignant disease in general;

Table 7.1 Tumour markers

Marker	Nature of marker	Malignant disease associated with rise in marker	Benign disease associated with rise in marker
α-Fetoprotein (AFP)	Protein secreted by fetal liver	Hepatocellular carcinoma and testicular teratoma	Viral hepatitis (e.g. hepatitis C) and cirrhosis; pregnancy esp. if spinal cord abnormality
β-Human chorionic gonadotrophin (β-HCG)	Protein normally produced by placenta	Testicular teratoma and chorion carcinoma	Pregnancy
Ca 15.3	Oncofetal antigen	Breast carcinoma	Hepatitis, cirrhosis, autoimmune diseases, benign lung disease
Ca 27.29	Glycoprotein mucin 1 (MUC1) on epithelial cells	Breast carcinoma	Benign breast disease, ovarian cysts, and liver and kidney disease
Ca 19.9	Intracellular adhesion molecule related to Lewis blood group	Hepatocellular and cholangiocarcinoma. Also other colorectal and ovarian carcinoma	Pancreatitis, cholestasis, cholangitis, cirrhosis
Ca 125	Glycoprotein on coelomic epithelium during fetal development	Ovarian carcinoma	Pregnancy, ovarian cysts, pelvic inflammation, ascites, cirrhosis, hepatitis, pancreatitis
Carcinoembryonic antigen (CEA)	Oncofetal protein (protein secreted by fetal gut)	Advanced colorectal, breast and lung carcinomas	Peptic ulcer, inflammatory bowel disease, pancreatitis
Prostate-specific antigen (PSA)	Glycoprotein produced by epithelium of prostatic duct	Prostatic carcinoma	Prostatitis, benign prostatic hypertrophy and prostatic trauma

in subsequent chapters, the management of specific tumours will be considered in more detail.

Curative treatment

1 *Surgery* (e.g. carcinoma of the lung or colon).
2 *Radiotherapy* alone (e.g. tumours of the mouth and pharynx).
3 *Cytotoxic chemotherapy* when the tumour is particularly sensitive to particular agents, such as teratoma of the testis to platinum compounds.
4 *A combination of treatment modalities* including surgery and/or radiotherapy and/or cytotoxic chemotherapy.

Palliative treatment

1 *Surgery.* The palliative excision of a primary lesion may be indicated, although secondary deposits may be present. For example, a carcinoma of the rectum may be excised to prevent pain, bleeding and mucus discharge, although secondary deposits may already be present in the liver. Irremovable obstructing growths in the bowel may be stented or bypassed. Inoperable obstructing tumours of the oesophagus or cardia of the stomach may also be stented so that dysphagia can be relieved. The bile duct may be stented endoscopically via the duodenal papilla for the relief of jaundice and pruritus in patients with inoperable carcinomas of the head of pancreas. Surgery may also be used for pain relief by interrupting nerve pathways, e.g. cordotomy in which the contralateral spinothalamic tract within the spinal cord is divided.

2 *Radiotherapy.* Palliative treatment may be given to localized secondary deposits in bone, irremovable breast tumours and inoperable

lymph node deposits, for example. It is particularly indicated for localized irremovable disease.

3 *Hormone therapy.* Applicable in carcinoma of the breast and prostate.

4 *Cytotoxic chemotherapy.* A wide range of drugs have anticancer action, but this action is not specific; all the drugs damage normal dividing cells, especially those of the bone marrow, the gut, the skin and the gonads. They may be classified into the following:

   a alkylating agents (e.g. cyclophosphamide, chlorambucil, busulphan);
   b antimetabolites (e.g. fluorouracil, methotrexate, gemcitabine);
   c plant alkaloids (e.g. vincristine, vinblastine);
   d cytotoxic antibiotics (e.g. bleomycin, doxorubicin);
   e platinum compounds (e.g. cisplatin, carboplatin);
   f epipodophyllotoxins (e.g. etoposide);
   g monoclonal antibodies (e.g. cetuximab, trastuzumab);
   h taxanes (e.g. paclitaxel, docetaxel);
   i protein kinase inhibitors (e.g. imatinib, erlotinib);
   j others (e.g. procarbazine).
      Multiple drugs are frequently used (combination chemotherapy) when their modes of action and toxicity profiles are different.
      A balance must be made between the chances of regression of the tumour in relatively fit patients with tumours likely to be sensitive (e.g. breast, ovary, testis) and the toxic effects of the drug regimen.

5 *Drugs.* These are administered for pain relief (non-steroidal analgesics, opiates), hypnotics, tranquillizers and anti-emetics (e.g. chlorpromazine).

6 *Nerve blocks,* with phenol or alcohol for relief of pain.

7 *Maintenance of morale.* This is often impossible, but might be improved by a cheerful and kindly attitude of medical and nursing staff.

Prognosis

The prognosis of any tumour depends on four main features:

1 extent of spread;
2 microscopic appearance;
3 anatomical situation;
4 general condition of the patient.

The extent of spread (staging)

The extent of the tumour (its staging) on clinical examination, at operation and on studying the excised surgical specimen, is of great prognostic importance. Obviously, the clinical findings of palpable distant secondaries or gross fixation of the primary tumour are serious. Similarly, the local invasiveness of the tumour at operation and evidence of distant spread are of great significance. Finally, histological study may reveal involvement of the nodes which had not been detected clinically, or microscopic extension of the growth to the edges of the resected specimen with consequent worsening of the outlook for the patient.

The TNM classification is an international system for tumour staging. Tumours are staged by scoring them according to the following:

• *T*umour characteristics – size and degree of invasion.
• *N*ode involvement – regional nodes and distant nodes.
• *M*etastases – presence or absence.

An example of TNM staging as it relates to breast cancer is illustrated on in Chapter 35, p. 304. Some tumours have additional classifications which are more familiar to the clinician. Examples are Breslow's staging of local invasion of malignant melanoma (Chapter 9, p. 55) and Dukes' staging of rectal carcinoma (Chapter 26, p. 228).

Microscopic appearance (histological differentiation)

As a general principle, the prognosis of a tumour is related to its degree of histological differentiation (its grading) on the spectrum between well differentiated and anaplastic.

The spread of the tumour and its histological differentiation should be considered in conjunction with each other. A small tumour with no apparent spread at the time of operation may still have a poor prognosis if it is highly anaplastic, whereas an extensive tumour is not incompatible with long survival of the patient after operation if the microscopic examination reveals a high degree of differentiation.

Anatomical situation

The site of the tumour may preclude its adequate removal and thus seriously affect the prognosis. For example, a tumour at the lower end of the oesophagus may be easily removable whereas an exactly similar tumour situated behind the arch of the aorta may be technically inoperable; a brain tumour located in the frontal lobe may be resected whereas a similar tumour in the brain stem will be a desperate surgical proposition.

General condition of the patient

A patient apparently curable from the point of view of the local condition may be inoperable because of poor general health. For example, gross congestive cardiac failure may convert what is technically an operable carcinoma of the rectum into a hopeless anaesthetic risk.

Screening

Screening is the process of testing individuals for a specific condition. It is commonly performed for tumours, but may be used in other contexts such as abdominal aortic aneurysm and hypertension. Effective screening for a given condition using a particular test has several prerequisites:

- The condition, if untreated, is sufficiently serious to warrant its prevention.
- The natural history of the condition should be understood.
- The condition has a recognizable early stage.
- Effective treatment is available.
- Treatment at an early stage could improve the prognosis, and is of more benefit than treatment started later in the disease.
- The screening test is simple, reliable and acceptable to the patient.
- The screening test should have minimal false-positive and false-negative outcomes (i.e. it should be both sensitive and specific). Incorrect diagnosis can have serious consequences.

In reality, cost-effective screening requires restricting the testing to those groups at highest risk of a condition. This may involve large-scale population screening or screening of families where a genetic predisposition exists.

Population screening

Examples of population screening include breast cancer screening by mammography, which is restricted to older women (over 50 years) and cervical cancer screening for women over 25 years. In cervical cancer, for example, a distinct progression exists from dysplasia through carcinoma *in situ* to invasive cancer. This progression may take 10 years. Hence, screening the population every 3–5 years by cervical smear cytology is cost-effective.

Screening for high-risk individuals

A number of cancer syndromes exist in which there is an inherited predisposition (e.g. familial adenomatous polyposis (FAP)) or a familial risk (e.g. breast and ovarian cancer).

Inherited cancer syndromes

Like FAP, most inherited cancers are autosomal and dominantly inherited. In at-risk families, early identification may be possible through either genetic mapping of the cancer or early recognition of a component of the syndrome. In FAP, early colonoscopy may identify villous adenomas (polyps) while they are still dysplastic and before they become malignant, at which stage prophylactic colectomy is indicated. Alternatively, identification of the gene (located on chromosome 5q21) will also signify carriage.

Familial clustering

Many of the familial cancers are now being associated with mutations of specific genes. Incomplete expression of the gene may account for the sporadic incidence of the tumour. For breast cancer, two genes have been identified, *BRCA1* (chromosome 17q21) and *BRCA2* (chromosome 13q12). Mutations of either gene confer an 80% risk of breast cancer by the age of 70 years, together with an increased risk of ovarian cancer. Screening tests based on the detection of these genes differ from the other screening tests mentioned above, as they identify a tendency to malignancy and not premalignant change or early curable malignancy. There is no consensus at present as to the best management of such patients.

Burns

Causes

- *Thermal burn*: the commonest cause of a burn, due either to direct contact with a hot object or flames or to hot vapour such as steam (scald).
- *Electrical burn*: severity depends on strength of current and duration of contact.
- *Chemical burn*: such as from caustic material. The chemical may penetrate deep into the skin and be difficult to remove.
- *Radiation burn*: due to exposure to radiation, as in the local erythema that may follow superficial radiotherapy.

Classification

Burns may be classified into partial thickness and full thickness, depending on whether or not the germinal epithelial layer of the skin is intact or destroyed (Figure 8.1; Table 8.1).

Partial thickness burns vary in appearance and severity:

1 *Erythema*: a superficial burn with erythema due to capillary dilatation and with or without areas of blistering produced by exudation of plasma beneath coagulated epidermis. The underlying germinal layer is intact, and complete healing takes place within a few days.
2 *Superficial partial thickness*: burn extends down through the epidermis to involve the germinal layer, but the dermal appendages such as sweat glands and hair follicles remain largely preserved. There is intense blistering followed by the formation of a slough. This separates after about 10 days, leaving healthy, newly formed, pink epithelium beneath.
3 *Deep partial thickness*: burn extends to the germinal layer and destroys a significant proportion of hair follicles, sebaceous glands and dermis. Healing is much slower and is associated with significant scarring.

Full thickness burns completely destroy the skin. There may be initial blistering, but this is soon replaced by a coagulum or slough; more often, this is present from the onset in an intense deep burn. Unlike the more superficial burns, this slough separates only slowly over 3–4 weeks, leaving an underlying surface of granulation tissue. Very small deep burns may heal from an ingrowth of epithelium from adjacent healthy skin; more extensive burns, unless grafted, heal by dense scar tissue with consequent contracture and deformity.

Clinical features

Pain

This is due to the stimulation of numerous nerve endings in the damaged skin. It is more severe in

Lecture Notes: General Surgery, 12th edition. © Harold Ellis, Sir Roy Y. Calne and Christopher J. E. Watson. Published 2011 by Blackwell Publishing Ltd.

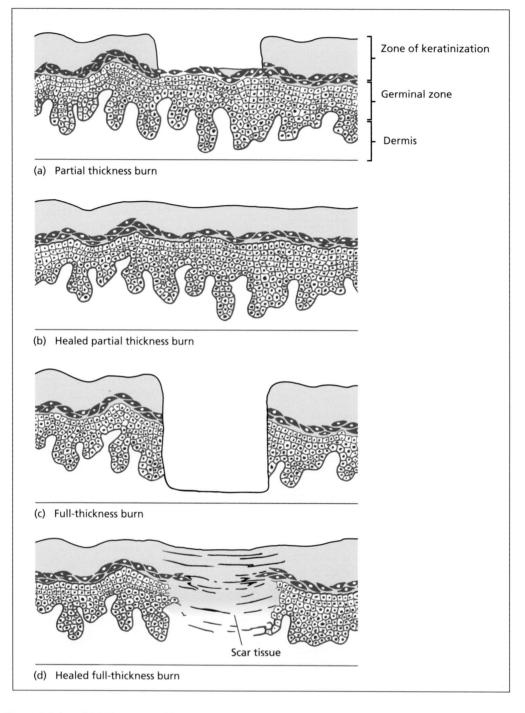

(a) Partial thickness burn

Zone of keratinization

Germinal zone

Dermis

(b) Healed partial thickness burn

(c) Full-thickness burn

Scar tissue

(d) Healed full-thickness burn

Figure 8.1 A partial-thickness burn (a) leaves part or the whole of the germinal epithelium intact; complete healing takes place (b). A full-thickness burn (c) destroys the germinal layer and, unless very small, can heal only by dense scar tissue (d).

Table 8.1 Burn comparison

	Partial thickness	Full thickness
Depth	Superficial	Deep
Underlying germinal layer	Intact	Destroyed
Sensation	Present	Absent
Healing	Complete	Scarring and contracture
Blistering	Prominent, followed by slough	Slight, slough dominates

superficial burns and, indeed, deep burns may be relatively painless owing to extensive destruction of nerve endings.

Plasma loss

Loss of the epidermis, together with the intense exudation of plasma through the damaged capillaries, which is especially marked in the first 24 hours after burning, results in an enormous loss of plasma. By the time a coagulum has formed (about 48 hours), this plasma loss ceases. The amount of this loss is proportional to the area of the burn and not its depth.

Hypovolaemic shock

Shock is a direct result of plasma loss. The intravascular volume is rapidly depleted as plasma is lost from the surface of the burn.

Anaemia

This results partly from destruction of red cells within involved skin capillaries and partly from toxic inhibition of the bone marrow if infection of the burnt area occurs.

Airway

Smoke inhalation or thermal injury of the respiratory tract may rapidly result in respiratory obstruction from pharyngeal or laryngeal oedema and is a common cause of death.

Stress reaction

The adrenocortical response of sodium and water retention, potassium loss and protein catabolism

occurs as in any severe injury. Peptic ulceration (Curling's ulcers[1]) may occur as a reaction to the stress.

Toxaemia

This is a combination of factors, which include biochemical disturbances, plasma loss and infection. It has also been postulated that the burnt tissues may produce a toxin. Toxaemia is less often seen now that burns are treated adequately.

Treatment

1 *Immediate first-aid treatment.* The immediate treatment of any burn is to stop the process straight away. This is done by removing the patient from the source of the burn, removing overlying clothing, which may contain the heat, and applying cold running water to cool the area and prevent continued damage.

   If the burn area is over 15% (10% if a child) admission and intravenous resuscitation is warranted. Less extensive burns can be managed by oral replacement.
2 *Subsequent treatment.* Thereafter, the principles of the treatment of burns are as follows:
   a management of the local condition – prevent infection and promote healing;
   b general treatment – mitigate the systemic effects of burns listed above;
   c reconstruction and rehabilitation.

Local treatment

- *Partial thickness burns* are managed with simple non-adherent dressings such as paraffin-impregnated gauze under several layers of absorbent gauze; dressings are changed every 2–3 days. When infection is suspected, or the patient presents late, a topical antibiotic such as silver sulfadiazine cream (Flamazine) may be applied to the burn. When the hands are involved, the burn may be covered by sulfadiazine cream and placed in a sealed polythene bag. Full thickness burns,

[1]Thomas Blizzard Curling (1811–1888), Surgeon to the London Hospital; also wrote the first accurate description of cretinism in adults (myxoedema) in 1850.

and some deep partial thickness burns, require total excision of the burn wound; smaller defects may be closed primarily whereas larger defects require application of split thickness skin grafts to hasten re-epithelialization of the defect. Any residual necrotic tissue will be a focus of infection.

- *Circumferential full thickness burns* affecting the chest or limb contract and may restrict breathing and impair blood flow to the limbs. Such contractions must be incised acutely to save the limb (escharotomy).
- *Inhalational burns* are indicated by burnt skin and soot around the face, particularly the mouth and nostrils. Burns to the airway produce oedema, particularly laryngeal oedema, which may necessitate intubation or tracheostomy. Evidence of hypoxia and pulmonary oedema should be treated by ventilation with humidified oxygen; antibiotics are given. The presence of carboxyhaemoglobin in the blood is further evidence suggesting inhalational burns.
- *Priority areas for skin grafting.* Skin grafting is carried out immediately if the eyelids are involved in order to prevent ectropion with the risk of corneal ulceration. The face, hands and the joint flexures are next in priority for skin grafting procedures, as scarring at these sites will obviously produce considerable deformity and disability.

General treatment

Pain

Relieve pain with intravenous opiates (e.g. morphine).

Hypovolaemic shock

Rapid fluid loss occurs, the rate of loss being quickest in the first 12 hours. Aggressive replacement of this fluid as soon as possible is essential. There are two underlying principles in this replacement: first, the correct amount of fluid should be replaced, and, second, the correct type of fluid is important.

1 *Amount of fluid replacement.* This depends upon the total area burnt. As a guide, the 'rule of nines' is helpful and readily calculated. The body is divided into zones of percentage of surface area as follows (Figure 8.2):

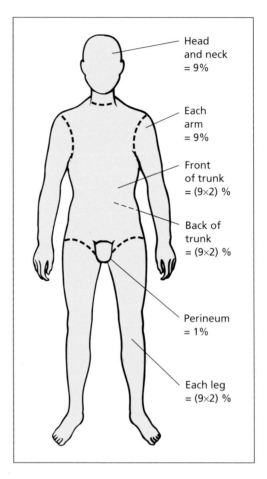

Figure 8.2 The 'rule of nines' – a useful guide to the estimation of the area of a burned surface. (Note also that a patient's hand represents 1% of the body surface area.)

	Percentage surface area
Head and neck	9
Each arm	9
Each leg	2 × 9 = 18
Front of the trunk	2 × 9 = 18
Back of the trunk	2 × 9 = 18
Perineum	1

As a rough rule, the patient's hand is approximately 1% of the body surface area.

An alternative is the Lund and Browder chart (Figure 8.3), which takes account of the differing surface areas of the body with age. For example, an infant's head has a proportionately greater surface area than an adult's. This chart tends to be more accurate than the 'rule of nines'.

In the figure:
Head and neck = 9%
Each arm = 9%
Front of trunk = (9×2) %
Back of trunk = (9×2) %
Perineum = 1%
Each leg = (9×2) %

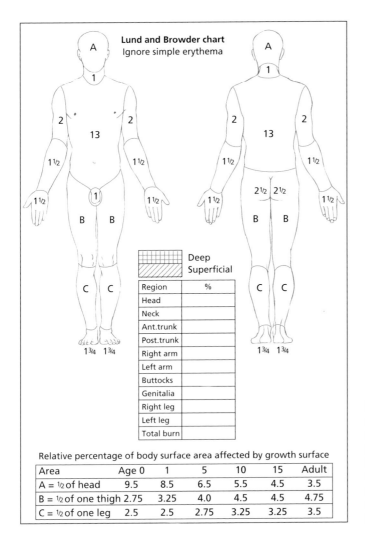

Region	%
Head	
Neck	
Ant.trunk	
Post.trunk	
Right arm	
Left arm	
Buttocks	
Genitalia	
Right leg	
Left leg	
Total burn	

Relative percentage of body surface area affected by growth surface

Area	Age 0	1	5	10	15	Adult
A = ½ of head	9.5	8.5	6.5	5.5	4.5	3.5
B = ½ of one thigh	2.75	3.25	4.0	4.5	4.5	4.75
C = ½ of one leg	2.5	2.5	2.75	3.25	3.25	3.5

Figure 8.3 The Lund and Browder chart allows more accurate estimation of burn surface area and is particularly useful in children. The extent of the burn is marked on the chart. The areas of burns on the head, thighs and lower legs (A, B and C on the chart) are calculated and multiplied by the age factor in the table.

The rate of fluid replacement must take into account that most fluid is lost in the first few hours after the burn, before a coagulum forms. The Parkland formula is now the most accepted way of estimating the volume of fluid to be given in the first 24 hours. Half the volume should be given in the first 8 hours; the remainder over the next 16 hours.

Fluid replacement (mL) in first 24 hours =

4 mL × weight (kg) × % burn area

For example, a 70 kg patient with a 40% burn would, using this formula, require a figure of 4 × 70 × 40 = 11 200 mL. Half of this (5600 mL) is given in the first 8 hours and the other half in the next 16 hours. This does not include the daily maintenance fluid requirement (3 litres in an adult).

During the resuscitation phase, careful clinical assessment of the patient should include monitoring hourly urinary output, pulse, blood pressure, central venous pressure and core temperature, together with regular haematocrit estimations. Fluid replacement may need to be adjusted according to these observations.

2 *Type of fluid used for replacement.* Ringer's lactate (Hartmann's solution) is the crystalloid of choice for the first 24 hours. This has been shown to cause less pulmonary oedema than colloid in the first

24 hours. At the end of 24 hours, colloid infusion such as albumen or fresh frozen plasma is begun, and free water in the form of 5% dextrose is given. If the burns are of full thickness, blood could be used as the colloid fluid replacement in order to replace the extensive red cell destruction that occurs within the affected area.

Antimicrobial chemotherapy

Topical agents are used in preference to systemic prophylactic antimicrobial therapy. Secondary infection of the burns may also require local application of antibiotics, and silver sulfadiazine is the commonest used. Invasive infection does require systemic administration of broad-spectrum antimicrobial treatment covering streptococcal and staphylococcal infection (including meticillin-resistant species, e.g. vancomycin) as well as *Pseudomonas* (e.g. gentamicin); prophylaxis against fungal infection (e.g. fluconazole) may also be appropriate in cases of extensive burns. When necrotic tissue is present, antibiotics will not eliminate infection, and there is the risk that resistant organisms will eventually proliferate. The best protection against infection is to excise the eschar and obtain skin cover.

Nutrition

The patient's nutrition should be maintained, especially when burns are extensive. If enteral nutrition is not possible, parenteral feeding should be instituted early (within 24 hours of the injury). Patients rapidly become catabolic, and adequate calorie and protein replacement are necessary to avoid a negative nitrogen balance.

Complications

Local

- Wound sepsis, usually with *Streptococcus pyogenes* or *Pseudomonas aeruginosa*.
- Scarring (full thickness).
- Wound contractures.

General

- Sepsis, particularly chest infection in inhalational injury, urinary tract infection resulting from catheterization and septicaemia directly from wound invasion.
- Acute peptic ulceration (Curling's ulcer).
- Seizures in children, owing to electrolyte imbalance.
- Renal failure resulting from the initial hypovolaemia due to plasma loss, precipitation of haemoglobin or myoglobin, or nephrotoxic antimicrobial agents.
- Psychological disturbance.

Prognosis

Prognosis depends on the extent and depth of the burns, and whether or not infection occurs. Young infants and the elderly carry a higher mortality than young adults. No matter which methods of treatment are used, few patients survive more than a 70% body area full thickness burn. As a very rough guide, if the patient's age + percentage body area of full thickness burn exceeds 100, the chances of survival are low.

9

The skin and its adnexae

Learning objective

✓ To know the range of lesions that may present in the skin, and in particular the different cancers of the skin, their presentation and management.

Sebaceous cyst

A sebaceous cyst (epidermoid cyst or wen) is a retention cyst produced by obstruction to the mouth of a sebaceous gland. Therefore, sebaceous cysts may occur wherever sebaceous glands exist and are not found on the gland-free palms and soles. They are especially common on the scalp, face, scrotum and vulva and on the lobe of the ear. The cyst is fluctuant and cannot be moved separately from the overlying skin. There may be a typical central punctum and the contents are cheesy with an unpleasant smell. The lining membrane consists of squamous epithelium.

Complications

- Infection.
- Ulceration, which may then resemble a fungating carcinoma ('Cock's peculiar tumour'[1]).
- Calcification, producing a hard subcutaneous tumour misnamed a 'benign calcifying epithelioma'.
- Keratin horn formation.
- Malignant change, which is very rare.

[1]Edward Cock (1805–1892), Surgeon, Guy's Hospital, London, UK.

Lecture Notes: General Surgery, 12th edition. © Harold Ellis, Sir Roy Y. Calne and Christopher J. E. Watson. Published 2011 by Blackwell Publishing Ltd.

Treatment

The uninfected sebaceous cyst should be removed to prevent possible complications. A small elliptical skin incision is made around the punctum of the cyst under local anaesthetic; the capsule is identified and the cyst removed intact. Failure to remove the cyst in its entirety may lead to recurrence.

If the cyst is acutely inflamed, incision and drainage will be required, followed later by excision of the capsule wall.

Dermoid cyst

There are two types of dermoid cyst: implantation dermoid and sequestration dermoid.

Implantation dermoid

This is a painless, subcutaneous, cystic swelling commonly found on the pulps of the fingers, attached neither to the skin nor to the deeper structures. It usually follows a puncture injury (e.g. from a rose thorn) with consequent implantation of epithelial cells into the subcutaneous tissues. The cyst typically contains a white, greasy material, which results from degeneration of the desquamated cells. An old healed scar over the cyst may help confirm the diagnosis.

Sequestration dermoid

This is a subcutaneous cystic swelling resulting from an embryological rest of epithelial cells along a line of fusion. The common sites are over the external angular process of the frontal bone (the external angular dermoid at the upper outer margin of the orbit), the root of the nose (internal angular dermoid) and in the midline. When in relation to the skull, the underlying bone is usually hollowed out around it. The possibility of communication with an intracranial dermoid or the meninges should be excluded by skull radiography or computed tomography (CT) scan prior to excision.

Verruca vulgaris (wart)

This is a well-localized horny projection that is common on the fingers, hands, feet and knees, particularly of children and young adults. Crops of warts may occur on the genitalia and perianal region, in many cases spread by sexual contact. Warts are often multiple and are due to a number of different strains of human papilloma virus.

Microscopically, there is a local hyperplasia of the prickle cell layer of the skin (acanthosis) with marked surface cornification.

Treatment

Untreated, warts usually vanish spontaneously within 2 years, hence the apparent efficacy of folklore 'wart cures'. Often, reassurance that these lesions will disappear is all that is required, but if treatment is demanded they can be burnt down by the application of a silver nitrate stick or podophyllin, frozen with liquid nitrogen, or curetted under local or general anaesthesia.

Plantar warts

Otherwise known as verrucas, these occur on the weight-bearing areas of the foot. Pressure forces the wart into the deeper tissues, producing intense local pain on walking. They may occur in epidemics in schools and other such places, where the hygiene of the communal bath or changing room is not of a high standard. They should be treated by podophyllin or curettage.

Keratoacanthoma (molluscum sebaceum)

This is a lesion that occurs in elderly patients, most commonly men, in sun-exposed areas such as the face and nose (75%), although it may occur on any skin surface. It appears as a rapidly growing nodule, which may reach 3 cm or more in diameter in a few weeks, with a characteristic central crater filled by a keratin plug. It closely resembles a squamous carcinoma or rodent ulcer in appearance, and it is only the history of very rapid growth that helps differentiate it from the latter.

Histologically, it consists of a central crater filled with keratin surrounded by hypertrophied squamous stratified epithelium. There is no invasion of the surrounding tissues.

If left untreated, the lesion disappears over a period of 4–5 months, leaving a faint white scar. It appears to be of hair follicle origin, and may be associated with a minor injury.

Treatment

It is safest to remove the lesion to establish histological proof of the diagnosis.

Ganglion

A ganglion presents as a cystic, subcutaneous swelling that transilluminates brilliantly. It most commonly occurs around the wrist and the dorsum of the foot (joint capsule origin), or along the flexor aspect of the fingers and on the peroneal tendons (tendon sheath origin). Although ganglia are among the commonest of surgical lumps, their origin is uncertain. They may represent a benign myxoma of joint capsule or tendon sheath, a hamartoma or a myxomatous degeneration due to trauma. They are thin-walled cysts with a synovial lining, and contain clear colourless material with the consistency of KY Jelly.

Treatment

The patient may complain of discomfort or of the cosmetic appearance; if so, the cyst should be excised under a general anaesthetic using a bloodless field produced by a tourniquet. The old-fashioned treatment of hitting the ganglion with the family bible ruptures the cyst, but recurrence usually occurs after some time. Unfortunately, recurrence is also common after surgical excision.

Pilonidal sinus

The majority of pilonidal sinuses occur in the skin of the natal cleft. They may be solitary or appear as a row in the midline. Frequently, tufts of hair are found lying free within the sinus (Latin *pilus*, hair; *nidus*, nest).

Usually, young adults are affected, males more than females, and more often dark-haired individuals; the sinuses are rarely seen in children and do not present until adolescence. They are an occupational disease of barbers, in whom sinuses occur in the clefts between the fingers. They are occasionally found in the axilla, at the umbilicus, in the perineum and on the sole of the foot as well as on amputation stumps.

Aetiology

The occurrence of pilonidal sinuses remote from the natal cleft, and the occurrence of such sinuses on the hands and feet of people working with cattle, where the contained hair is clearly of animal origin, supports the hypothesis that these sinuses occur by implantation of hair into the skin; these set up a foreign-body reaction and produce a chronic infected sinus. It may be that, in some cases, post-anal pits act as traps for loose hairs, thus combining both the congenital and acquired theories of origin. The hair enters the skin follicles from its distal end and works its way in due to tapered lateral hair extensions angled proximally, rather as a grass seed migrates up one's sleeve.

Clinical features

The pilonidal sinus is asymptomatic until it becomes infected; there is then a typical history of recurrent abscesses, which either require drainage or discharge spontaneously.

Treatment

1 *Acute abscess.* This is drained in the usual way.
2 *Quiescent sinus.* The track is excised or simply laid open and allowed to heal by granulation.

Recurrence is diminished by keeping the surrounding skin free from hair by rubbing with fine sandpaper, shaving or the use of depilatory creams.

The nails

The nails are the site of some common and important surgical conditions.

Paronychia

Paronychia denotes infection of the nail fold, usually of the finger, but it may complicate an ingrowing toenail (see below).

Diagnosis of acute paronychia is obvious; the nail fold is red, swollen and tender, and pus may be visible beneath the skin.

Treatment

If seen before pus has formed, at the cellulitic stage, infection may be aborted by a course of flucloxacillin or other appropriate anti-staphylococcal antibiotic together with immobilization by a splint to the finger and elevation of the arm in a sling. If pus is present, drainage is performed through an incision carried proximally through the nail fold, combined with removal of the base of the nail if pus has tracked beneath it.

Chronic paronychia is seen in those whose occupation requires constant soaking of the hands in water, but it may also occur as a result of fungal infection (*Candida*) of the nails and where the peripheral circulation is deficient, e.g. Raynaud's phenomenon (Chapter 12, p. 94).

Ingrowing toenail

This is nearly always confined to the hallux and is usually due to a combination of tight shoes (particularly 'trainers') and the habit of paring the nail downwards into the nail fold, rather than transversely; the sharp edge of the nail then grows into the side of the nail bed, producing ulceration and infection.

Treatment

If seen before infection has occurred, advice is given on correct cutting of the nails; nylon socks and trainers are vetoed. A pledget of cotton wool tucked daily into the side of the nail bed, after preliminary soaking of the feet in hot water to soften the nails, enables the nail to grow up out of the fold.

If an acute paronychia is present, drainage will be required by means of removal of the side of the nail or avulsion of the whole nail. For recurrent cases when the infection has settled, the affected side may be excised together with the nail root (wedge excision), or the entire nail may be obliterated completely by excision of the nail root (Zadik's operation[2]) or by treating the nail bed with liquefied phenol, or a combination of the two techniques.

Onychogryphosis

The nail is coiled like a 'ram's horn'. It may affect any of the toes, although the hallux is the commonest site. It may follow trauma to the nail bed and is usually found in elderly subjects.

Treatment

Relatively mild examples can be kept under control by trimming the nail with bone-cutting forceps. Merely avulsing the nail is invariably followed by recurrence, and the only adequate treatment is excision of the nail root.

Lesions of the nail bed

It is convenient to list a number of relatively common conditions that affect the nail bed.

Subungual haematoma

As a result of crush injury to the terminal phalanx, with or without fracture of the underlying bone, a tense, painful haematoma may develop beneath the nail. Relief is afforded by evacuating the clot through a hole made either by a dental drill or by a red-hot needle; both procedures are painless. Occasionally, a small haematoma may develop after a trivial or forgotten injury and clinically may closely simulate a subungual melanoma.

Subungual exostosis

This is nearly always confined to the hallux and is especially found in adolescents and young adults.

It appears as a reddish-brown area under the nail, which is tender on pressure. The exostosis may ulcerate through the overlying nail, producing an infected granulating mass. The diagnosis is confirmed by X-ray of the toe, and treatment is to remove the nail and excise the underlying exostosis.

Subungual melanoma

The nail bed is a common site for malignant melanoma (see p. 52). There is a long history of slow growth and often a misleading history of trauma. The lesion should be confirmed by excision biopsy followed by amputation of the digit. If the regional lymph nodes are involved, block dissection is performed.

Glomus tumour

The nail beds of the fingers and toes are a common site of this extremely painful lesion, which is a benign tumour arising in a subcutaneous glomus body (highly innervated arteriovenous anastomoses in dermis responsible for temperature regulation). It is considered on p. 57.

Tumours of the skin and subcutaneous tissues

Classification

1 Epidermal.
  a Benign: papilloma, senile keratosis, seborrhoeic keratosis.
  b Malignant: Bowen's disease, squamous cell carcinoma, basal cell carcinoma, secondary deposits (e.g. from carcinoma of breast and lung, leukaemia, Hodgkin's disease).
2 Benign and malignant melanomas.
3 Tumours of sebaceous and sweat glands.
4 Dermal tumours from blood vessels, lymphatics, nerves, fibrous tissue or fat.

Epidermal tumours

Papilloma

This is a common, benign, pedunculated tumour, often pigmented with melanin. Microscopically, it comprises a keratinized papillary tumour of squamous epithelium.

---

[2]Frank Raphael Zadik (1914–1995), Orthopaedic Surgeon, Leigh and Wigan, UK.

Seborrhoeic keratosis (basal cell papilloma)

This is a common tumour occurring after the age of 40 years. It appears as a yellowish or brown raised lesion on the face, arms or trunk and is often multiple. It often appears greasy, and its surface is characterized by a network of crypts.

Microscopically, there is hyperkeratosis, proliferation of the basal cell layer and melanin pigmentation.

The lesion is quite benign, but differential diagnosis from a melanoma can only be made with certainty by excising the lump and submitting it to histological examination.

Solar (actinic) keratosis

This is a small, hard, brown, scaly tumour on sun-exposed areas of skin (e.g. the forehead, ears and backs of hands) of the elderly. Keratoses are more common in individuals with fair skin, and after prolonged exposure to ultraviolet light.

Microscopically, hyperkeratosis is present, often with atypical dividing cells in the prickle cell layer.

The lesions may be treated with liquid nitrogen cryotherapy or curettage; large areas may require topical chemotherapy (e.g. 5-fluorouracil). Imiquimod has also been used, and acts as an immune modifier, stimulating an immune response with resolution of the lesions.

The importance of this lesion is that it may undergo change into a squamous cell carcinoma.

Bowen's disease[3]

This appears as a very slowly growing, red, scaly plaque, and represents 'squamous carcinoma *in situ*'. It may be mistaken for a psoriatic plaque. Human papilloma virus (HPV) DNA (particularly HPV16, but also HPV2) has been found in some lesions.

Microscopically, atypical keratinocytes with vacuolization, mitoses and multinucleated giant cells are prominent in the epidermis but the basal layer is intact.

Treatment is excision; if left untreated, eventually a squamous cell carcinoma will supervene.

Squamous cell carcinoma (epithelioma)

Occurs usually in the elderly male, especially in skin areas exposed to sunshine, e.g. the face and backs of the hands. Like solar keratoses, it is relatively common in white subjects who live in the tropics.

Predisposing factors

These include the following:

- solar keratosis;
- Bowen's disease;
- exposure to sunshine or ultraviolet irradiation;
- exposure to ionizing irradiation;
- infection with human papilloma virus types 6, 11, 16 and 18;
- carcinogens, e.g. pitch, tar, soot, mineral oils;
- chronic ulceration, particularly in burns scars (Marjolin's ulcer – see below);
- immunosuppressive drugs.

Pathology

Macroscopically, it presents as a typical carcinomatous ulcer with indurated, raised everted edges and a central scab. Microscopically, there are solid columns of epithelial cells growing into the dermis with epithelial pearls of central keratin surrounded by prickle cells. Occasionally, anaplastic tumours are seen in which these pearls are absent.

Spread occurs by local infiltration and then by lymphatics. Blood spread occurs only in very advanced cases.

Treatment

Treatment consists of either wide excision or radiotherapy, depending on the site of the lesion. If the regional lymph nodes are involved, block dissection is indicated.

Marjolin's ulcer[4]

The name applied to malignant change in a scar, ulcer or sinus, e.g. a chronic venous ulcer, an unhealed burn or the sinus of chronic osteomyelitis. It has the following characteristics:

- *slow growth*, because the lesion is relatively avascular;

---

[3]John Templeton Bowen (1857–1941), Dermatologist, Harvard Medical School, Boston, MA, USA.

[4]Jean Nicholas Marjolin (1780–1850), Surgeon, Hôpital Sainte-Eugénie, Paris, France.

- *painless*, because the scar tissue does not contain cutaneous nerve fibres;
- *lymphatic spread is late*, because the scar tissue produces lymphatic obliteration.

Once the tumour reaches the normal tissues beyond the diseased area, rapid growth, pain and lymphatic involvement take place.

Basal cell carcinoma (rodent ulcer)

This is the most common form of skin cancer in white people. It occurs usually in elderly subjects, in males twice as commonly as in females. Ninety per cent are found on the face above a line joining the angle of the mouth to the external auditory meatus, particularly around the eye, the nasolabial folds and the hair line of the scalp. The tumour may, however, arise on any part of the skin, including the anal margin. Predisposing factors are exposure to sunlight or irradiation.

Pathology

Macroscopically, the tumour has raised, rolled, but not everted edges. It consists of pearly nodules over which fine blood vessels can be seen to course (telangiectasia). Starting as a small nodule, the tumour very slowly grows over the years with central ulceration and scabbing.

Microscopically, solid sheets of uniform, darkly staining cells arising from the basal layer of the skin are seen. Prickle cells and epithelial pearls are both absent.

Spread is by infiltration with slow but steady destruction of surrounding tissues; in advanced cases, the underlying skull may be eroded or the face, nose and eye may be destroyed, hence the name 'rodent'. Lymphatic and blood spread occur with extreme rarity.

Treatment

Treatment is by excision, where this can be done with an adequate margin and without cosmetic deformity. It is also indicated in late cases where the tumour has recurred after irradiation or has invaded the underlying bone or cartilage. In the majority of cases, however, superficial radiotherapy gives excellent results. Where the tumour occurs on or near the eyelid, the conjunctiva must be protected by means of a lead shield during irradiation therapy.

Melanoma

Aetiology

Melanomas develop from melanocytes, which are situated in the basal layer of the epidermis and which originate from the neuroectoderm of the embryonic neural crest. Some melanocytes contain no visible pigment, but all are characterized by a positive dihydroxyphenyl alanine (DOPA) reaction – they can all convert DOPA into melanin. While most melanomas arise in the skin, they may also occur at other sites to which neural crest cells migrate, in particular the pigmented choroid layer of the eye.

Classification

Melanomas may be classified into the following:

- intradermal melanoma or naevus (the common mole);
- junctional melanoma or naevus;
- compound melanoma or naevus;
- juvenile melanoma;
- malignant melanoma.

Nearly everyone possesses one or more moles; some have hundreds, although they may not become apparent until after puberty. Those moles that are entirely within the dermis remain benign, but a small percentage of the junctional naevi, so called because they are seen in the basal layer of the epidermis at its junction with the dermis, may undergo malignant change (Figure 9.1).

Intradermal melanoma or naevus

This is the commonest variety of mole. The naevus may be light or dark in colour and may be flat or raised, hairy or hairless. A hairy mole is nearly always intradermal. They may be found in any place in the body except the palm of the hand, the sole of the foot or the scrotal skin.

Histologically, there is a nest of melanocytes situated entirely within the dermis where the cells form non-encapsulated masses. They never undergo malignant change, and need no treatment unless the diagnosis is uncertain.

Junctional melanoma or naevus

The junctional naevus is pigmented to a variable

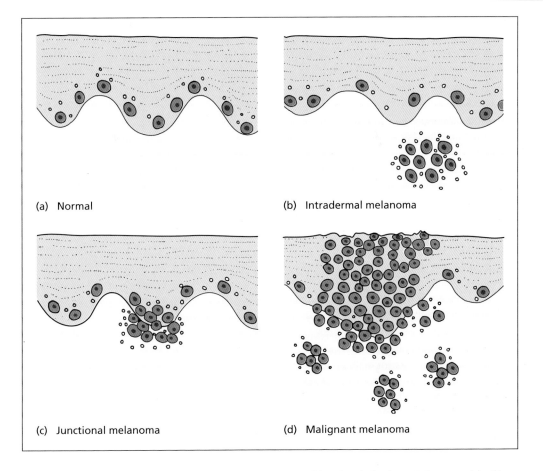

(a) Normal

(b) Intradermal melanoma

(c) Junctional melanoma

(d) Malignant melanoma

Figure 9.1 (a) The normal skin contains melanocytes (shown as cells) and melanin pigment shown as dots. The pigment increases in sunburn and freckles. (b) A benign intradermal naevus; the melanocytes are clumped together in the dermis to form a localized benign tumour. (c) A junctional naevus with melanocytes clumping together in the basal layer of the epidermis. These are usually benign but may occasionally give rise to an invasive malignant melanoma (d).

shade from light brown to almost black. It is nearly always flat, smooth and hairless. It may occur anywhere on the body and, unlike the intradermal naevus, may be found on the palm of the hand, sole of the foot and the genitalia.

Histologically, naevus cells are seen in the basal layers of the epidermis from which the cells may spread to the surface.

Only a small percentage of junctional naevi undergo malignant change, but it is from this group that the vast majority of malignant melanomas arise.

Compound melanoma or naevus

Clinically, this is indistinguishable from the intradermal naevus, but histologically it has junctional elements that make it potentially malignant.

Juvenile melanoma

Melanomas before puberty are relatively unusual, and may present as a dark nodule. Microscopically, they may be indistinguishable from malignant melanoma; yet fortunately and surprisingly, these usually pursue a completely benign course. Melanomas in children should therefore always be dealt with by conservative surgery in spite of their frightening histological appearance.

Malignant melanoma

Malignant melanomas arise in pre-existing naevi, either junctional naevi or compound naevi where there is a junctional component. They occur in white people on light-exposed areas, hence the higher incidence on the legs of females. It is rarely found in the pigmented skin of dark-skinned races, tending to be found in the non-pigmented skin on the sole of the foot or, less commonly, the palm. A premalignant form, the lentigo maligna, also exists.

Presentations

The two main presentations of malignant melanoma are the superficial spreading type, and the nodular type.

- *Superficial spreading melanoma.* The commonest presentation of malignant melanoma is of a previously dormant naevus starting to spread superficially. The surface has patches of deep pigmentation.
- *Nodular melanoma.* The naevus is nodular and deeply pigmented and may bleed or ulcerate. Such a nodule may occur on a pigmented background such as the lentigo maligna. It tends to invade deeply rather than spread superficially, and carries a poorer prognosis with earlier lymphatic involvement.

In addition to the common types of malignant melanoma above, less common forms include the following:

- *Lentigo maligna.* This is a brown pigmented patch with an irregular outline and is usually found on the cheeks of elderly women, often called a Hutchinson's freckle.[5] The pale patch appears over several years; malignant change is indicated by deeper pigmentation or nodule formation.
- *Acral melanoma.* These are so called because they occur at the extremities, commonly on the palms and soles of the feet. It is this type

that also occurs in dark-skinned races. The subungual melanoma is a variant of acral melanoma (see p. 50).

- *Mucosal melanoma.* Malignant melanoma may be found on the mucous membranes of the nose, mouth, anus and intestine.
- *Choroid melanoma.* Melanomas may arise from melanocytes in the pigment layer of the retina. These are renowned for presenting many years after enucleation with hepatic metastases; hence, the aphorism 'beware the patient with the large liver and the glass eye'.
- *Amelanotic melanoma.* Paradoxically, melanomas are not always pigmented, but they remain DOPA positive.

Signs of malignant change in a melanoma

- Increase or irregularity in size.
- Increase or irregularity in pigmentation.
- Bleeding or ulceration.
- Spread of pigment from the edge of the naevus.
- Itching or pain.
- Formation of daughter or satellite nodules.
- Lymph node or distant spread.

Pathology

Microscopically, pleomorphic cells are seen, which spread through the layers of the epidermis and which are usually pigmented (occasionally the cells are amelanotic).

Spread

As well as local growth and ulceration, malignant melanomas seed by lymphatic permeation, which produces cutaneous nodules by progressive proximal spread, and by lymphatic emboli to the regional lymph nodes. There is also widespread dissemination by the bloodstream to any and every organ in the body. Free melanin in the blood may produce generalized skin pigmentation and melanuria in late cases.

Staging

The prognosis of malignant melanoma depends upon its degree of invasion, which is measured by the depth of invasion. The depth may be measured either by reference to the normal skin layers (Clark's levels) or, more simply and accurately, according to its measured depth (Breslow depth[6]).

[5]Sir Jonathan Hutchinson (1828–1913), Surgeon, The London Hospital, London, UK. Described numerous conditions and was first to perform a successful operation for reduction of an intussusception in a child.

[6]Alexander Breslow (1928–1980), Pathologist, George Washington University Hospital, Washington, DC, USA.

Because of its simplicity, Breslow's method is now routinely adopted.

Treatment of pigmented lesions

The following is a general guide to the management of pigmented lesions of the skin.

Prophylactic removal

Any pigmented tumour on the hand, sole or genitalia, or any that, in other situations, are subjected to trauma should be excised; these are the commonest among the small percentage of naevi to undergo malignant change. In addition, pigmented lesions should be removed for cosmetic reasons or if the patient is acutely anxious about their presence – this is a particularly common phenomenon among doctors, nurses and medical students. Such lesions are sent for careful histological examination and should always be removed in their entirety.

Suspicious naevi

If the pigmented lesion shows any of the features already listed that suggest that malignant change has taken place, the naevus is first removed for urgent histological examination (frozen section). If malignant melanoma is confirmed, a wide local excision of the area is performed, with a margin of clearance proportional to the depth of invasion (Breslow depth). Traditionally this was translated into a centimetre margin for every millimetre of invasion; primary skin grafting may be required.

Sentinel lymph nodes

The sentinel node, the primary lymphatic drainage of the tumour, is identified and excised for histological examination. Identification of the sentinel node is by injection of vital blue dye around the primary melanoma, combined with preoperative lymphoscintigraphy to map the lymphatic drainage. If the sentinel node is involved, the regional nodes are excised by block dissection.

Adjuvant therapy

Malignant melanoma deposits often show regression when the primary lesion is excised, implying an immunological component. Immunotherapy with high dose interferon-α2b may be effective at prolonging survival. Interleukin 2 administration has also had some success.

Melanomas are generally radioresistant. Results of chemotherapy, including high-dose isolated perfusion of a limb with cytotoxic chemotherapeutic agents, have been disappointing.

Table 9.1 Five year survival according to Breslow depth

Depth	5 year survival
<0.75 mm	>95%
0.75–1.5 mm	90%
1.5–4.0 mm	70%
>4.0 mm	<50%

Prognosis

Prognosis depends on a large number of factors.

- *Breslow depth* of the primary lesion, measured vertically from the top of the granular layer to the deepest point of tumour invasion. This is the most important prognostic factor. Prognosis is good when this depth is less than 1.5 mm. The deeper the lesion, the greater the risk of lymph node metastasis and the worse the 5 year survival (Table 9.1).
- *Type of lesion.* A superficial spreading melanoma has a better prognosis than a penetrating and ulcerating lesion.
- *The anatomical site.* Tumours on the trunk and scalp have a poor prognosis.
- *Lymph node metastases.* They indicate poor prognosis, more so if there are cutaneous deposits. The presence of sentinel node involvement, or satellite lesions, reduces 5 year survival to under 30%.

Tumours of sweat glands and sebaceous glands

Benign and malignant tumours of these glandular adnexae of the skin are rare.

Sebaceous adenomas

These are more in the nature of a hyperplasia of the glands than true tumours. They occur as pink or yellow papules on the nose, cheek and forehead. Microscopically, they are merely overgrowths of sebaceous glands.

Sebaceous carcinoma

Found rarely on the face and scalp in elderly subjects, it is an uncommon but aggressive cancer. Carcinomatous change may rarely occur in sebaceous cysts.

Sweat gland adenomas or carcinomas

These may occur on the face and scalp and in the apocrine sweat glands of the axilla, vulva and scrotum. They are composed of columns or cylinders of clear cells and the descriptive term 'cylindroma' is applied to these tumours for this reason. On the scalp, they may form masses of large nodules ('turban tumour'), but tumours of similar appearance may also be of basal cell origin.

Blood vessel tumours

Tumours of blood vessels usually lie in the dermis, although the underlying muscles and soft tissues may be involved. The abdominal viscera, central nervous system and bone may also be the sites of these lesions. The terminology of blood vessel tumours is confusing and is bedevilled with picturesque descriptive terms. Most benign blood vessel 'tumours' are indeed congenital malformations or hamartomas.

Classification

- Capillary haemangioma.
- Cavernous haemangioma.
- Sclerosing angioma (fibrous histiocytoma).
- Glomus tumour.
- Haemangiosarcoma.
- Kaposi's sarcoma.

Capillary haemangioma

A variety of types of congenital capillary malformation may be found in the skin, usually at birth.

- A *salmon pink patch* is a common blemish on the head or neck of a newborn child and rapidly disappears spontaneously.
- A *strawberry naevus* is bright red and raised, and usually disappears during the first few years of life, although there may at first be a rapid alarming enlargement, even with ulceration, before involution occurs.
- A *port-wine stain*, flush with the skin, usually on the face, lips and buccal mucosa, produces an extensive area of dark red, blue or purple discolouration. It is present from birth and shows no tendency to regress with age.

  Note that port-wine stain of the face may have a segmental distribution corresponding to the cutaneous branches of the trigeminal nerve and may be associated with angiomas of the cerebral pia–arachnoid, which may manifest themselves by focal epileptic attacks (the Sturge–Weber syndrome[7]).

- *Campbell de Morgan spots*[8] are found on the trunk of middle-aged and elderly subjects. They are bright red aggregates of dilated capillaries, which can be emptied by pressing on them with the tip of a pencil. They are of no significance.
- *Spider naevus* is another example of a capillary haemangioma. Isolated 'spiders' are present in normal people, but they are more common during pregnancy and in chronic liver disease. They comprise a central arteriole from which radiate capillaries. Pressure on the central arteriole with a pinhead causes the lesion to disappear while pressure is maintained.

Treatment

Most strawberry naevi disappear spontaneously, but diathermy coagulation, application of CO_2 snow or excision and grafting may be required. The port-wine stain may respond to cutaneous laser therapy, but the simplest treatment remains camouflage with cosmetics.

Cavernous haemangioma

These are made up of large blood spaces lined with endothelium. They occur on the skin and lip and, quite commonly, as multiple nodules in the liver. They are usually present at birth, and grow to keep pace with normal body growth.

The lesions are blue, may be raised and may partly empty on pressure. They may infiltrate the underlying tissues and may be associated with unsightly overlying cutaneous thickening.

Treatment

This is often difficult. The condition may be disguised by the use of cosmetics, or thrombosis can be encouraged by injection of sclerosing agents. Very unsightly small lesions may be excised and skin grafted.

---

[7]William Allen Sturge (1850–1919), Physician, Royal Free Hospital, London, UK. Frederick Parkes Weber (1863–1962), Physician, London, UK, with a life-long interest in rare diseases.
[8]Campbell de Morgan (1811–1876), Surgeon, Middlesex Hospital, London, UK.

Sclerosing angioma (fibrous histiocytoma)

This is a pigmented tumour of the skin that may easily be confused with a malignant melanoma with which it has a close macroscopic resemblance. Palpation, however, reveals a typically hard consistency due to the dense fibrous stroma. It is probably produced as a result of fibrosis of a capillary haemangioma. The pigment is due to iron and not to melanin; this is easily shown with specific histological staining.

Glomus tumour

Glomus bodies are found in the subcutaneous tissues of the limbs, particularly the fingers, the toes and their nail beds. They are convoluted arteriovenous anastomoses with a cellular wall comprising a thick layer of cuboidal 'glomus' cells, which are modified plain muscles; between these cells are abundant nerve fibres. These structures are perhaps concerned with cutaneous heat regulation. Glomus tumours are blue or reddish, small, raised lesions, which occur in young adults at the common sites of glomus bodies. Their characteristic is exquisite tenderness, which makes the slightest touch agonizing.

Treatment

Treatment is excision of the lesion, which is rewarded by the heartfelt gratitude of the patient.

Kaposi's sarcoma[9]

This tumour has a multicentric origin. It used to be most common in the elderly in central Europe, particularly Ashkenazi Jews;[10] now it is a common tumour in patients with acquired immune deficiency syndrome (AIDS), and also occurs more commonly in immunosuppressed organ transplant recipients. DNA extracted from Kaposi's sarcoma tissue has been found to contain human herpes virus type 8 (HHV8), now known as Kaposi sarcoma herpes virus (KSHV), indicating a significant aetiological role for this virus. It presents as a number of bluish red or dark blue nodules scattered over the extremities of one or more of the limbs. The nodules spread centrally along the limb, may ulcerate and can metastasize to the liver and lungs. In the aggressive form, which occurs in the immunosuppressed, visceral involvement occurs with bowel perforation, haemorrhage or intussusception.

Histologically, there are two components: blood vessels and fibroblasts. The latter show the malignant features, thus distinguishing this tumour from a haemangiosarcoma. Treatment involves control of HIV infection with highly active antiretroviral treatment (HAART) or reduction of immunosuppression in transplant recipients, together with local radiotherapy or cytotoxic drugs.

Telangiectasia

Telangiectases, although not truly tumours, are conveniently mentioned in this section. They are dilatations of normal capillaries and are seen in a number of circumstances, e.g. on the weatherbeaten faces of country people and on the legs of young women, who may complain of their cosmetic appearance.

Hereditary haemorrhagic telangiectasia (HHT; Osler–Weber–Rendu syndrome[11]) is an inherited autosomal dominant disease characterized by tiny capillary angiomas of the skin, lips and mucous membranes; they may give rise to repeated nose bleeds and gastrointestinal haemorrhage. The genetic abnormality is a mutation of either endoglin (HHT type 1) or activin receptor-like kinase (HHT type 2) genes. Typically, the telangiectases are visible around the mouth and in the fauces, and present with nose bleeds. Occult arteriovenous malformations are common.

Lymph vessel tumours

Lymphangiomas are congenital in origin and similar to haemangiomas; they are lined by endothelium but contain lymph. They are relatively uncommon, but occur mainly on the lips, tongue and cheek, resulting in macrocheilia or macroglossia.

---

[9]Moriz Kaposi (1837–1902), Professor of Dermatology, Vienna, Austria.
[10]Ashkenazi Jews: contrast Sephardic and Oriental Jews. Migrated to Germany, Poland and Russia.

[11]Sir William Osler (1849–1919), Professor of Medicine, successively at McGill University, Montreal, Canada; Johns Hopkins University, Baltimore, MD, USA; and the University of Oxford, Oxford, UK. Frederick Parkes Weber (1863–1962), Physician, London, UK. Henri Rendu (1844–1902), Physician, Hôpital Necker, Paris, France.

Cystic hygroma

A form of lymphangioma, the aetiology of cystic hygromas is thought to relate to a combination of a failure of lymphatics to connect to the venous system, abnormal growth of embryonal lymphatics and sequestered lymphatic rests. Most occur in the neck, usually the left side, and were thought to be related to the embryonic precursor of the jugular part of the thoracic duct. They consist of a multilocular cystic mass, which is often present at birth or noticed in early infancy. Characteristically, they are supremely transilluminable. They may respond to injection of sclerosant agents such as alcohol or doxycycline. Surgical treatment consists of excision, but this is a difficult procedure as the cysts ramify throughout the structures of the neck.

Nerve tumours

Tumours of the peripheral nerves arise from the neurilemmal sheath of Schwann;[12] hence, the terms neurilemmoma, neurofibroma or schwannoma. They push the fibres of the nerve to one side or actually grow within the substance of the nerve. The tumours may be solitary or multiple and may involve any peripheral nerve in the body. Of the cranial nerves, the eighth is most commonly involved, often as a solitary tumour (the acoustic neuroma; see Chapter 14). Tumours may arise within the spinal canal, particularly from the dorsal nerve roots, resulting in an extramedullary, intrathecal, slow-growing spinal tumour (see Chapter 16). Part of this tumour may protrude through the intervertebral foramen, producing a dumb-bell tumour, which projects into either the thoracic cavity or the abdominal cavity.

In the skin and subcutaneous tissues, there is a wide range of presentations from a solitary tumour arising from a peripheral nerve to uncountable numbers involving the whole of the body (*von Recklinghausen's disease*;[13] his name is also applied to the osteitis fibrosa cystica of hyperparathyroidism – see Chapter 38).

Clinical features

The tumours may appear in childhood and there is often a family history. Three types of neurofibromatosis are recognized, and all are autosomal dominant. von Recklinghausen's disease is type 1 neurofibromatosis[14] and results from a mutation in the neurofibromin gene. The cutaneous lesions are soft and often pedunculated. They are usually painless, although pressure may produce pain along the line of the nerve, particularly when larger nerve trunks are involved. The tumour is mobile from side to side but not longitudinally, in the line of the nerve to which is it attached. There may be associated café-au-lait patches of pigmentation. In some cases, there are disfiguring masses of neurofibromatous tissue over which the thickened skin hangs in ugly folds. The 'elephant man' of the London Hospital was a gross example of the disease.

Treatment

Where the neurofibromas are solitary or few in number, removal can be performed, either by enucleation, if the nerve fibres are pushed to one side, or by resection with suture of the divided nerve. Incomplete removal must not be performed, as sarcomatous change may follow. Where the whole body is covered by these lesions, some cosmetic improvement can be effected by excising the more noticeable lesions from the face and hands.

Neurofibrosarcomas are uncommon. They may arise *de novo* or as malignant change in a neurofibroma. Clinical features are pain, rapid growth and peripheral anaesthesia or paralysis. Treatment is wide excision.

Fatty tumours

Lipoma

Lipomas are the commonest of benign tumours. They usually occur in adults, and the sex distribution is equal, although females are more likely to present to the surgeon for cosmetic removal of these lesions. Lipomas may arise in any connective tissue but especially in the subcutaneous fat, particularly around the shoulder and over the trunk. They do not occur in the palm, sole of the foot or the scalp, because in these areas the fat is

---

[12]Theodor Schwann (1810–1882), Professor of Anatomy, Louvain and then Liège, Belgium.

[13]Friederich Daniel von Recklinghausen (1833–1910), Professor of Pathology, successively at Königsberg, Germany; Würzburg, Germany; and Strasbourg, France.

[14]Type II neurofibromatosis (mutation in neurofibromin 2 gene) is characterized by eighth nerve tumours, meningiomas and schwannomas of the dorsal roots of the spinal cord; type III neurofibromatosis has features of both type I and type II, with café-au-lait spots, cutaneous lesions and intracranial neurofibromas and meningiomas.

contained within dense fibrous septa. Occasionally, lipomas appear in large numbers subcutaneously and are tender (adiposis dolorosa or Dercum's disease[15]) and it is sometimes quite difficult to differentiate them from neurofibromas. Elsewhere it is useful to remember that 'lipomas occur beneath everything'; thus, in addition to being subcutaneous, they may be subfascial, subperiosteal, subperitoneal, submucosal and subpleural.

The diagnosis is rarely in doubt with this soft, lobulated, fluctuant tumour. The fluctuation is interesting; it is often said to be due to the fat being liquid at body temperature, but anyone observing an operation will notice that fat within the body certainly does not flow out in liquid form over the surgeon's boots when the skin is incised. The fluctuation can be explained by the histological structure of the lipoma, which consists of aggregates of typical fat cells; each cell itself forms a microscopic cyst. This is very much like the fluc-tuation that can be elicited in a colloid goitre made up of thyroid vesicles distended with colloid material.

Treatment

Treatment consists of excision if the lipoma is cosmetically troublesome.

Liposarcoma

A rare tumour, which probably arises as an unusual event in a pre-existing benign lipoma. The retroperitoneal site is commonest, but it may also occur around the thigh region and should be suspected if the tumour is very large, firmer than usual, vascular or rapidly growing.

Treatment

Treatment comprises wide excision if this is possible.

---

[15]Francis Xavier Dercum (1856–1931), Professor of Clinical Neurology, Jefferson Medical College, Philadelphia, PA, USA.

10

The chest and lungs

Learning objectives

✓ To have a knowledge of the types of chest injury and their management.

✓ To have a knowledge of lung cancer and its management; this is particularly important as it is the commonest cancer cause of death in the UK.

Injury to the chest

Ventilation of the lungs depends on a patent main airway and pulmonary alveoli, the rigid bony skeleton of the thorax and the integrity of the nerves and muscles that control the movements of the ribs and diaphragm. Traumatic disruption of the chest wall is likely to be lethal unless treatment is instituted rapidly. Dangerous complications of chest injury are:

- paradoxical respiration;
- pneumothorax;
- penetration of the lung;
- haemothorax;
- cardiac tamponade due to laceration of the heart;
- large-vessel damage.

Serious harm can also result from blunt (crush) injuries that do not penetrate the chest; thus, a main bronchus or the aorta may be ruptured, the lung contused and papillary muscles of the heart or the coronary arteries may be damaged.

Fractures of the ribs

Clinical features

The commonest injury to the chest is fracture of the ribs by a direct blow. The most commonly affected ribs are the seventh, eighth and ninth, in which the fracture usually occurs in the region of the midaxillary line. The patient complains of pain in the chest overlying the fracture and this pain is intensified by springing the ribs with gentle but sharp pressure on the sternum.

Special investigations

- *Chest X-ray* may confirm rib fractures, and will identify underlying lung damage or haemorrhage that might not have been suspected from the trivial nature of the patient's symptoms. A chest X-ray may not always demonstrate a fracture; if the patient has clinical signs of fractured ribs, he or she should be treated for this condition in spite of a negative X-ray. A repeat X-ray at 2 weeks may show fracture callus and confirm the diagnosis.
- *Bone scans* are more sensitive at detecting fractures, especially pathological fractures, when they may also reveal metastatic tumour deposits elsewhere in the skeleton, or be suggestive of metabolic bone disease.

Lecture Notes: General Surgery, 12th edition. © Harold Ellis, Sir Roy Y. Calne and Christopher J. E. Watson. Published 2011 by Blackwell Publishing Ltd.

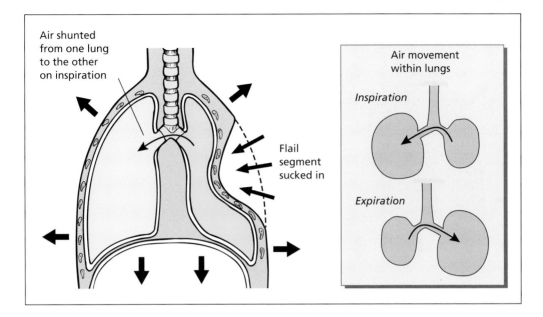

Figure 10.1 Flail chest. On inspiration, the detached segment of the chest wall is sucked inwards, producing paradoxical movement, and inhaled air shunts back and forth between lungs.

Complications

Flail chest (Figure 10.1)

Crush injuries of the chest, in which the whole sternum is loosened by fractured ribs on either side or several ribs are fractured in two places, result in the condition of flail chest. On inspiration, the flail part of the chest wall becomes indrawn by the negative intrathoracic pressure, as it is no longer in structural continuity with the bony thoracic cage. Similarly, in expiration the flail part of the chest is pushed out while the rest of the bony cage becomes contracted. This is termed *paradoxical movement*. The patient becomes grossly hypoxic due to failure of adequate expansion of the affected side and also because of shunting of deoxygenated air from the lung on the side of the fracture into the opposite side. The pendulum movements of the mediastinum also produce cardiovascular embarrassment so that the patient becomes rapidly and progressively shocked.

Pneumothorax

If a bony spicule penetrates the lung, air escapes into the pleural cavity and will result in a pneumothorax.

A *tension pneumothorax* (Figure 10.2) results if the pleural tear is valvular, allowing air to be sucked into the pleural cavity at each inspiration but preventing air returning to the bronchi on expiration. A tension pneumothorax produces rapidly increasing dyspnoea; the trachea and the apex beat are displaced away from the side of the pneumothorax; and, on the left side, cardiac dullness may be absent. The chest on the affected side gives a tympanitic percussion note with bulging of the intercostal spaces.

Subcutaneous emphysema (surgical emphysema)

When a fractured rib tears the overlying soft tissue and allows air from the pneumothorax to enter the subcutaneous tissues, subcutaneous emphysema will result. The skin over the trunk, neck and sometimes face gives a peculiar crackling feel to the examining fingers (*crepitation*) and, in severe cases, the face and neck may become grossly swollen. The alternative name, surgical emphysema, is misleading as it is rarely caused by surgeons.

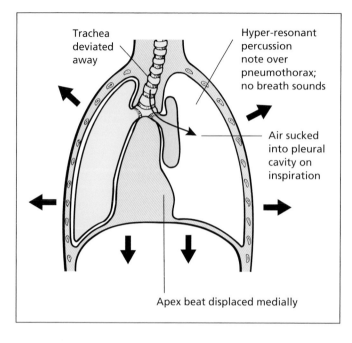

Trachea deviated away

Hyper-resonant percussion note over pneumothorax; no breath sounds

Air sucked into pleural cavity on inspiration

Apex beat displaced medially

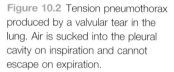

Figure 10.2 Tension pneumothorax produced by a valvular tear in the lung. Air is sucked into the pleural cavity on inspiration and cannot escape on expiration.

Sucking wound of the chest

A pneumothorax will also result from a penetrating wound of the chest wall produced, for example, by a knife stab or gunshot wound. The lips of the wound may also have a valvular effect so that air is sucked into the cavity at each inspiration, but cannot escape on expiration, thus resulting in another variety of tension pneumothorax, which has been vividly named a sucking wound of the chest.

Haemothorax

A haemothorax often accompanies a chest injury and may be associated with a pneumothorax (*haemopneumothorax*). The bleeding is usually from an intercostal artery in the lacerated chest wall or from underlying contused lung, but on occasions may result from injury to the heart or great vessels. Retropleural bleeding may compress the thoracic viscera without breaching the pleural cavity.

Traumatic asphyxia

With severe crush injuries of the chest, the sudden sharp rise in venous pressure produces extensive bruising and petechial haemorrhages over the head, neck and trunk. There are often subconjunctival haemorrhages and nasal bleeding. Any area of the skin that has been subjected to compression at the time of injury (e.g. from a tight collar, braces or spectacles) is protected and these areas remain mapped out on the body as strips of normal skin, giving a characteristic appearance to the patient.

Other visceral injury

It is important to remember that penetrating wounds of the chest may also injure the underlying diaphragm and thence the abdominal viscera. Thus, it is not uncommon for a knife or bullet wound of the left chest to penetrate the spleen or, on the right side, to damage the liver – incorrect placement of a chest drain may do the same.

Treatment

The priorities in the management of chest injuries are as follows:

- *Airway control.* This may involve the passage of an endotracheal tube, particularly where a head injury coexists with chest trauma. Aspiration of vomit is prevented by passing a nasogastric tube to empty the stomach.
- *Breathing.* Ensure the patient is breathing and maintaining adequate oxygenation. A saturation monitor should be employed and

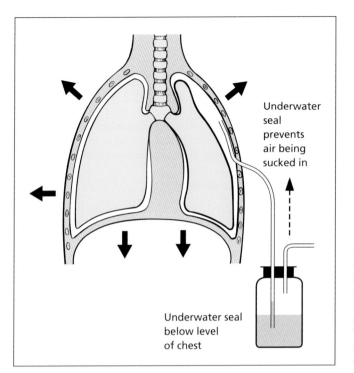

Underwater seal prevents air being sucked in

Underwater seal below level of chest

Figure 10.3 Underwater seal chest drain in the treatment of a pneumothorax. Air escapes from the pleural cavity on expiration but cannot be sucked back through the water seal on inspiration (as shown here). The water bottle is placed below the level of the chest to ensure fluid does not reflux into the thoracic cavity.

intubation and ventilation considered when the oxygen saturation is below 80% or $P\text{co}_2$ above 7.3 kPa (55 mmHg).

- *Sucking wounds.* These should be closed. In an emergency, a dressing pad should be applied over the hole and secured in place.
- *Lung expansion.* This should be achieved by insertion of an intercostal drain with underwater drainage.
- *Stop bleeding.* A haemothorax should be drained, and large haemothoraces may require multiple drains, all placed on underwater seals as for a pneumothorax (Figure 10.3). Continued bleeding is an indication for an exploratory thoracotomy.

Simple rib fracture

- *Pain relief* may be achieved by analgesics, particularly non-steroidal anti-inflammatory drugs (NSAIDs), by the injection of local anaesthetic in the paravertebral region to block the intercostal nerves or by a thoracic epidural block, which can be maintained by means of an infusion into an indwelling plastic catheter.
- *Vigorous physiotherapy* is administered to encourage deep breathing.

- *Strapping of the chest wall* inhibits thoracic movement and encourages pulmonary collapse; it should be avoided.

Flail chest

- *Support the flail segment* in an emergency by means of a firm pad held by strapping. This stops the paradoxical movement and air shunting.
- *Endotracheal intubation* and *positive-pressure ventilation* on admission to hospital will stop the paradoxical movement, as the chest wall now moves as a single functional unit. The treatment is continued for about 10 days until fixation of the chest wall occurs. In cases of gross instability, wire fixation of the chest wall may be necessary.
- *Tracheostomy* may be indicated for prolonged periods of intubation.

Pneumothorax

A traumatic pneumothorax requires insertion of a chest drain, in contrast to a spontaneous pneumothorax, which may resolve without intervention.

Tension pneumothorax

Urgent emergency treatment is required by inserting an *intercostal tube drain*.

A *chest drain* is inserted into the pleural cavity via an intercostal space, the fifth space being preferred. After cutting through the overlying skin in the midaxillary line, the remaining insertion is done by blunt dissection into the pleural cavity, at which point the drain is inserted and connected to an underwater seal. When the pressure in the pleural space is increased on expiration, the air escapes through the water but air cannot enter the chest at inspiration as this is prevented by the water seal. This essential safety valve has been a most important step in the development of safe thoracic surgery (Figure 10.3).

A *bronchopleural fistula*, due to rupture of a bronchus into the pleural space, should be suspected if the pneumothorax persists. It may require a thoracotomy to repair.

Penetrating wounds of the chest

Immediate application of a dressing is required in order to prevent suction of air into the pleural space. Minor cases require only wound toilet with an underwater intercostal drain to allow escape of any accumulated blood or air in the pleural space. Large wounds demand formal exploration with excision or repair of damaged lung tissue, repair of any diaphragmatic tear and exclusion of injury to underlying abdominal viscera.

Cardiac tamponade

This may follow open or closed injuries to the chest or upper abdomen. It is characterized by a rise in venous pressure and a fall in arterial pressure. The heart sounds are distant and the cardiac shadow enlarged on chest X-ray. Treatment is emergency surgical exploration; the pericardium is opened, the blood is evacuated and the cardiac laceration sutured.

Lung abscess

Aetiology

- Bronchial obstruction secondary to carcinoma of the lung.
- Inhalation pneumonitis, e.g. inhaled vomit or pus.
- Inhaled foreign body, e.g. at dental extraction.
- Infected cyst.
- Infected pulmonary infarct.
- Blood borne, secondary to staphylococcal septicaemia.
- Secondary to pulmonary infection, e.g. pneumonia, bronchiectasis or tuberculosis, especially in immunocompromised patients.

Clinical features

The history may suggest the primary cause. There is usually acute fever and toxaemia, although the disease may sometimes run a more chronic course. If the abscess ruptures into the bronchus there is a foul productive cough.

Complications

- Empyema.
- Metastatic cerebral abscess (a feared complication of all pulmonary sepsis).

Special investigations

- *Chest X-ray* shows a solid opacity or a fluid level if the abscess communicates with the bronchus.
- *Bronchoscopy* may demonstrate the primary cause if this is a foreign body or carcinoma.
- *Computed tomography* (CT) will accurately locate the abscess and confirm the diagnosis. Percutaneous CT-guided drainage may be possible and effective.

Treatment

The underlying cause may itself require treatment. The mainstay of therapy for lung abscess is postural drainage combined with antibiotics. Surgical excision is required only for the small percentage who fail to respond to this therapy, when some underlying cause needs to be treated, or when, in a late case, there is a complicating empyema that requires drainage.

Empyema

An empyema (pyothorax) is a collection of pus in the pleural cavity.

Aetiology

- Underlying lung disease: pneumonia, bronchiectasis or carcinoma of the lung; tuberculous empyema is now uncommon.
- Penetrating wounds of the chest wall or infection following a transthoracic operation.
- Perforation of the oesophagus.
- Transdiaphragmatic infection from a subphrenic abscess.
- Haematogenous.

Complications

- Rupture into a bronchus (bronchopleural fistula).
- Discharge through the chest wall (empyema necessitans).
- Cerebral abscess.

Clinical features

There is usually a history of the underlying cause. The patient is febrile, toxic and may be anaemic. There are signs of fluid in the chest on the affected side. In chronic cases, finger clubbing may be present.

Special investigations

- *Full blood count* will reveal a leucocytosis.
- *Chest X-ray* demonstrates an effusion and there may be evidence of the underlying lung disease.
- *Bronchoscopy* is useful in determining the primary pathology.
- *Aspiration* of the chest confirms the diagnosis and identifies the responsible bacteria. The infecting organisms are usually *Pneumococcus*, *Streptococcus* or *Staphylococcus*.

Treatment

An acute empyema may respond to repeated aspirations together with antibiotic therapy, based on the sensitivity of the responsible organism and given both systemically and into the pleural cavity. If the condition fails to respond to this treatment, drainage by means of excision of a rib overlying the empyema becomes necessary. An intercostal tube is inserted and progress followed by repeated sinograms to ensure adequate drainage and ultimate obliteration of the empyema cavity. In more chronic cases, the fibrous wall of the empyema cavity may require excision (decortication).

Lung tumours

Classification

Benign

- Adenoma.
- Carcinoid (occasionally malignant).
- Hamartoma.
- Haemangioma (rare).

Malignant

1 Primary
   a squamous cell carcinoma;
   b adenocarcinoma;
   c small-cell carcinoma;
   d large-cell carcinoma;
   e carcinoid.
2 Secondary
   a carcinoma (especially breast, kidney);
   b sarcoma (especially bone);
   c melanoma.

Adenoma

Pathology

Adenomas account for about 4% of lung primary tumours. Two-thirds of the patients are female, and the average age is 40 years.

The tumour arises from the mucosa usually of the main bronchus as a cherry-red swelling, which ulcerates and bleeds (hence the common presenting symptom of haemoptysis). The growth may eventually block the bronchus with resulting pulmonary collapse and infection. Although slow growing, it cannot be considered benign, as infiltration and metastases may eventually take place.

Occasionally, serotonin (5-hydroxytryptamine) is secreted, producing attacks of flushing and dyspnoea (carcinoid syndrome; see Chapter 23, p. 197).

Treatment

Removal by local resection, lobectomy or pneumonectomy.

Carcinoma

This is the second commonest cancer affecting men (after prostate) and accounts for 17% of all new male cancers; it is responsible for some 40 000 deaths per year in the UK, with an age-standardized incidence for men of around 61 per 100 000 per year, and 37 per 100 000 for women. In women, it accounts for 11% of all new cancers, and is the third commonest cancer in women after breast (31%) and colorectal cancer (12%).

Aetiology

In the UK, the main aetiological factor is the smoking of cigarettes. Passive smoking, air pollution with diesel, petrol and other volatile hydrocarbon fumes, asbestos exposure and exposure to radioactive gases such as radon in uranium mines are also predisposing factors. The incidence is higher in urban than in rural populations.

Carcinoma of the lung has an extremely poor prognosis, and the gravity of this condition should be impressed on all patients who are inveterate smokers. The decision whether or not to continue smoking depends on the patient, but there is no doubt that the doctor's advice should be against it. There is an increased incidence of carcinoma of the lung even in patients who smoke only a few cigarettes a day, and this danger is greatly increased in patients smoking more than 20 cigarettes a day for a number of years.

Pathology

There used to be a considerable predominance of men over women in this disease (6:1 in the 1950s), but the ratio is decreasing as women tend to smoke more and men less. In 1975 the age-standardized incidence of lung cancer in men was 113 per 100 000, falling to 59 in 2007; in women, it has risen from 23 to 38 per 100 000 over the same period.

Macroscopic appearance

About half the tumours arise in the main bronchi (particularly squamous carcinoma), and 75% are visible at bronchoscopy. The growth may arise peripherally (particularly adenocarcinoma) and some appear to be multifocal.

The bronchial wall is narrowed and ulcerated. Surrounding lung tissue is invaded by a pale mass of tumour, which may undergo necrosis, haemor-rhage or abscess formation. The lung segments distal to the occlusion may show collapse, bronchiectasis or abscess formation.

Microscopic appearance

- *Squamous cell carcinoma (40%)*. Mostly poorly differentiated and arising in an area of squamous metaplasia of bronchial epithelium. Following successful resection, new primaries are common (10%), reflecting the 'field change'.
- *Adenocarcinoma (30%)*. Very rapidly growing tumour often found in the periphery of the lung, associated with a large fibrotic (desmoplastic) reaction. This type of lung primary often occurs in non-smokers.
- *Large-cell carcinoma (10%)*. Large cells containing abundant cytoplasm and without evidence of squamous or glandular differentiation.
- *Small-cell carcinoma (20%)* (also known as oat-cell carcinoma). This has neuroendocrine properties and produces peptides giving rise to paraneoplastic syndromes (Chapter 7, p. 37). The tumour comprises small cells with little cytoplasm. It has a poor prognosis, has generally spread by the time of diagnosis and is best treated by chemotherapy.

Spread

- *Local*: to pleura, left recurrent laryngeal nerve, phrenic nerve, pericardium, oesophagus (broncho-oesophageal fistula), sympathetic chain (Horner's syndrome[1]) and brachial plexus (Pancoast's tumour[2]).
- *Lymphatic*: to mediastinal and cervical nodes. Compression of the superior vena cava by massive mediastinal node involvement produces gross oedema and cyanosis of the face and upper limbs (superior vena cava syndrome).
- *Blood*: to bone, brain, liver and suprarenals.
- *Transcoelomic*: pleural seedlings and effusion.

Clinical features

Carcinoma of the lung may present with the following features:

[1]Johann Horner (1831–1886), Professor of Ophthalmology, Zurich, Switzerland.
[2]Henry Pancoast (1875–1939), Professor of Radiology, University of Pennsylvania, Philadelphia, PA, USA.

- *Local features*, namely cough, dyspnoea, haemoptysis or lung infection. Chest pain suggests spread to pleural surface.
- *Secondaries*, which are especially likely to occur in the brain, suprarenal, liver and bones; thus, the patient may present with evidence of a space-occupying lesion within the skull, pathological fracture, jaundice and hepatomegaly, or adrenocortical failure.
- *Paraneoplastic syndromes* due to the remote effects of a hormone or cell product produced by the tumour. Small-cell carcinomas often produce adrenocorticotrophic hormone (ACTH), while squamous carcinomas may produce parathormone (PTH) and present with hypercalcaemia.
- *The general effects of neoplasm*: loss of weight, anaemia, cachexia and endocrine disturbances. Patients may also present with bizarre neuropathies and myopathies.

Unfortunately, by the time carcinoma of the lung is diagnosed, most cases are incurable. About half the patients will be found to have inoperable growths when they have had no symptoms at all, with a lesion discovered on routine chest X-ray. Certainly, any middle-aged or elderly person presenting with a respiratory infection that has continued for more than 2 weeks should have a chest X-ray, and, if the symptoms persist and nothing shows on the chest X-ray, he or she should undergo bronchoscopy.

Cancer of the lung is likely to lead to pulmonary infection and the patients often develop clubbing of the fingers, which are usually nicotine stained.

On examination, special attention should be paid to evidence of stridor or hoarseness of the voice due to recurrent laryngeal nerve involvement by the cancer. The heart may be invaded, resulting in atrial fibrillation or cardiac failure. There may be enlarged lymph nodes, especially at the root of the neck, and signs in the chest of consolidation, fluid or collapse.

Special investigations

- *Chest X-ray* and *thoracic CT scan* may show an opacity in the lung and enlargement of the hilar lymph nodes. The differential diagnosis of a mediastinal mass on radiological examination of the chest is listed in Box 10.1. There may be paralysis of one side of the diaphragm due to involvement of the phrenic

---

> **Box 10.1 Abnormal shadow in the mediastinum**
>
> - Retrosternal thyroid
> - Aneurysm of the thoracic aorta
> - Thymic tumour and cysts
> - Carcinoma of the lung with a mediastinal mass
> - Heart enlargement: cardiac failure; valve incompetence; pericardial effusion; left–right shunts; cardiomyopathies
> - Enlarged lymph nodes: sarcoid; Hodgkin's disease; non-Hodgkin's lymphoma; leukaemia; secondary deposits
> - Oesophageal enlargement: tumour; hiatus hernia; mega-oesophagus in achalasia of the cardia
> - Paravertebral abscess, particularly due to tuberculosis
> - Scoliosis
> - Dumb-bell tumour of neurofibroma
> - Dermoid cyst or teratoma

---

nerve. In addition to imaging the chest, a CT scan should also image the liver and suprarenal glands for evidence of secondary spread.
- *Cytology* of the sputum may identify malignant cells, a particularly sensitive test in proximal exuberant bronchial growths.
- *Bronchoscopy and biopsy.* Bronchoscopy may reveal an ulcerating or exuberant growth, and involved lymph nodes may widen the carina. Brushings and washings may be taken for cytology in addition to biopsy of a visible tumour.
- *Fine-needle aspiration cytology* of a peripherally placed lesion under X-ray guidance.
- *Mediastinoscopy*, performed through a small suprasternal incision, may be indicated to remove lymph nodes from the region of the carina for histological examination to aid in staging. Video-assisted thoracoscopic surgery (VATS) may also be helpful.
- *Pulmonary function tests* to determine lung reserve and hence capacity to withstand surgery. Chronic obstructive pulmonary disease is common in this patient group. Patients with a forced expiratory volume in 1 second (FEV_1) >2.5 litres can usually tolerate

pneumonectomy; those with an FEV_1 >1.1 litres can usually tolerate lobectomy.

Treatment

Surgery

Overall, 80% of patients with non-small-cell lung cancer die within 1 year of diagnosis. The possibility of curative surgery is assessed by biopsy of all suspicious nodes to exclude spread, as well as radiological imaging and bronchoscopy. Removal of a lobe, or of the whole lung, is performed when there is a possibility of cure, i.e. small tumours with no spread; in these highly selected cases, the 5 year survival rate of this disease is of the order of 40–60%. Increasingly resection is performed by video-assisted thoracoscopy rather than thoracotomy.

Sometimes, with a technically resectable early tumour, the patient's general respiratory reserve is so limited by years of tobacco abuse as to make resection impossible.

Radiotherapy

Radiotherapy may give useful palliation for inoperable cases. Although it may not prolong life, it may stop distressing haemoptysis, relieve the pain from bone secondaries and produce dramatic improvement in a patient with acute superior vena caval obstruction. It may also give some relief from the irritating cough and dyspnoea resulting from early bronchial obstruction.

Cytotoxic chemotherapy

Cyclical cytotoxic therapy combined with radiotherapy is the treatment of choice for small-cell tumours; there is increasing evidence that this approach with cisplatin-based regimens, together with agents such as gemcitabine and paclitaxel for advanced disease, is also helpful in the treatment of unresectable non-small-cell cancers.

Secondary tumours

The lung is second only to the liver as the site of metastases, which may be from carcinoma (especially breast, kidney), sarcoma (especially bone) or melanoma. Spread may be as a result of either vascular deposits or retrograde lymphatic permeation from involved mediastinal nodes – lymphangitis carcinomatosa.

Pulmonary metastases are so common that it should be routine practice to image the chest by plain X-ray or CT scan in every case of malignant disease to aid staging the primary.

11

The heart and thoracic aorta

Learning objectives

✓ To know the principal surgical conditions of the heart and thoracic aorta, and how they are treated.

✓ To know the surgically remediable causes of hypertension.

Cardiopulmonary bypass

Background

Prior to the development of cardiopulmonary bypass, surgery on the heart was limited to procedures that could be performed rapidly on a beating heart, such as mitral valvotomy to relieve mitral stenosis, where a finger is passed blindly through the left atrial appendage and through the stenotic mitral valve. If the circulation is temporarily stopped at normal body temperature, organs suffer ischaemic damage owing to lack of oxygen, the extent varying according to the metabolic demand of the organ. The brain is the most sensitive tissue in this respect and is liable to irreversible changes after 3 minutes of ischaemia. The spinal cord is next, followed by heart muscle, which will tolerate between 3 and 6 minutes of ischaemia at normal temperature. The tolerance to ischaemia can be increased slightly by lowering the metabolic rate by hypothermia; at 28°C, up to 10 minutes of circulatory arrest can be tolerated.

Following the development of cardiopulmonary bypass, it is now possible to stop the heart for prolonged periods while a machine is used to take over the pumping and oxygenation of the blood. Generally, a combination of hypothermia and cardiopulmonary bypass is used.

Technique (Figure 11.1)

After full heparinization, cannulae are inserted into the venae cavae via the right atrium to siphon off the venous return from the systemic circulation. The blood is then pumped through an oxygenator and a heat exchanger before returning to the systemic circulation via a cannula in the ascending aorta or femoral artery. This form of bypass will perfuse the whole body with oxygenated blood at an adequate pressure while diverting it from the heart and lungs. The heart may now be stopped and cooled by infusion via the coronary arteries of cold 'cardioplegic' solution containing potassium to produce rapid cardiac arrest in diastole. If the aorta is cross-clamped, the heart may be opened in a bloodless field with access to all chambers.

Complications

- *Emboli*. Air entrapped during formation of the bypass circuit or entering during bypass, or thrombus forming in the bypass circuit, may embolize into the cerebral and peripheral circulation with catastrophic results.
- *Haemorrhage* postoperatively may result in cardiac tamponade. Passage through the

Lecture Notes: General Surgery, 12th edition. © Harold Ellis, Sir Roy Y. Calne and Christopher J. E. Watson. Published 2011 by Blackwell Publishing Ltd.

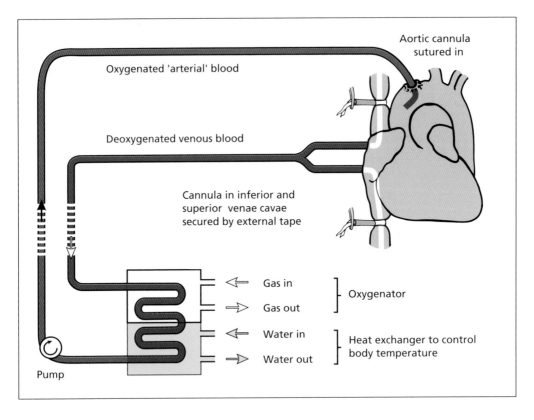

Figure 11.1 Cardiopulmonary bypass.

bypass circuit activates the clotting cascade and consumes platelets, thus increasing the risk of haemorrhage.

- *Hypothermic injury and ischaemia* may result in pancreatitis and contribute to the occurrence of peptic ulceration and mesenteric ischaemia.

Valvular disease

Valve repair and replacement

With the advent of cardiopulmonary bypass, it has become possible to remove diseased valves and replace them with artificial ones – prosthetic, human or xenograft. In mitral valve regurgitation, if the valve is not heavily distorted or calcified, repair may be undertaken in preference to replacement.

Prosthetic valves

Many examples exist, such as the St Jude bileaflet valve, where the valve comprises two semicircular tilting leaflets. Prosthetic valves may become obstructed by thrombus owing to turbulent flow across the valve leaflets; recipients should therefore be anticoagulated indefinitely. Prosthetic valves have a risk of catastrophic failure such as when tilting discs dislodge or fracture.

Allograft and xenograft valves

These are taken from fresh human cadaver hearts or from pig hearts. The valve is suspended on a prosthetic ring to allow it to be sewn in place; once implanted, the recipient does not require anticoagulation. The lifetime of such valves is generally shorter than prosthetic valves, but the avoidance of anticoagulation makes them the preferred choice in the elderly.

Complications of valve replacement

- *Valve thrombosis and embolus formation,* especially if not on anticoagulation.
- *Mechanical failure* with embolus of valve fragments, outflow obstruction or massive valve incompetence.
- *Anticoagulation* with the risks of haemorrhage due to over-anticoagulation.
- *Paraprosthetic leaks,* where blood leaks between the artificial valve ring and the outflow tract.
- *Infection of valve,* a situation akin to infective endocarditis of a native valve.

Aortic stenosis

Stenosis of the aortic valve may be congenital or acquired. The acquired variety may be due to rheumatic heart disease, but in older patients it is more commonly due to calcification of congenitally bicuspid valves – 1% of the population have only two aortic valve leaflets owing to fusion of two adjacent valve cusps. Unfortunately, no matter what the cause, the aortic valve, when stenosed, is usually grossly distorted and calcified and unsuitable for valve repair; replacement is the treatment of choice.

Clinical features

The three presenting symptoms of aortic stenosis are angina, dyspnoea due to cardiac failure and syncope (occasionally sudden death). Examination reveals a slow rising pulse, a low blood pressure and left ventricular hypertrophy, as shown on electrocardiogram (ECG) and echocardiogram. Chest X-ray may show valve calcification and post-stenotic dilatation of the aorta. Once the gradient across the valve exceeds 50 mmHg, or the patient is symptomatic, surgery is advised.

Treatment

Valve replacement on cardiopulmonary bypass. Coincidental coronary artery disease may be treated at the same time. Percutaneous aortic valve replacement, via the femoral artery, is currently being evaluated for the unfit elderly patient.

Mitral stenosis

Rheumatic fever occasionally followed throat infection with the group A β-haemolytic *Streptococcus*. Antigens on this organism cross-react with various body tissues, with manifestations that included serial involvement of large joints (hence the name), the basal ganglia (Sydenham's chorea[1]) and, most importantly, the heart muscle and valves. Rheumatic fever has now become much less common in Western nations, perhaps because of decreased virulence of the organism and the widespread use of antibiotics in throat infections, but is still seen commonly in developing countries.

Pathology

Pathological changes consist of fusion of the valve commissures with shortening of the chordae tendinae. As the mitral valve opening narrows, blood flow across the valve is impaired and the left atrium, particularly the atrial appendage, dilates and, with the dilatation, atrial fibrillation follows. Thrombus may form in the atrial appendage. In time, the valve narrows critically and prevents adequate ventricular filling, resulting in exertional dyspnoea.

Clinical features

Patients usually present between the 20th and 40th year, women more commonly than men. The usual presenting feature is increasing dyspnoea due to progressive cardiac failure. There may be nocturnal dyspnoea and episodes of pulmonary oedema with recurrent lung infections.

On examination, the patient may have the typical malar flush. There is a mid-diastolic murmur in the mitral area and the opening snap of the mitral valve may be audible and palpable as a tapping apex beat. Atrial fibrillation is common and this is accompanied by the disappearance of the presystolic murmur as effective atrial contraction ceases.

---

[1]Thomas Sydenham (1624–1689). After serving under Cromwell in the Civil War, he became a distinguished London physician.

Complications

- Right heart failure.
- Peripheral arterial embolism (particularly in atrial fibrillation).
- Infective endocarditis – likely wherever there is a valve abnormality.

Treatment

In the absence of mitral regurgitation, evidence of valve calcification or a history of emboli, an open valvotomy is performed to split the fused commissures. If this is unsuccessful, or in the presence of calcified and distorted valves or regurgitation, valve replacement is performed.

Ischaemic heart disease

Severe angina, due to myocardial ischaemia, may be alleviated by increasing the arterial supply to the muscle. Two treatment options exist: endoluminal intervention with balloon angioplasty and stenting, or surgical revascularization.

Aetiology

The risk factors for coronary artery disease are those for atheroma in general (see Box 12.2). In particular, raised serum cholesterol, hypertension and cigarette smoking each double the risk of coronary artery disease. The presence of all three increases the risk eightfold.

Special investigations

- *Exercise ECG* shows whether there is myocardial ischaemia on exercise.
- *Myocardial perfusion imaging.* In patients unfit for treadmill exercise, myocardial stress can be induced pharmacologically using dobutamine or adenosine while imaging with magnetic resonance or methoxyisobutylisonitrile (MIBI).
- *Stress echocardiography* is an alternative to myocardial perfusion imaging. The contraction of different segments of the heart wall is studied before and during pharmacologically induced stress.
- *Coronary arteriography* is performed on patients with ischaemic responses to exercise.

It is important for accurate anatomical diagnosis, and may be combined with endoluminal therapy.

Treatment

- *Angioplasty.* Isolated stenoses in proximal vessels are most appropriate for percutaneous transluminal coronary angioplasty (PTCA), often combined with endoluminal stenting to prolong patency.
- *Surgical revascularization.* For total occlusions or stenoses in multiple vessels, the procedure of choice is surgery. This involves joining an internal mammary (internal thoracic) artery to the diseased coronary artery distal to the blockage. For multiple grafts, autogenous reversed saphenous vein or radial artery can also be used as aortocoronary bypass conduits (Figure 11.2).

As with all arterial surgery for atherosclerosis, there is a tendency for recurrent disease with the passage of time. This may require repeat surgery, or may be amenable to endoluminal procedures. In young patients crippled by angina in whom direct bypass surgery is impossible or in those with gross myocardial disease, cardiac transplantation may be indicated to give relief of symptoms and to enable a return to normal life.

Surgery for the complications of myocardial infarction

1 *Acute ventriculoseptal defect.* When the infarcted ventricular muscle is part of the septum and undergoes necrosis, septal rupture may occur. This occurs 1–2 weeks after myocardial infarction in 0.5% of patients and requires urgent repair, which may be achieved surgically or via an endovascular approach. Mortality is high.
2 *Ventricular aneurysm.* If the infarcted ventricular wall is apical, it may necrose and rupture, leading to rapid death by tamponade. Alternatively, it may heal with fibrosis, and subsequently a ventricular aneurysm may form. This may require excision if paradoxical movement or thrombus become symptomatic.

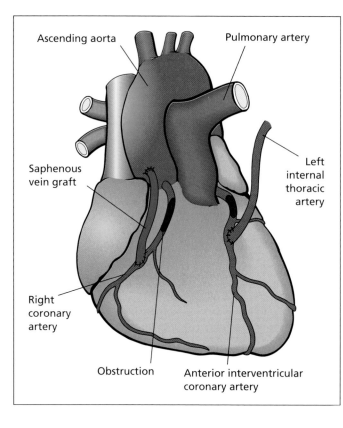

Ascending aorta

Pulmonary artery

Saphenous vein graft

Left internal thoracic artery

Right coronary artery

Obstruction

Anterior interventricular coronary artery

Figure 11.2 A saphenous vein graft from the aorta to the right coronary artery and a direct left internal mammary (thoracic) artery graft to the anterior interventricular coronary artery (also known as the left anterior descending (the 'LAD') artery).

Thoracic aortic disease

Persistent ductus arteriosus (Figure 11.3)

Pathology

If the channel between the aorta and pulmonary artery fails to close at the time of birth, blood will be shunted from the systemic circulation with its higher pressure into the pulmonary circulation, resulting in pulmonary hypertension. In time, pulmonary vascular resistance increases and exceeds peripheral resistance, at which time the shunt reverses, deoxygenated blood from the pulmonary artery passes into the systemic circulation and the patient becomes cyanosed. It carries a risk of development of infective endarteritis.

Clinical features

In neonates with a large duct, shunting may progress rapidly and cardiac failure may occur in infancy. A duct with moderate flow tends to present later with exertional dyspnoea. Most commonly, the patient is asymptomatic and the condition is diagnosed on finding the characteristic machinery-like continuous murmur with systolic accentuation best heard over the second left space anteriorly. In infants, the bruit may be purely systolic.

Special investigations

- *Chest X-ray* will usually show left ventricular hypertrophy and increased pulmonary arterial markings.
- *Echocardiography and angiography* will demonstrate the persistent ductus and indeed the cardiac catheter can often be manipulated through the ductus into the aorta.

Treatment

Operative ligation and division of a persistent ductus should be undertaken on diagnosis, and before irreversible pulmonary hypertension or cardiac failure has occurred. Percutaneous

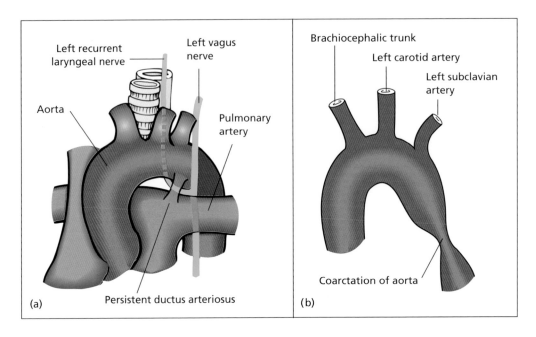

Figure 11.3 (a) A persistent ductus arteriosus – note its close relationship to the left recurrent laryngeal nerve. (b) Coarctation of the aorta. (Reproduced from Ellis H, Mahadevan V. (2010) *Clinical Anatomy*, 12th edn. Oxford: Wiley-Blackwell.)

endovascular insertion of an occlusive device into the ductus may achieve a cure without surgery.

Coarctation of the aorta

Pathology

This is a congenital narrowing of the aorta which, in the majority of cases, occurs in the descending aorta just distal to the origin of the left subclavian artery close to the obliterated ductus arteriosus. Indeed, the pathogenesis of coarctation formation may be related to the presence of abnormal ductus tissue. Coarctation can rarely occur in other sites up and down the aorta. The stenosis is usually extreme, only a pinpoint lumen remaining. There is often a coexistent cardiac anomaly.

Blood reaches the distal aorta via collateral connections between branches of the subclavian, scapular and intercostal arteries, and by the anastomosis between the internal thoracic and inferior epigastric arteries. Although the blood supply to the lower part of the body is diminished, patients with coarctation seldom have peripheral gangrene, although occasionally they complain of intermittent claudication. The danger of coarctation is due to the effects of hypertension proximal to the coarctation. This is often severe and is likely to result in cerebral haemorrhage or left ventricular failure. The mechanism of the hypertension is probably due to the relatively poor blood supply to the kidneys, which results in release of renin and renal hypertension (see Figure 11.5).

Patients also run the risk of developing infective endarteritis at the stenosis, and the lesion may also be the origin of an aortic dissection.

Clinical features

The diagnosis is considered in any child or young adult with hypertension. In addition to the hypertension, the most characteristic physical sign is absent, diminished or delayed femoral pulsations in relation to the radial pulse, and is confirmed by a large difference in the blood pressure between the arm and leg. A systolic murmur is sometimes present posterior in the left chest, and large collateral blood vessels may be seen or felt in the subcutaneous tissues of the chest wall.

Special investigations

- *Chest X-ray* will show left ventricular hypertrophy, and often the ribs are notched by the large intercostal collateral blood vessels bypassing the stenotic area.
- *Echocardiography* in an infant to exclude coexisting cardiac anomalies.
- *Angiography* will confirm the diagnosis.

Treatment

This is desirable before complications arise and consists of excision of the stenotic segment and either end-to-end anastomosis of the proximal and distal aorta or, if the gap to bridge is too great, an arterial graft interposed between the two aortic ends. Balloon angioplasty is an alternative treatment.

Thoracic aortic aneurysms

Aneurysms can occur in any place in the body (see Chapter 12) but the aorta is particularly liable to be affected. Aneurysms of the arch of the aorta were once commonly syphilitic but now are mainly due to Marfan's syndrome,[2] medial degeneration or atherosclerosis. Aneurysms of the descending thoracic aorta may be traumatic, syphilitic or atherosclerotic. With the exception of aneurysms with a very narrow neck, those involving the thoracic aorta require some form of vascular bypass in order to treat them surgically.

A thoracoabdominal aneurysm is an aneurysm extending across the diaphragm and involving the coeliac, superior mesenteric and renal artery origins.

Clinical features

Aneurysms of the ascending aorta may present with chest pain, aortic regurgitation, obstruction of the superior vena cava, obstruction of the right main bronchus and eventually a pulsating mass in the front of the chest, which may even ulcerate through the chest wall, resulting in exsanguination.

Aneurysms of the arch of the aorta may compress the trachea or ulcerate into it; they are liable to stretch the left recurrent laryngeal nerve leading to hoarseness and may obstruct the left lower lobe bronchus, producing an area of collapse.

Aneurysms of the descending thoracic aorta may produce pain in the back, erosion of vertebrae or may press on the oesophagus, producing dysphagia and even rupture into it. Not surprisingly, this is the most lethal cause of haematemesis.

Special investigations

- *Chest X-ray* may show the extent of the aneurysm due to calcification in its walls.
- *Computed tomography (CT) and magnetic resonance (MR) imaging* are useful in demonstrating the size and extent of the aneurysm and its relation to the major vessels of the neck.
- *Aortography* may be dangerous and often does not help in establishing the diagnosis, as the lumen of the aneurysm is narrowed by thrombus.
- *Echocardiography* is important to diagnose aortic incompetence caused by aneurysmal dilatation of the valve ring.

Treatment

Aneurysms of the ascending aorta and arch require total cardiopulmonary bypass for adequate surgical treatment, which consists of partial excision of the aneurysm and insertion of a prosthetic graft with appropriate junction limbs to the main aortic branches. Aneurysms of the descending thoracic aorta require a left heart bypass for their surgical treatment, which is similar in principle to those of the arch. More recently, endovascular stenting of thoracic aneurysms has proved to be a promising alternative.

Complications

- *Spinal ischaemia* is due to loss of flow in the great radicular artery (of Adamkiewicz[3]), which arises from the aorta near T10 and supplies the lower part of the spinal cord. This results in paraplegia.

[2]Antonine Marfan (1858–1942), Professor of Paediatrics, Hôpital des Enfants Malades, Paris, France. Marfan's syndrome is due to a mutation in the fibrillin-1 gene on chromosome 15, and manifests with cardiovascular, skeletal and ocular abnormalities.

[3]Albert Adamkiewicz (1850–1921), Professor of Pathology, Cracow, Poland.

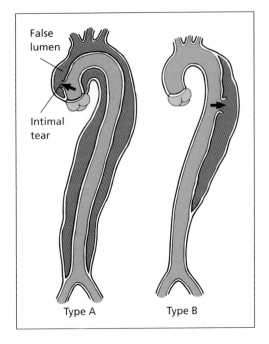

False lumen

Intimal tear

Type A   Type B

Figure 11.4 Classification of aortic dissection.

Aortic dissection (Figure 11.4)

Pathology

An aortic dissection (dissecting aneurysm) consists of a tear in the wall of the aorta, usually in the region of its arch, which allows blood to dissect along a plane of cleavage in the media. The false passage thus formed may rupture internally into the true lumen, thus decompressing itself and resulting in an aorta with a double lumen. Such a patient may survive. More commonly, the aneurysm ruptures externally into the pericardium, producing cardiac tamponade, or into the mediastinum or abdominal cavity with fatal haemorrhage.

Aetiology

Cystic medial degeneration weakens the wall of the aorta and enables the splitting to occur. It is usually found in atherosclerotic, hypertensive subjects.

Classification

Aortic dissection has been classified into type A and type B (Stanford classification[4]).

- *Type A dissection* affects the ascending aorta and arch and occurs in two-thirds of cases.
- *Type B dissection* has an initial tear distal to the origin of the left subclavian artery and only the descending aorta is affected. It occurs in one-third of cases.

Clinical features

The patient usually presents with a sudden severe pain in the chest, which may radiate to the arms, neck or abdomen, or with a tearing interscapular pain. In addition, there may be signs of shock, either from cardiac tamponade or from external rupture of the aneurysm. Patients with aortic dissection are often initially diagnosed as suffering from coronary thrombosis, and an ECG may not help differentiate between the two conditions. Indeed, if the coronary sinus is involved, coronary occlusion may have occurred. In type A dissections, the aortic valve may become incompetent as the root dilates.

As the dissection in the wall of the aorta progresses, the origins of the main arterial branches may become blocked, producing progression of symptoms and the disappearance and reappearance of peripheral pulses. If the renal vessels are involved, there may be haematuria or anuria. One or both femoral pulses may disappear with leg ischaemia. Mesenteric ischaemia is usually diagnosed late.

Neurological abnormalities may also occur, ranging from hemiparesis, as a result of occlusion of the carotid and subclavian artery origins, to paraesthesia, as a result of peripheral nerve ischaemia; Horner's syndrome[5] (see Chapter 17, p. 142) may occur owing to interruption of the cervical sympathetic chain, and hoarseness may complicate recurrent laryngeal nerve involvement.

---

[4]Stanford University School of Medicine, Stanford, CA, USA. The Stanford classification was described in 1970 by Norman Shumway and colleagues in the Division of Cardiovascular Surgery.
[5]Johann Horner (1831–1886), Professor of Ophthalmology, Zurich, Switzerland.

Special investigations

- *Chest X-ray* shows widening of the mediastinum in two-thirds of patients and a small left pleural effusion.
- *Contrast-enhanced CT* shows a flap across the aortic lumen with distal aneurysmal change.
- *Echocardiography* may also demonstrate a flap and aortic regurgitation. *Transoesophageal echocardiography (TOE)* is probably the investigation of choice.

Treatment

Once the diagnosis is made, treatment depends largely upon the type of dissection.

Type A dissections should be managed surgically because of the risk that the dissection may extend back across the aortic root resulting in tamponade, and to correct aortic incompetence where present. The surgery aims to interpose a prosthetic tube graft at the aortic root to prevent further dissection (and tamponade), and carries a high mortality.

Type B dissections are usually treated conservatively, and hypotensive drugs are used, reducing systolic pressure to 100–120 mmHg to prevent further extension of the dissection. The dissected portion may then thrombose. Any organ, limb or mesenteric ischaemia resulting from the dissection is treated by revascularization. An aneurysm resulting from a chronic dissection may require treatment if it enlarges or produces pressure symptoms. In cases where there is evidence of impending aortic rupture or non-perfusion of a visceral artery, endovascular placement of a covered stent (a stent–graft) is appropriate. The stent is placed to cover the proximal entry into the false lumen, and to re-establish blood flow through the collapsed true lumen.

Hypertension

This section summarizes raised blood pressure in its surgical aspects.

Classification

- Primary (cause unknown).
- Secondary (causes at least partially understood).

Primary hypertension

Primary hypertension is a disease of middle-aged and elderly patients, which tends to run in families. It is a very common condition and may be compatible with few symptoms and a long life. There is an increase in the peripheral resistance due to arteriolar thickening or spasm, but, as arteriolar thickening is a consequence of hypertension, the argument as to which is the primary factor has not been resolved in this disease.

The kidney may be an important contributor to the hypertension when its blood supply is impaired owing to arteriolar narrowing. There is a vicious circle of arteriolar spasm, arteriolar thickening, renal ischaemia and further hypertension, which leads to a progressive increase in the severity of this condition.

Secondary hypertension

This may be due to the following factors:

1 Renal disease.
2 Coarctation of the aorta (p. 74).
3 Endocrine causes:
   a phaeochromocytoma (Chapter 40, p. 333);
   b Cushing's syndrome (Chapter 40, p. 331);
   c Conn's syndrome (Chapter 40, p. 332).
4 Raised intracranial pressure (Chapter 15, p. 117).
5 Toxaemia of pregnancy.

Renovascular hypertension

Mechanism of renal hypertension (Figure 11.5)

Ever since the experiments of Goldblatt,[6] it has been known that impairment of blood perfusion to the kidneys can result in hypertension which, if the renal perfusion remains impaired, may become permanent, owing to the vicious circle that has already been mentioned. The mechanism of renal hypertension appears to be the release of the hormone renin from the juxtaglomerular cells in the renal cortex. Renin acts on the serum protein angiotensinogen to give rise to a physiologically inactive decapeptide, angiotensin I. Angiotensin I is then converted to the octapeptide

[6]Harry Goldblatt (1891–1977), Professor of Experimental Pathology, University of Southern California, Los Angeles, CA, USA.

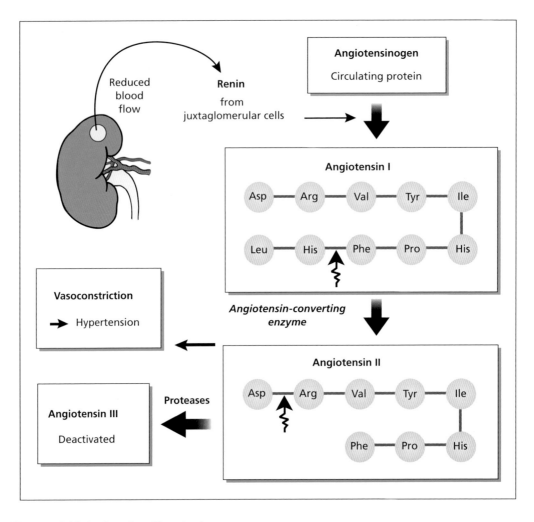

Figure 11.5 Mechanism of renal hypertension.

angiotensin II by the action of angiotensin-converting enzyme (ACE). Angiotensin II is a potent vasoconstrictor and causes an increase in peripheral resistance (and thus hypertension) and acts on the suprarenal cortex to release aldosterone (which causes sodium retention). The features of hypertension are thus set in motion. This renin mechanism is protective as far as the kidney is concerned and is one method by which the kidney maintains its circulation. How important renin is in the maintenance of normal blood pressure has not been established. All forms of renal parenchymal disease are likely to produce hypertension. Especially common are chronic glomerulonephritis and chronic pyelonephritis.

ACE inhibitors, such as captopril, are effective at reducing blood pressure in patients with renal disease. However, when renal insufficiency is due to renal artery stenosis, their use will exacerbate the impaired perfusion and result in deterioration in renal function.

Unilateral renal diseases producing hypertension

These are of particular surgical importance, as they may sometimes be amenable to curative treatment either by nephrectomy or by reconstructive procedures on the kidney or on its blood supply.

Unilateral pyelonephritis

Rarely, pyelonephritis may affect one kidney only, especially if this kidney has been the site of previous trauma or of congenital malformation, if the ureter on that side has been blocked or if there is unilateral hydronephrosis. If the condition is diagnosed early, before the hypertension has reached the chronic established stage and before hypertensive changes have taken place in the opposite kidney, removal of the affected kidney may result in a return to normal blood pressure. Presence of a functioning contralateral kidney should be confirmed first.

Renal artery stenosis

This is a fairly common cause of secondary hypertension. It occurs in two age groups: the elderly (70%), in whom the cause of the narrowing is atherosclerosis, and young people, especially women, in whom the cause appears to be the thickening of the intima and media by hyperplasia of collagen and muscle – fibromuscular dysplasia.

Special investigations

- *Arteriography* should be performed in young patients, in whom fibromuscular dysplasia characteristically shows up as a string of beads in the distal part of the renal artery and is bilateral.
- *Duplex scanning* may permit diagnosis of a significant stenosis.
- *Renin estimation* should be performed by selective renal vein catheterization. Renin concentration is at least 1.5 times higher on the affected side.

- *Diethylene-triamine-penta-acetic acid (DTPA) radionuclide scan* will show renal blood flow difference, especially if the patient has been given an ACE inhibitor such as captopril to exaggerate the condition.

Treatment

- *Angioplasty.* In suitable cases, a localized stenosis can be dilated by a balloon angioplasty. This is particularly successful in fibromuscular dysplasia.
- *Renal artery bypass.* If the stenosis is fairly proximal and the distal vessels relatively healthy, it may be possible to remove the stenotic portion of the artery or bypass it, e.g. on the left side by joining the splenic artery to the renal artery distal to the blockage.
- *Autotransplantation* of the kidney may be performed after excising the stenosed portion of the artery.
- *Unilateral nephrectomy* is appropriate when the small intrarenal branches of the renal artery are also diseased.

Other lesions of the renal arteries, for instance aneurysm and congenital bands, may also result in hypertension, which can be cured by unilateral nephrectomy or direct arterial surgery.

It should be noted that, since the introduction of effective antihypertensive drugs (in particular ACE inhibitors), enthusiasm for surgery in unilateral renal disease has waned, apart from patients in whom the kidney's function is grossly impaired.

Other unilateral renal diseases can cause hypertension, including hydronephrosis, tuberculosis of the kidneys or tumours of the kidney; nephrectomy is indicated in these conditions.

12

Arterial disease

Learning objectives

✓ To know the types of arterial trauma and their management.

✓ To know the causes of arterial aneurysms, their manifestation and treatment.

✓ To have knowledge of occlusive arterial disease (including thromboembolic disease), its risk factors, manifestations and treatment options.

Arterial trauma

Traumatic arterial injuries are due to either closed (blunt) trauma or open (penetrating) trauma.

Closed injuries

The artery is injured by extraneous compression such as a crush injury, fractures of adjacent bones with displacement of the artery (e.g. supracondylar fracture of the humerus in children) or joint dislocation. Iatrogenic causes include a tight plaster of Paris cast in which no allowance has been made for post-traumatic oedema.

Penetrating injuries

Penetrating arterial injuries may result from gunshot wounds, stabbing, penetration by bone spicules in fractures or iatrogenic injury.

Types of arterial injury

- *Mural contusion* with secondary spasm.
- *Intimal tear*. This injury is usually a result of distraction, in which the artery is stretched and the intimal layer tears, while the surrounding adventitia remains intact. The intima then buckles and causes a localized stenosis, which may or may not result in thrombosis or dissection.
- *Full thickness tear*. All layers of the artery are divided, and this may be partial or complete. Partial tears bleed copiously, while complete division of the artery often results in contraction and spasm of the divided vessel with surprisingly little blood loss.

Consequences of injury

- *Haemorrhage*. This may be concealed or overt.
- *Thrombosis*. Immediate or delayed.
- *Arteriovenous fistula formation*.
- *False (pseudo-) aneurysm formation* (see p. 81).
- *Arterial dissection*.
- *Compartment syndrome*. Ischaemic muscle swells and if the muscle is contained by a fibrous fascial compartment, such as in the forearm or in the lower leg, the swelling further exacerbates the ischaemia by an increased compartment pressure. Volkmann's[1] ischaemic contracture (Chapter 17, p. 141) is a result of compartment syndrome.

Lecture Notes: General Surgery, 12th edition. © Harold Ellis, Sir Roy Y. Calne and Christopher J. E. Watson. Published 2011 by Blackwell Publishing Ltd.

[1]Richard von Volkmann (1830–1889), Professor of Surgery, Halle, Germany.

Clinical features

The features of arterial injury may be those of acute ischaemia, haemorrhage or often both. Acute ischaemia is characterized by:

- pain (in the limb supplied, starting distally and progressing proximally);
- pallor;
- pulselessness;
- paraesthesiae;
- paralysis;
- coldness.

Haemorrhage may be overt (bright red blood) or concealed (e.g. closed limb fractures). Symptoms are those of rapidly developing hypovolaemic shock (cold, clamminess, tachycardia, hypotension, loss of consciousness, oliguria progressing to anuria).

Treatment

Closed injuries

- *Treat causative factors.* If the cause of ischaemia is a tight plaster cast, remove or split the cast. If it is due to a supracondylar humeral fracture, the peripheral pulses should return when the fracture is reduced; if the radial pulse does not return rapidly, surgical exploration is indicated.
- *Angiography.* An angiogram will reveal whether ischaemia is due to spasm, intimal tear or arterial disruption. It may be performed in a radiology suite or intraoperatively. Partial tears in large vessels may be amenable to intravascular stenting.
- *Operative exploration.* If a limb fails to reperfuse after a fracture or dislocation is reduced, and angiography is unhelpful or shows a tear or block, exploration is mandatory. Either the affected vessel is repaired directly or a segment of saphenous vein interposed to replace the injured area.
- *Fasciotomy.* Muscle ischaemia leads to swelling and compartment syndrome. The fascial compartments should be opened by splitting the deep fascia widely to relieve compartment pressure.

Open injuries

- *Direct compression.* Primary measures to staunch haemorrhage should include direct pressure. The use of a proximal tourniquet usually exacerbates blood loss, as it seldom generates sufficient pressure to occlude arterial flow, but does block venous return, which results in increased blood loss.
- *Resuscitation.* Replace blood loss.
- *Exploration.* Small vessels that are part of a large collateral supply may be sacrificed and ligated above the site of injury. Partial tears may be directly sutured or closed with a vein patch; complete division often requires interposition of reversed saphenous vein. The use of prosthetic material after trauma is avoided if possible owing to the risk of contamination and graft infection.

Aneurysm

An aneurysm is an abnormal permanent dilatation of an artery or part of an artery or the heart. Morphologically, it may be fusiform or saccular. The term aneurysm is also used to describe any condition in which there is a sac communicating with an arterial lumen, in which case the aneurysms are false or pseudo-aneurysms. These false aneurysms may also involve arteriovenous fistulae (arteriovenous aneurysms) or arterial dissections (also known as dissecting aneurysms).

Aneurysm types (Figure 12.1)

Saccular aneurysms

A dilated portion of the artery joins the main lumen by a narrow neck. Mycotic aneurysms are often of this sort, in which infection causes a local weakness of the wall, which gives way to aneurysmal dilatation.

Fusiform aneurysm

A generalized dilatation of the artery exists, and this is the commonest type of aneurysm to affect the abdominal aorta.

False (pseudo-) aneurysm

Blood leaks out of an artery and is contained by the surrounding connective tissue lined with thrombus. The resultant blood collection communicates with the artery so it is pulsatile and

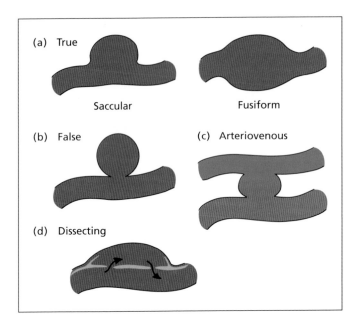

(a) True

Saccular   Fusiform

(b) False   (c) Arteriovenous

(d) Dissecting

Figure 12.1 (a–d) Types of aneurysms.

expansile. It will either thrombose spontaneously or enlarge and rupture.

Arteriovenous aneurysm

A communication between adjacent artery and vein; this is a false aneurysm intervening between artery and vein.

Aneurysm complicating arterial dissection

Blood forces a passage through a break in the intima of a vessel, creating a separate 'false' channel between the external layers of the arterial wall. This false channel may then either rupture back into the lumen, or rupture out of the adventitia externally. Over the arterial segment where flow is extraluminal, vessels taking their origin from the true lumen will be deprived of blood (see aortic dissection, Chapter 11, p. 76).

Aetiology

Congenital

The small berry (or saccular) aneurysms that occur intracranially on the circle of Willis[2] (see

---

[2]Thomas Willis (1621–1675), Physician and Anatomist, first in Oxford then in London, UK.

p. 110) are thought to result from congenital weakness of the cerebral arteries. Arteriovenous aneurysms and fistulae in the limbs may also be congenital.

Degenerative

Atheromatous degeneration of the vessel wall is the commonest cause of a true aneurysm.

Traumatic

Penetration or weakening of the arterial wall by a penetrating wound such as a bullet or knife, or iatrogenic injury during catheterization for angiography and angioplasty, may result in a true aneurysm or false aneurysm, possibly with an associated arteriovenous fistula.

Infection

Mycotic aneurysms, previously seen in the thoracic aorta of patients with tertiary syphilis, are now more commonly seen in the abdominal aorta or femoral artery as a consequence of salmonellosis, or resulting from mycotic emboli in patients with infective endocarditis. Patients with immunodeficiency, whether as a result of immunosuppression for organ transplantation or as a result of human immunodeficiency virus (HIV) infection, are prone to mycotic aneurysms from unusual bacteria or fungi.

Inflammatory

This is a subtype of atherosclerotic and mycotic aneurysms in which there is an immune response to components in the aneurysm wall resulting in a dense inflammatory response with a rind of inflammatory tissue surrounding the lumen. In non-infective cases, this may subside with corticosteroid treatment. It is also associated with retroperitoneal fibrosis and ureteric obstruction. The erythrocyte sedimentation rate is raised.

Clinical features of true aneurysms

The clinical features of an aneurysm depend on its location, and it may present with symptoms far distant from the aneurysm itself. Abdominal aortic aneurysms may present with back pain but they are frequently asymptomatic and picked up incidentally during the course of investigation for some other condition. The patient may feel a sensation of abdominal bloating or may have noticed the pulsatile swelling, or may present with distal emboli from the sac contents. When the peripheral arteries are involved, it is more common to find a complaint of a pulsatile mass or distal ischaemia. On examination there is a dilatation along the course of the artery. The aneurysm itself is both pulsatile and expansile. In smaller peripheral aneurysms, direct compression may empty the sac or diminish its size, and pressure on the artery proximal to the aneurysm may reduce its pulsation. If the feeding vessel has a narrow orifice, there may be a thrill and bruit, and if there is an arteriovenous communication, a machinery murmur is audible.

Differential diagnosis

- A dilated, tortuous, atheromatous artery; commonly seen in the carotid and brachial arteries of elderly subjects.
- A mass overlying or displacing the artery superficially. In the abdomen, for example, the palpable mass of a carcinoma of the pancreas may have a transmitted pulsation from the underlying aorta but will not be expansile, distinguishing it from an aneurysm.

Complications

- *Rupture.* The likelihood of rupture increases as the diameter of the artery increases relative to its normal size.

- *Thrombosis.* Thrombus lines the wall of the aneurysm, and may dislodge or extend to completely occlude the artery. This results in acute impairment of the distal circulation.
- *Embolism.* Lining thrombus may detach and embolize to distal circulation, either as small emboli resulting in digital ischaemia or as a large mass of thrombus threatening the entire limb.
- *Pressure.* Adjacent structures may be eroded or displaced. Hence backache and sciatica are common in patients with large abdominal aortic aneurysms, and occlusion of the femoral vein is common with large femoral aneurysms.
- *Infection.* An aneurysm may become infected or arise secondary to infection and consequent weakening of the arterial wall.

Special investigations

- *Abdominal X-ray.* This may show calcification in the wall of the aneurysm. A lateral film is particularly helpful in demonstrating aortic aneurysm calcification.
- *Computed tomography (CT), magnetic resonance (MR) and ultrasound scanning* may delineate the size and extent of an aneurysm, its relationship to other structures and provide evidence of leakage.
- *Angiography* underestimates the size and extent of a true aneurysm, as it images the lumen, which is usually narrowed by thrombus. In addition, it may be dangerous, as the guidewire or cannula may perforate the aneurysm wall. It is useful in false aneurysms to identify the connection between the artery and the sac.

Treatment

The treatment of an arterial aneurysm depends on its nature (true or false), location, size and symptoms. Abdominal aortic aneurysms should be resected or stented when they become symptomatic or reach a size at which the risk of rupture outweighs the likely operative mortality for the individual. Aneurysms of other large vessels, such as the femoral and popliteal arteries, may be replaced with a prosthetic graft or saphenous vein, whereas a small peripheral aneurysm can usually be excised without endangering the distal circulation, assuming an adequate collateral circulation. False aneurysms and mycotic aneurysms are more prone to rupture and require urgent attention.

Abdominal aortic aneurysm

Dilatation of the abdominal aorta is a common finding in older males, and in those with a positive family history. Around 10% will have a coinciden-tal popliteal aneurysm. Small aneurysms (less than 4 cm) are generally benign and grow slowly (1–2 mm per annum). As they enlarge, the growth rate increases, and the risk of symptoms increases. The most feared complication is rupture. This has an incidence of around 5% per annum once the aneurysm reaches 6 cm in anteroposterior diam-eter. With operative mortality at or below 5%, resection of the aneurysm is advised at 5.5–6 cm as prophylaxis against rupture.

Management

Patients with small asymptomatic aortic aneu-rysms are followed up by regular ultrasound scans to monitor the rate of growth. Once the threshold diameter is reached, or if the aneurysm becomes symptomatic, elective surgical resection is advised. Preoperative assessment includes eval-uating the patient's operative risk by screening for coincident cardiac disease (by resting and exercise ECG or echocardiography) and for carotid arterial disease. This information may affect the decision to operate.

Operative management

Surgery involves replacement of the aneurysmal aorta with an artificial graft, usually made of Dacron. Increasingly aortic aneurysms are treated electively by endovascular stent–graft placement. The prosthetic graft is introduced via a femoral artery and positioned across the aneurysm. It is secured in the normal diameter aorta above and below the aneurysm with self-expanding stents. The aneurysm sac is thus excluded from aortic blood flow and any residual blood in the sac thromboses. When there is not a sufficient length or normal diameter aorta below the aneurysm either a bifurcated graft is deployed with compo-nents via both femorals or a unilateral aortoiliac graft is deployed and a subsequent femorofemoral bypass graft is performed. This minimally invasive approach is ideal for patients who are otherwise unfit for surgery, such as the elderly or those with other significant comorbidity such as obstructive pulmonary disease.

Complications of surgery

- *Renal failure.* The renal arterial ostia are often compressed when the aorta is clamped, thus rendering the kidneys ischaemic for the duration of cross-clamping. The left renal vein may be ligated as it passes across the front of the aorta to enter the inferior vena cava and divided as part of the operative procedure. Hypotension pre- or postoperatively may exacerbate the renal injury.
- *Distal embolization.* Thrombus from the sac may disperse distally and block the small vessels in the foot and lower leg causing acute ischaemia, in this context called 'trash foot'.
- *Myocardial infarction.* Coronary artery disease is common in the population who develop aortic aneurysms. Cross-clamping the aorta during surgery dramatically increases the peripheral resistance against which the heart must work, and this extra stress, coupled with the metabolic stress that occurs when the legs are reperfused, may precipitate a myocardial infarct.
- *Graft infection.* This occurs in about 1% of cases and may lead to an aortoenteric fistula.

Ruptured abdominal aortic aneurysm

A patient with a ruptured aneurysm usually presents with severe back pain, frequently with radiation to the groin, and the diagnosis is often confused with renal colic, although renal colic is less likely in the elderly population (60 years and over) than a ruptured aneurysm. Occasionally, only groin or iliac fossa pain may be the present-ing symptom. Sometimes, the pain is confined to the epigastrium, leading to the mistaken diagnosis of myocardial infarction.

Fifty per cent of patients die from the initial rupture and never reach hospital. Those who do reach hospital are usually profoundly shocked (cold, clammy, tachycardic, hypotensive) with generalized abdominal tenderness. A pulsatile mass is an indication for immediate laparotomy. In most patients reaching hospital, the rupture is contained by the retroperitoneum, helped by the hypotension following rupture. Injudicious fluid replacement to restore normal blood pressure prior to surgery may lead to further bleeding and breaching of the retroperitoneum, resulting in haemoperitoneum and exsanguination. Occasionally, the aortic aneurysm may rupture into the inferior vena cava (aortocaval fistula, diagnosed by a machinery murmur and pulsatile veins) or into the duodenum (aortoduodenal fistula, diagnosis suggested by coexistence of an aneurysm and brisk haematemesis or melaena).

Acute aortic expansion

The aneurysm may expand acutely and result in the typical pain of rupture but without the haemodynamic consequences of a bleed. Indeed, some patients are paradoxically hypertensive during this phase. At laparotomy, the aneurysm sac is found to be oedematous or a local rupture is found.

Special investigations

Investigation of a patient with a suspected rupture should be performed only if there is reasonable doubt about the diagnosis, as delay may be fatal. Investigation should answer two questions:

1 *Does the patient have an aneurysm?* Often an aneurysm is difficult to feel because of hypotension and a large retroperitoneal haematoma masking the sac. A plain X-ray will frequently show calcification in the wall of an aneurysm, especially in an aortic aneurysm. A dorsal decubitus film is particularly valuable, showing the calcified sac displacing the bowel anteriorly.
2 *Is the aneurysm bleeding?* A patient known to have an aneurysm presents with abdominal pain and is normotensive. In this context, a CT is useful to identify a leak, but no modality will distinguish an uncomplicated aneurysm from one that has acutely expanded and that may imminently rupture.

Treatment

Urgent surgery is indicated in anyone with a high suspicion of a ruptured abdominal aortic aneu-rysm. Prior investigations are indicated only when doubt exists. Even with prompt surgery there is a significant mortality rate, together with morbidity, including acute renal failure, myocardial infarction and distal embolization.

Popliteal aneurysm

Popliteal aneurysms are the most common peripheral aneurysms, and historically were the first to be diagnosed and treated surgically. They are usually associated with other aneurysms, and are frequently bilateral.

Clinical features

Popliteal aneurysms are generally asymptomatic. When they do present, it is either in association with distal embolization of sac contents leading to claudication or digital infarction, acute occlusion or rupture (uncommon). Examination confirms a prominent pulsation in the popliteal fossa, often extending proximally. Distal pulses should be sought for evidence of embolization.

Special investigations

• *Duplex ultrasonography.* Delineates the extent and size of the aneurysm.
• *Angiography.* To examine the arterial tree distal to the aneurysm.

Treatment

Symptomatic aneurysms should be treated by femoral to distal popliteal bypass, with ligation of the feeding vessels. Aneurysms containing clot should be repaired electively. Distal emboli may be treated by embolectomy and direct intra-arterial thrombolysis at the time of surgery.

Assessing the patient with arterial disease

Diseases of the arteries may result in impaired blood supply to the limbs. It is important to remember when assessing a particular patient that arterial disease is rarely localized to the peripheries; involvement of other organs, particularly the heart, central nervous system (CNS) and abdominal viscera, must be kept in mind.

The vascular diseases to be considered are the following:

- atherosclerosis;
- diabetic microangiopathy;
- thromboembolism;
- Raynaud's phenomenon;
- Buerger's disease;
- ergot poisoning – usually iatrogenic from migraine therapies;
- arterial injury due to trauma (see p. 80);
- cold or chemical injury.

By far the commonest of these is atherosclerosis, which may often be complicated by coexisting diabetes.

Clinical features

Accurate pathological and anatomical diagnosis can often be made by careful history taking and clinical examination.

History

The time-course of the symptoms is important, ranging from the insidious progression of intermittent claudication of the calves over a period of months or years to the acute onset of ischaemia following an embolus. Sudden onset of pain in the leg suggestive of an embolus should prompt the student to seek a likely source such as atrial fibrillation, recent myocardial infarction or aortic aneurysm. Acute deterioration in a patient with claudication is suggestive of thrombosis on the background of atherosclerotic occlusive disease. A history of cold, painful hands since childhood, especially in the female, will be suggestive of Raynaud's disease, and coexistence of connective tissue disorders, such as systemic lupus erythematosus (SLE) or systemic sclerosis (scleroderma), favours Raynaud's phenomenon. The change in colour (pale and deathly white, then blue and finally a dusky red) precipitated by cold immersion is typical.

Symptoms of atherosclerosis occurring in a young person, especially a heavy smoking male, is typical of Buerger's disease.

Ergot poisoning is occasionally seen in patients with migraine who are consuming large doses of ergotamine.

It is important to determine the degree of handicap produced by the symptoms, for the selection of patients for reconstructive surgery will depend on this. Similarly, if a patient has angina pectoris as well as intermittent claudication, there may be more handicap from the angina than from the claudication, and more benefit from coronary revascularization (Chapter 11, p. 72).

Atherosclerosis is a generalized disease, and the cerebral circulation is often affected in addition to the circulation in the legs. Thus, a history of intermittent loss of consciousness, blindness and hemiparesis is of importance and may indicate coexisting carotid artery disease.

Examination

Careful clinical examination will usually provide a very clear indication of the severity and nature of the ischaemic disease. It is important that attention should be directed to other systems of the body, especially the heart, and blood pressure (is the poor circulation due to a poor cardiac output?).

- *Heart rhythm.* The presence of atrial fibrillation or other cardiac arrhythmias should be noted, particularly if there is a history of acute limb ischaemia (Box 12.1) or stroke. The heart should be examined with particular attention to the apex beat (ventricular aneurysm) and auscultated for evidence of valvular disease (e.g. mitral stenosis).
- *Inspection of limbs.* Attention is then directed to the legs. Inspection may reveal marked skin pallor, an absence of hairs, ulcers (usually lateral malleolus and often in the interdigital clefts) and gangrene, all being evidence of impaired circulation. Fixed staining (purpuric areas not blanching on pressure) in the context of an acutely ischaemic limb is a sign of irreversible tissue injury. A tense, tender calf with impaired dorsiflexion in acute ischaemia

---

Box 12.1 Acute limb ischaemia

- Pain
- Pallor
- Pulselessness
- Paraesthesiae
- Paralysis
- Perishingly cold

signifies compartment compression and requires urgent fasciotomy in addition to revascularization.

- *Venous guttering.* The veins of the foot and leg in a patient with diminished arterial supply are often very inconspicuous compared with normal veins. Indeed, the veins may be so empty that they appear as shallow grooves or gutters, especially in the elevated limb.
- *Buerger's test.*[3] Buerger's test involves raising the legs to 45° above the horizontal and keeping them there for a couple of minutes. A poor arterial supply is shown by rapid pallor. The legs are then allowed to hang dependent over the examination couch. The feet reperfuse with a dusky crimson colour in contrast to a normally perfused foot, which has no colour change. In severe cases, the foot may remain pale and some time may pass before the reactive hyperaemia appears.
- *Capillary return.* The speed of return of capillary circulation after the blanching produced by pressure on the nails is a very useful gauge of the peripheral circulation.
- *Skin temperature.* In addition to the pulses, skin temperature can be readily assessed by palpation, which is especially sensitive when the dorsum of the hand is used. A difference between the temperatures of one part of the leg and another or between the two legs can be ascertained when it is as small as 1°C. A clearly marked change of temperature may reveal the site of blockage of a main artery.
- *Peripheral pulses.* The peripheral pulses throughout the body should be examined. Whereas normal pulsation can be appreciated easily, palpation of weak pulsation requires practice, care and, above all, time. The presence of a weak pulse that is definitely palpated is of considerable significance diagnostically and can be important prognostically, as even a weak pulse means the vessel is patent.

   Careful recording of the peripheral pulses will often clearly delineate a blockage in the arterial system. For instance, the presence of a good femoral pulse and absence of pulses distal to the femoral suggests a superficial femoral arterial block. Ischaemia of the digits in the presence of all pulses including the radial and ulnar pulses is a typical finding in Raynaud's phenomenon.

- *Aortic pulsation.* The abdomen should be examined for any evidence of abnormal aortic pulsation; the popliteal and femoral arteries are also often aneurysmal and should be examined with this in mind. If distal pulses are absent, then it is possible that no aortic pulsation will be felt owing to thrombosis of the terminal aorta.
- *Auscultation of vessels.* In all areas where pulses are felt, auscultation should be performed. Partial blockage of arteries very often causes bruits, which are usually systolic in timing. They may even be felt as thrills. Arteriovenous communications will produce continuous bruits with systolic accentuation (machinery murmur) and pulsating dilated veins.
- *Ankle brachial pressure index (ABPI).* The ABPI should be measured in each leg as part of the routine examination. A Doppler[4] probe is held over the brachial artery and a blood pressure cuff inflated to occlude the blood flow. As the blood pressure cuff is deflated, a Doppler signal reappears and a systolic pressure can be recorded. Similar pressure readings are taken from the dorsalis pedis and posterior tibial arteries with a cuff just above the ankle. The ABPI is the ratio of pressure at the foot pulse to that at the brachial artery. Values less than 0.5 indicate significant ('critical') ischaemia. Heavily calcified vessels, as are common in patients with diabetes, may be incompressible and give false high readings.
- *Exercise test.* If it is difficult to obtain a clear history of the exact severity of intermittent claudication, the patient should be taken for a walk with the doctor, who observes the time and nature of the onset of symptoms. Measurement of the ABPI before and after exercise may show a significant fall from normal after exercise, indicating a critical stenosis in the proximal vessels.

Special investigations

- *Urine test for sugar and blood glucose* to exclude diabetes, a common accompaniment of peripheral artery disease. If necessary, a fasting blood glucose estimation or

---

[3]Leo Buerger (1879–1943), born in Vienna; Urologist, Mount Sinai Hospital, New York, NY, USA.

[4]Christian Doppler (1803–1853), Professor of Physics, University of Vienna, Austria.

glycosylated haemoglobin (HbA1c) may be necessary.

- *Haemoglobin estimation* to exclude anaemia or polycythaemia. Anaemia may sometimes precipitate angina or claudication.
- *Erythrocyte sedimentation rate (ESR)* and *C-reactive protein (CRP)*[5] are raised in inflammatory and mycotic aneurysms.
- *Serum cholesterol* is often raised in atherosclerosis, and is treatable.
- *Electrocardiogram (ECG)* to exclude associated coronary disease.
- *Echocardiogram* to confirm valvular lesions, mural thrombus on an akinetic ventricular wall, ventricular aneurysm and atrial myxoma.
- *Chest X-ray.* Bronchial carcinoma is a common finding in end-stage vascular disease, both being caused by smoking. Chest X-ray also allows assessment of the cardiac silhouette.
- *Doppler ultrasound.* The Doppler ultrasonic probe can be used to generate a waveform of the arterial pulse in the peripheral vessels in addition to allowing the measurement of pressure and derivation of the ABPI. The waveform is biphasic in normal elastic arteries, but becomes monophasic in hardened arteries.
- *Duplex ultrasonography.* Combining Doppler ultrasound with real time produces duplex scanning, which is a sensitive method of imaging blood vessels. By measuring flow patterns, it can quantify the degree of stenosis of a vessel because the blood velocity increases as it crosses a stenosis in order to maintain the same flow rate. Summation of scans produces a result similar to angiography, but non-invasively. It is particularly useful in assessing carotid artery disease.
- *Arteriography* is used to determine the site and extent of a blockage, and is performed if reconstructive surgery or angioplasty is contemplated to identify the severity and distribution of disease, whether atheromatous plaques, stenoses or complete blocks as well as demonstrating run-off (Figure 12.2).
- *Angioplasty.* At the time of arteriography, a stenosed segment of artery may be dilated using a specially designed balloon catheter. This percutaneous transluminal angioplasty (PTA) is now commonly undertaken for

coronary as well as peripheral arteries. It may be combined with endoluminal stenting to maintain the patency of the dilated segment.

- *CT and ultrasound scanning.* These are useful in determining the presence and extent of aneurysmal disease, and their relation to other structures.

Principles of treatment

There are two treatment principles underlying the management of patients with vascular disease; both come under the adage of *primum non nocere* (first do no harm).

1 *Treat handicap not disability.* Treatment must be tailored to the patient. If a patient claudicates at 500 m (the disability) but seldom needs to walk that distance, there is no handicap with this disability and therefore the patient needs no treatment. However, if the patient is young and work requires him or her to walk 500 m (e.g. on a post round) then the patient is handicapped by the disability and merits treatment.

There are usually two treatment options: conservative management and surgery. Reconstructive surgery can produce dramatic results but at a risk.

2 *Prophylactic surgery is appropriate only when the risk of the event outweighs the risk of the procedure.* For example, surgical repair of an aortic aneurysm is advised when the risk of rupture (which is usually fatal) outweighs the operative mortality. If the patient is a poor operative risk then the threshold for surgery increases.

Atherosclerotic arterial disease

Arterial disease may be divided into occlusive disease and aneurysmal disease (see p. 81), the commonest cause of both being atherosclerosis. Both manifestations may coexist; hence, patients with an abdominal aortic aneurysm frequently also have coronary artery disease.

Aetiology

Many factors have been shown to contribute to the genesis of atherosclerosis. While there is a

---

[5]A marker of inflammation, C-reactive protein was so named because it reacts with the C polysaccharide in the wall of *Pneumococcus.* It is not related to protein C or C-peptide.

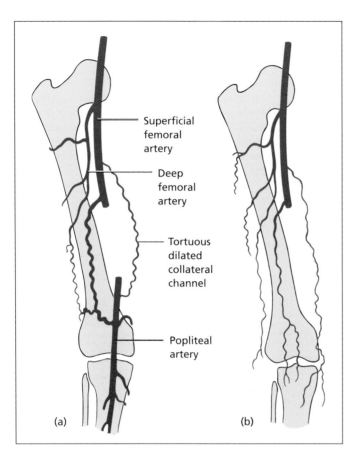

(a)

(b)

Superficial
femoral
artery

Deep
femoral
artery

Tortuous
dilated
collateral
channel

Popliteal
artery

Figure 12.2 Tracings of arteriograms. (a) An example of a good 'run-off' from the occluded superficial femoral artery, with a patent popliteal artery; this is suitable for reconstructive surgery. (b) The main arterial tree is obliterated and reconstruction cannot be carried out.

familial tendency to the disease, the most common aetiological factors are smoking, hyperlipidaemia and hypercholesterolaemia, hypertension and diabetes (Box 12.2). It is a disease that predominantly affects men, although, with increasing age, women become more susceptible.

Box 12.2 Risk factors for atherosclerotic disease

- Smoking
- Hyperlipidaemia
- Hypertension
- Diabetes mellitus
- Male sex
- Increasing age
- Family history

Smoking

There are three components of the serious effects of smoking in atherosclerotic disease.

1 Nicotine, which induces vasospasm.
2 Carbon monoxide, present in inhaled smoke, which is taken up by haemoglobin to form carboxyhaemoglobin, which dissociates slowly and is, therefore, unavailable for oxygen carrying, resulting in relative tissue hypoxia.
3 Increased platelet stickiness, with increased risk of thrombus formation.

Hyperlipidaemia

Raised cholesterol and raised triglycerides are both implicated in vascular disease and cholesterol-lowering agents have been shown to reduce the risk of death from coronary artery disease in patients with hypercholesterolaemia.

Diabetes

Diabetic patients are prone to higher incidence of atherosclerosis, and also are at risk of diabetic microangiopathy, resulting in poor tissue perfusion, ulceration and gangrene, owing to both tissue perfusion and the neuropathy that accompanies diabetes. Two clinical manifestations of diabetic arterial disease should be distinguished:

1 The young diabetic patient with peripheral gangrene but with good pulses in the limb. Control of infection with the appropriate antibiotic and improved diabetic control, together with local debridement of the gangrenous tissue, usually results in limb salvage.
2 The elderly patient with atherosclerosis (as shown by absent peripheral pulses) who is also diabetic. Here, the diabetes makes the prognosis of the disease much worse.

Atherosclerotic occlusive arterial disease

Occlusive disease results in ischaemia of the end-organ or tissue that is supplied. In the peripheral arteries, the three cardinal features are exercise-induced pain (*intermittent claudication*), which may progress, as the disease progresses, to *pain at rest* and *gangrene*. The progression is not necessarily a smooth one in the early stage, with deterioration in claudication distance, followed by some improvement as collateral circulation develops, before further deterioration due to thrombosis.

Parallels to peripheral artery occlusive disease are present in the other circulatory systems.

Coronary occlusive disease

Angina pectoris is the coronary circulation's equivalent of intermittent claudication, with pain on exertion as oxygen demand exceeds supply, and rest pain being analogous to unstable angina with resultant infarction if the coronary circulation is not revascularized by either thrombolysis or bypass surgery.

Mesenteric occlusive disease

Mesenteric angina occurs when the blood supply to the gut is impaired and follows the ingestion of food. Patients present with pain after meals, a history of marked weight loss and fear of eating because of pain. Acute occlusion results in bowel infarction.

Cerebral occlusive disease

In the cerebral circulation, progressive occlusive disease manifests as dementia, while small emboli causing occlusion of small vessels may appear as transient ischaemic attacks, complete occlusion resulting in cerebral infarction in the absence of a collateral circulation.

Intermittent claudication

Intermittent claudication manifests as a gripping, tight, cramp-like pain in the calf on exercise, and usually affects one leg in advance of the other. The pain disappears on resting. Pain that is present on standing and that requires the patient to sit down before it is relieved is more typical of cauda equina compression (spinal claudication) (Chapter 16, p. 133).

The pathology lies in one of the main arteries supplying the leg. Calf claudication is usually due to a lesion in the thigh, whereas buttock claudication is due to a reduced blood flow down the internal iliac arteries, owing to a lesion either there or higher up in the common iliac artery or the aorta. Bilateral buttock claudication is associated with impotence, as both internal iliac arteries are compromised (Leriche's syndrome;[6] absent femoral pulses, intermittent claudication of the buttock muscles, pale cold legs and impotence).

[6]René Leriche (1879–1955), Professor of Surgery, successively at Lyon, Strasbourg and Paris, France.

> **Box 12.3 Treatment of claudication**
>
> **Conservative**
>
> - Stop smoking
> - Exercise to increase the collateral circulation
> - Learn to live within a claudication distance, involving a change in lifestyle and perhaps employment
> - Weight loss – less effort for the muscles
> - Raising the heel of the shoe – less effort for the calf muscles
> - Foot care to prevent minor trauma that may lead to gangrene
> - Treat coexisting conditions such as diabetes, hypertension and hyperlipidaemia
>
> **Interventional**
>
> - Angioplasty
> - Endoluminal stenting
> - Bypass surgery, but only if severely handicapped

Management (Box 12.3)

Conservative treatment

If patients stop smoking and continue exercise, or better still are enrolled into a programme of supervised exercise, over one-third of patients will extend their claudication distance owing to the development of collateral vessels that bypass the blockage. Only one-third will deteriorate. In addition to cessation of smoking, the other risk factors for the development of arterial disease should be treated, so diabetes should be sought and treated aggressively and hyperlipidaemia if present should be treated.

The work performed by the legs is greater if the patient is overweight, so strict dieting may well improve exercise tolerance. If the claudication is limited to the calf, raising the heels of the shoes 2 cm will relieve the work performed by the calf muscles, and therefore allow the patient to walk a greater distance. Careful chiropody is important. Gangrene can commence from a minor trauma such as faulty nail or corn cutting and may result in limb loss.

Interventional treatment

If claudication is a significant handicap to the patient, the possibility of reconstructive surgery or angiographic intervention should be considered.

Special investigations

The special investigations detailed above should be arranged, including the following in particular.

- *Arteriography*, either with an intra-arterial cannula or by MR scan. This should include the aorta and iliac, femoral, popliteal and distal arteries on the affected side. In particular, this should look for short (less than 10 cm) occlusions or significant (greater than 70%) stenoses, which would be amenable to angioplasty.
- *Duplex sonography*. Duplex scanning is now replacing angiography in many centres. It takes longer to perform and is more subjective but can give better information as to the significance of stenoses and has the benefit of being non-invasive.

Treatment choices (Box 12.3)

- *Angioplasty.* Angioplasty involves inflating a balloon within the vessel to stretch and fracture the stenosis or blockage, and allow more blood to pass through. This is most successful with concentric stenoses or blocks in the iliac system and is less successful with long blocks over 10 cm, particularly in the distal femoral and popliteal arteries. An endovascular stent may be used to maintain patency. Angioplasty carries the risk of distal embolization and vessel perforation.
- *Thrombolysis.* When there has been an acute deterioration in claudication distance because of thrombosis occurring on a background of pre-existing disease, thrombolysis may be appropriate. A fibrinolytic enzyme such as streptokinase or tissue plasminogen activator (TPA) is infused into the clot, which it dissolves. Complete dissolution of thrombus takes time, so the technique is not appropriate when limb viability is acutely threatened.
- *Bypass surgery.* Bypass surgery should not be undertaken for minimal symptoms and is now generally reserved for limiting claudication or rest pain. Complications include intimal dissection, distal embolization and graft thrombosis, which worsen the initial situation.

Critical ischaemia

Critical ischaemia may be defined as rest pain, ulceration or gangrene associated with absent pedal pulses. An ABPI of less than 0.5 also signifies critical ischaemia (see p. 87).

Rest pain

Rest pain occurs when the blood supply to the leg is insufficient. Initially, the pain occurs at night after the foot has been horizontal for a few hours in bed. The patient gains relief by sleeping with the leg hanging out of bed. As the disease progresses, the pain becomes continuous.

Gangrene

The presence of gangrene indicates a severe degree of vascular impairment. Typically, it occurs in the toes or at pressure areas on the foot, particularly the heel, over the malleoli or on the plantar aspect of the ball of the hallux. Gangrene results from infection of ischaemic tissues. Minimal trauma, such as a nick of the skin while cutting the toenails or an abrasion from a tight shoe, enables ingress of bacteria into the infarcted tissues; the combination of these two factors results in clinical gangrene.

Investigation

Critical ischaemia needs investigating with great urgency to relieve the patient's pain and to prevent irreversible damage leading to limb loss. The investigations are the same as those used to evaluate claudication.

Treatment

Non-operative treatment

- *Arteriography and angioplasty.* Arteriography should be performed with a view to angioplasty or stenting when possible, and to identify surgically reconstructable disease.
- *Lumbar sympathectomy.* Palliation may be achieved by lumbar sympathectomy, which increases the blood supply to the skin, and which can be performed percutaneously. The small increase in blood supply may be sufficient to allow an ulcer to heal but will not generally improve rest pain.

Operative treatment

- Reconstructive surgery. Successful surgical reconstruction demands four things:
  1 *Inflow.* A good arterial supply up to the area of blockage is necessary to ensure that enough blood can be carried distally via the conduit to the ischaemic area.
  2 *Outflow (run-off).* There should be good vessels below the area of disease onto which a conduit can be anastomosed. If there is nowhere for the blood to go, the conduit will occlude.
  3 *The conduit.* A graft of saphenous vein, reversed or used *in situ* with valve destruction, or an inert prosthetic material such as polytetrafluoroethylene (PTFE), may be used for the conduit to take blood from the proximal to the distal segment of the artery beyond the blockage. In grafts that start and finish above the knee, there is little to choose between PTFE and vein in terms of long-term patency, but a graft that crosses the knee is much more likely to remain patent if it is saphenous vein rather than PTFE. Infection is less likely with autologous vein.
  4 *The patient.* Critical ischaemia is often the first sign of the end-stage vascular disease, which inevitably results in death. Surgery for critical ischaemia has a high mortality reflecting this general deterioration.
- *Amputation.* Pain that is not controlled by sympathectomy or reconstructive surgery, and gangrene that is associated with life-threatening infection are indications for amputation of the limb or part of the limb. The general principle is to achieve a viable stump that heals primarily, and a secondary goal is to make the stump as distal as possible.

Carotid artery disease (Figure 12.3)

Atheroma usually affects the bifurcation of the carotid artery into the internal and external carotid arteries. Atheromatous plaques may ulcerate and thrombus form on their surface. If this thrombus breaks off, it forms an embolus comprising

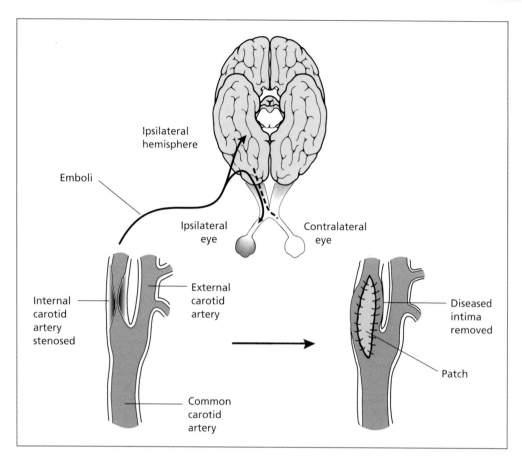

Figure 12.3 Symptoms and treatment of carotid artery stenosis.

platelet clumps or atheromatous debris. This may impact in the ipsilateral retinal artery, producing ipsilateral blindness, or the cerebral arteries of the ipsilateral hemisphere, producing contralateral paralysis. Alternatively, the atheroma may so narrow the artery that blood flow is critically limited or totally occluded, producing similar symptoms.

Clinical features

- *Amaurosis fugax.* The patient commonly complains of a loss of vision like a curtain coming down across his or her visual field. The blindness is unilateral, ipsilateral to the diseased carotid, and usually lasts a few minutes.
- *Cerebrovascular accidents (stroke).* Emboli in the carotid territory of the cerebral circulation

of the ipsilateral hemisphere will result in symptoms affecting the contralateral side of the body, commonly loss of use of the arm. If the dominant hemisphere is involved, speech may be affected.
- *Transient ischaemic attack (TIA).* By definition, these mimic strokes, but last less than 24 hours.
- *Cerebral hypoperfusion.* Bilateral severe stenoses may result in critical ischaemia in the brain such that cerebral or physical exertion may result in relative hypoperfusion and confusion or TIA.

Examination may reveal a bruit over the affected side (although very tight stenoses are often silent) and evidence of vascular disease elsewhere. During an attack, unilateral weakness affecting the arm or leg, dysphasia, and retinal emboli and infarction may be noted.

Differential diagnosis

Other causes of focal neurological deficits include hypoglycaemia, focal epilepsy, migraine, intracerebral neoplasm and emboli secondary to cardiac arrhythmias and valve disease.

Special investigations

- *Duplex ultrasonography*. This gives a non-invasive assessment of the degree of stenosis and is useful to screen for the disease.
- *Angiography* allows accurate assessment of the degree of stenosis, but carries the risk of dislodging thrombus and precipitating an embolic stroke.
- *MR angiography* can also give good images of the carotid vessels and allows good visualization of the vertebral system to assess the complete cerebral perfusion. It is less accurate in the measurement of the degree of stenosis.
- *MR/CT of the brain* is indicated if any doubt over symptoms exists, since intracranial tumours may mimic carotid artery disease, and may coexist.
- *Cerebral reactivity*. If cerebral perfusion is marginal, with bilateral stenoses or an occlusion on one side and stenosis on the other, the haemodynamic response to stress can be gauged by measuring the change in cerebral blood flow using intracranial duplex scanning while the patient breathes CO_2, which causes vasodilatation, so intracranial blood flow should increase. If there is a critical stenosis affecting the carotid artery, and the collateral cerebral circulation provided by the circle of Willis is not intact or sufficient, there will be no reactive increase in perfusion.
- *ECG/echocardiography*. This may be necessary to exclude a cardiac cause of cerebral symptoms.

Treatment

Patients who have had a recent TIA, amaurosis fugax or stroke with full recovery in the presence of an internal carotid stenosis of 70% or more are at high risk of a subsequent stroke in the months following. These patients benefit from endarterectomy to remove the diseased intima and re-establish normal carotid flow. All patients should be started on aspirin upon diagnosis, and this should be continued indefinitely as prophylaxis against further events. Patients with asymptomatic stenoses may also benefit from surgery, but here the risk/benefit ratio is not as favourable.

Carotid endarterectomy is performed as prophylaxis against future stroke. The diseased intima is removed, and peroperatively a shunt may be used to keep blood flowing to the brain. Increasingly carotid angioplasty is being performed in place of surgery.

Complications of carotid endarterectomy

- *Death and disabling stroke.* Up to 5% of patients will suffer a stroke, some of whom will die as a consequence.
- *Haemorrhage.* Bleeding is common, as the patients are on aspirin therapy. Occasionally, postoperative haemorrhage requires re-exploration.
- *Hypoglossal neuropraxia.* The hypoglossal nerve crosses the upper part of the incision and may be damaged during surgery, resulting in a hypoglossal palsy, manifested by protrusion of the tongue to the ipsilateral side.
- *Reperfusion syndrome.* The sudden increase in blood flow to the brain may result in cerebral oedema and fitting or haemorrhage. Good postoperative blood pressure control is therefore vital.
- *Restenosis.* The vessel may restenose at the site of the arteriotomy. To overcome this, a patch is usually used, made from saphenous vein or prosthetic material such as PTFE or Dacron.

Raynaud's phenomenon[7]

Clinical features

The syndrome occurs as a result of intermittent spasm of the small arteries and arterioles of the hands (and feet). Spasm is usually precipitated by cold exposure. During the spasm, the hands go white. As the vasospasm resolves, the pallor changes to cyanosis and then crimson red as reperfusion and hyperaemia occurs, the process commonly taking 30–45 minutes.

[7]Maurice Raynaud (1834–1881), Physician, Paris, France.

Aetiology

This may be primary Raynaud's disease, almost invariably in women, or Raynaud's phenomenon, secondary to some other lesion, particularly connective tissue disorders such as scleroderma and polyarteritis nodosa, the other symptoms of which it may precede by several years. It may occur in patients with cryoglobulinaemia or it can result from work with vibrating tools. It is important to exclude other causes of cold, cyanosed hands, for instance pressure on the subclavian artery from a cervical rib (sometimes complicated by multiple emboli arising from the damaged artery wall at the site of rib pressure), or blockage of a main artery in the upper limb due to atherosclerosis or Buerger's disease.

Treatment

Conservative

The management should initially be conservative. Patients should be exhorted to keep their hands and feet warm, to wear gloves and fur-lined boots in the winter, and to make sure that the house, especially the bed, is warm at night. They should also avoid immersion of the limbs in cold water. Treatment with vasodilator drugs is usually tried but the results are often disappointing. Smoking must be stopped.

Surgery

Sympathectomy almost invariably produces a dramatic improvement in the symptoms, but unfortunately may not be long-lasting in the upper limbs. Rarely, Raynaud's phenomenon or disease leads to actual necrosis of tissues and gangrene of the digits. If this occurs, local amputation may be necessary, but, as the circulation of the proximal part of the hand is usually satisfactory, major amputations are seldom required.

Buerger's disease

Buerger's disease (thromboangiitis obliterans) is a rather poorly defined entity, usually affecting men (90%), the salient features of which are similar to atherosclerosis but the age incidence is much younger and the association with heavy smoking is almost invariable. Peripheral vessels tend to be affected earlier in Buerger's disease and the veins may be inflamed together with the arteries. It is more an inflammatory condition than atherosclerotic, although the symptoms of distal claudication and ischaemic ulceration of the toes are similar. It tends to affect the hands and fingers more commonly than atheroma.

Embolism (Figure 12.4)

An embolus is abnormal undissolved material carried in the bloodstream from one part of the vascular system to impact in a distant part. While the embolus may comprise air, fat or tumour (including atrial myxoma), it is most commonly thrombus that becomes dislodged from its source, usually the heart or the major vessels.

Emboli tend to lodge at the bifurcation of vessels; their danger will depend upon the anatomical situation. Blockage of arteries of the CNS, retina and small intestine will produce dramatic effects. Emboli in the renal arteries will produce haematuria and pain in the loin. Emboli in the splenic artery will produce pain under the left costal margin. Large emboli straddling the aortic bifurcation (a saddle embolus) may cause bilateral signs.

The late results of embolism in limb vessels are similar to those of atherosclerosis and may, in fact, be associated with or caused by this condition. However, acute embolism is a surgical emergency and prompt adequate treatment may produce a complete recovery.

Clinical features

The limb

With an acute blockage of the principal artery to a limb, the history is usually one of sudden pain in the limb, which soon becomes white and cold. Sensation may disappear and the muscles may become rapidly paralysed. As time progresses, the limb becomes anaesthetic and fixed muscular contractures develop. On examination, the site of the block will usually be considerably proximal to the site at which pain is experienced. It is fairly common for the level of occlusion to move distally in the course of the first few hours, owing to the embolus being dislodged or fragmented. In time, skin staining appears, which does not blanch on

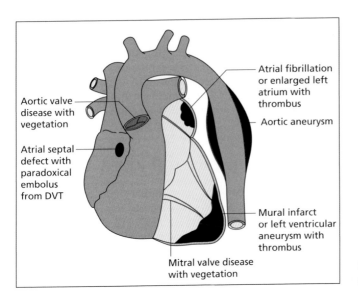

Figure 12.4 Source of peripheral emboli. DVT, deep vein thrombosis.

Box 12.4 Potential sources of emboli

- *Left atrium:* atrial fibrillation and mitral stenosis, atrial myxoma
- *Heart valves:* infective endocarditis
- *Left ventricular wall:* mural thrombus after myocardial infarction or from ventricular aneurysm
- *Aorta:* from aneurysm or atheroma
- *Interventricular septum:* rare paradoxical embolus via a septal defect, originating in the systemic veins

---

pressure (fixed staining); this is a sign of irreversible tissue damage.

The underlying cause

The history and physical signs may reveal a cause for the embolus (Box 12.4).

- *Atrial fibrillation* is by far the most common cause of arterial emboli. The atrial fibrillation may be due to rheumatic heart disease or myocardial ischaemia.
- A *mural thrombus*, typically following a myocardial infarction, may also dislodge and embolize. This typically occurs around 10 days after infarct.

- *Aortic dissection* is an uncommon differential diagnosis, when ischaemia may progress down the body, often with spontaneous recovery corresponding to the intimal flap dissecting away from the true lumen (Chapter 11, p. 76).
- *Paradoxical emboli* are also uncommon. In patients with a patent foramen ovale, or other septal defect, a clot originating in the veins may pass up towards the chest. In addition to impacting in the pulmonary arterial tree, the clot may pass across the septal defect and lodge in the arterial system. This is particularly likely after a pulmonary embolus, as the resultant raised pulmonary artery pressure results in increased shunting across a septal defect if present.
- An *atrial myxoma* is rare, but may present with distal embolization of adherent clot or tumour fragments.

Treatment

1 *Assessment.* The limb is exposed to room temperature and observed for signs of impairment to the circulation. If the block seems to be resolving, with the appearance of pulses that had previously been absent, the collateral circulation may produce adequate distal arterial blood supply and surgery may not be required; thrombolysis may be an appropriate alternative. If the distal limb has apparently no blood supply and there are

neurological changes, urgent surgery is indicated. Absent femoral, popliteal or aortic pulsations are indications that operation will probably prove necessary.

The likelihood of surgical removal of an embolus successfully restoring viability to a limb is inversely proportional to the time since the onset of the arterial occlusion; after 24 hours have elapsed, successful revascularization of the limb becomes unlikely. Fixed staining of the skin is a sign that it is too late.

2 *Heparinization.* As soon as the diagnosis is made, the patient should be systemically heparinized, so as to prevent propagation of clot from the site of blockage.

3 *Surgical embolectomy.* The approach to the involved vessel will depend on physical findings indicating the level of the block. The operative treatment is relatively simple: the vessel is exposed, opened and the clot removed. A special balloon catheter (designed by Thomas Fogarty[8] when he was a medical student) is passed into the vessel with the balloon collapsed. The balloon is then inflated and pulled back, the clot being expelled by the balloon via the arteriotomy. Poor results will be due to propagation of clot beyond the embolus, particularly down the branches of the popliteal artery, and local thrombolysis may be required. Emboli in the upper limb vessels usually produce less disability than those in the lower limb, as a collateral circulation in the upper limb is better. Surgery is therefore indicated less often.

4 *Thrombolysis.* When there is no obvious cause for an embolus, a spontaneous thrombosis *in situ* must be considered. This is more likely if the patient has a previous history of occlusive symptoms such as claudication. In this case, collaterals have already developed and the limb remains viable. Thrombolysis may restore patency, followed by angioplasty to treat the underlying disease. Occasionally, *in situ* thrombosis may be a manifestation of malignancy.

It is most important that, after the successful outcome of an embolectomy, the cause of the embolism be treated if this is possible.

Cold injury

Frostbite may result from prolonged exposure to cold and results from a combination of ice crystal formation in the tissues, capillary sludging and thrombosis within small vessels of the exposed extremities. Treatment comprises gentle warming, anticoagulation with heparin to prevent further thrombosis, and antibiotics to inhibit infection of necrotic tissues. Local amputation to remove necrotic digits is performed once clear demarcation develops. Raynaud's phenomenon may be experienced as a late complication.

[8]Thomas Fogarty (b. 1934), Surgeon, Portland, OR, USA.

13

Venous disorders of the lower limb

Learning objective

✓ To know the causes and treatment of varicose veins and deep venous insufficiency of the lower limb.

Anatomy of the venous drainage of the lower limb

In order to understand the various manifestations of venous disease in the lower leg, it is essential to understand the functional anatomy of the venous system. There are two venous systems taking blood from the skin and muscles of the lower limb back to the trunk: the deep system and the superficial system (Figure 13.1).

The deep venous system

This comprises a network of veins which accompany the main arteries of the lower limb, lying deep to the deep fascia that envelops the muscular compartments of the leg. Smaller tributaries drain into the popliteal vein behind the knee, which then ascends as the femoral vein to the inguinal ligament, where it becomes the external iliac vein. From there, blood passes up the common iliac vein, via the inferior vena cava, to the right atrium.

The superficial venous system

This comprises the medially placed great (long) saphenous vein, draining from the dorsum of the foot to the saphenofemoral junction in the groin, and the small (short) saphenous vein, which drains the lateral aspect of the lower limb into the popliteal vein behind the knee. The superficial system lies outside the deep fascia, and drains the skin and superficial tissues.

Perforating veins

Besides the saphenofemoral and saphenopopliteal junctions, there are additional communications between superficial and deep veins with valves allowing blood in the superficial system to pass into the deep system, and preventing blood flowing out from deep to superficial. These are called perforating veins, or perforators. Typically, there is one mid-thigh (called the hunterian perforator on account of its relationship to Hunter's canal[1]), and several running up the medial and lateral aspect of the tibia just above the ankle.

The calf pump

All the major leg veins have valves that prevent blood flowing away from the heart. As the calf muscles contract, the deep veins within them are squeezed and emptied, the blood passing upwards, directed towards the heart by the non-return valves. As the muscles relax, blood flows in from the superficial system via perforators as well as from more distal segments of the

Lecture Notes: General Surgery, 12th edition. © Harold Ellis, Sir Roy Y. Calne and Christopher J. E. Watson. Published 2011 by Blackwell Publishing Ltd.

[1]John Hunter (1728–1793), Surgeon, St George's Hospital, London, UK.

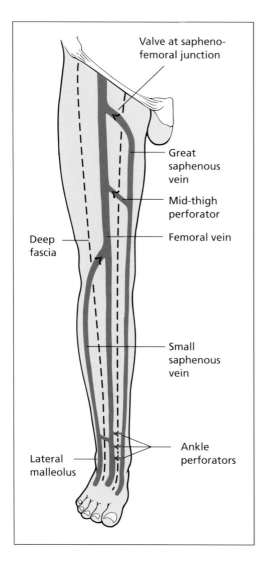

Valve at sapheno-femoral junction

Great saphenous vein

Mid-thigh perforator

Femoral vein

Deep fascia

Small saphenous vein

Ankle perforators

Lateral malleolus

Figure 13.1 The superficial and deep veins of the leg. Note the two superficial systems – the great saphenous and small saphenous – each of which communicates with the deep veins by piercing the deep fascia.

vein, only to be forced upwards again by the next contraction of the calf muscles, which are thus acting as a pump.

Pathology of venous disease

Venous disorders, whether in the superficial veins (e.g. varicose veins) or in the deep veins (venous insufficiency), share the same underlying pathology: valvular incompetence resulting in a disturbance of the normal flow of blood (Figure 13.2). This haemodynamic disturbance is due either to a physical obstruction, such as a thrombosis, or to a functional obstruction leading to high pressure as occurs when valves are incompetent or, rarely, when an arteriovenous fistula exists. When valves are incompetent, there is a greater resistance to return flow (the functional obstruction). One incompetent valve will put extra pressure on the next and will tend to make this incompetent; so, once defects have arisen, there is a tendency for the condition to get worse as further valves are involved.

There are no valves in the vena cava, and none in the common iliac veins. The first valve usually occurs in the external iliac vein. Congenital absence of this, or destruction following disease, imposes increased pressure on the next in line, commonly the one guarding the saphenofemoral junction. The pressure on this valve is then equivalent to a column of blood from the saphenofemoral junction to the right atrium. This absence of valves and the tendency to develop varicose veins is the unfortunate legacy from the days before humans adopted the upright posture.

Varicose veins

Definition

Varicose veins are abnormally dilated and lengthened superficial veins. They should be distinguished from prominent normal veins, which are most obvious over the muscular calves of an athlete, and venous flare, the clusters of small, dilated venules that occur subcutaneously as a result of hormonal change, pregnancy or trauma.

Classification

Primary or idiopathic

The great majority of cases are idiopathic. This probably represents a primary valve defect and may be familial. Women are affected twice as commonly as men. Symptoms are often accentuated by pregnancy, partly as a result of pressure of the enlarged uterus on the iliac veins and partly as a result of relaxation of smooth

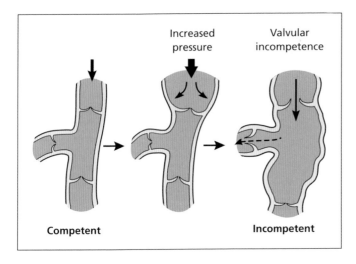

Increased pressure

Valvular incompetence

Competent

Incompetent

Figure 13.2 Normal veins and incompetent varicose veins. Note that the vein dilates under pressure and the valve becomes incompetent.

muscle under the influence of hormones such as progesterone.

Secondary

- *Previous deep vein thrombosis.* Occluded veins may subsequently recanalize but their valves are rendered incompetent.
- *Raised venous pressure* due to compression (e.g. by a pelvic tumour including a pregnant uterus), congenital venous malformation (e.g. Klippel–Trenaunay syndrome[2]), arteriovenous fistula (congenital or acquired following trauma) or severe tricuspid incompetence. The last two cause pulsating varicosities.

Clinical features

History

Varicose veins are prominent and unsightly, and patients may seek treatment on account of the unpleasant appearance. Other symptoms are of tiredness, aching or throbbing in the legs and swelling of the ankles, particularly after long periods of standing. Other points to note are a history of deep vein thrombosis, or a history

[2]Maurice Klippel (1858–1942), French Neurologist, Salpêtrière Hospital, Paris, France. Paul Trenaunay (b. 1875), French Neurologist. The syndrome involves multiple congenital venous malformations producing varicose veins together with hypertrophy of bones and soft tissues and extensive cutaneous haemangiomas, usually affecting the lower limbs.

suggestive of thrombosis such as swelling and pain postoperatively, during pregnancy, or after a long period of immobilization. If the deep veins are still blocked, the varicose veins that are visible may represent the sole venous drainage of the leg. A history of any complications arising from the veins (e.g. thrombophlebitis) should be sought.

Examination

A patient with varicose veins must be examined while standing. Examination of the legs should include inspection of the medial gaiter area for evidence of deep venous insufficiency (haemosiderosis, eczema, lipodermatosclerosis – see later). Overlying port-wine stains or similar pigmentation may suggest underlying arteriovenous malformation, especially in young patients. Auscultation over such areas may be diagnostic.

A *saphena varix*, a prominent dilatation of the vein (varicosity) at the saphenofemoral junction, may be present. It gives a characteristic thrill to the examining fingers when the patient coughs, quite different from a femoral hernia. It disappears when the patient lies flat.

The *tap test* involves placing the fingers of one hand over the saphenofemoral (or saphenopopliteal) junction and, with the patient standing, tapping over distally placed varicosities. In the absence of valves, there will be a continuous column of blood and a transmitted thrill will be palpated proximally.

Trendelenburg's test[3] detects reflux from deep into superficial veins, and when carefully performed can identify the site of the incompetent connections. The patient lies flat and the leg is elevated to empty the superficial veins. A tourniquet is placed around the upper thigh and the patient stands up. If saphenofemoral junction incompetence is the cause of the superficial venous reflux, this high thigh tourniquet will control it and the varicose veins will remain empty. If this high tourniquet does not control the varices, the tourniquet test can be repeated with progressively lower placement of the tourniquet until the varicosities are controlled, and the level of the incompetent connection between deep and superficial veins identified.

Special investigations

- A *hand-held Doppler probe* is useful to diagnose reflux at saphenofemoral and saphenopopliteal junctions. Identifying perforating veins is more difficult, and the device is not as sensitive as duplex scanning or venography; it is superior to clinical examination.
- *Duplex scanning* can accurately map the veins in the leg and diagnose both valvular and perforator incompetence, as well as occlusion of large veins. Like the hand-held Doppler probe, it allows accurate preoperative localization of perforating veins.
- *Venography* involves placing a tourniquet around the ankle to occlude superficial veins and injecting contrast medium into the dorsum of the foot such that it will pass through the deep system up the leg. Its progress is followed on sequential X-rays. Reflux through perforating veins and deep vein occlusion are readily detected.

Treatment

Graded compression stockings

Indicated for minor varicosities, and for the elderly, the pregnant and the unfit. The stocking is elasticated and specially fitted to ensure that it delivers graduated compression along its length, such that at the ankle the elastic compression of the lower leg is much higher than that at the thigh.

[3]Friedrich Trendelenburg (1844–1924), Professor of Surgery, successively at Rostock, Bonn and Leipzig, Germany.

Sclerotherapy

Superficial varicosities that are cosmetically undesirable may be obliterated by injection of a small volume of sclerosant with the vein emptied. The vein is kept compressed with firm pressure bandaging for a period of 2 weeks to enable fibrosis to take place. This outpatient treatment is used for small- or moderate-sized varices below the knee. Recurrences can be treated by further injections. Complications include bruising, phlebitis with unsightly skin staining, ulceration and deep vein thrombosis.

Surgical treatment

Varicose vein surgery is one of the most commonly performed elective surgical procedures in the UK. More recently, the indications for the procedure have come under fresh scrutiny on account of their cosmetic nature, the need for the great saphenous vein as a conduit for future arterial surgery, such as coronary artery bypass, and the cost.

Indications for varicose vein surgery include the following:

- *haemorrhage* occurring from a varicosity;
- *varicosities* being grossly dilated or otherwise symptomatic;
- *skin changes*, typically in the medial gaiter area, which may suggest coincident deep venous insufficiency;
- *incompetent perforator veins*, which should be identified preoperatively and ligated by a conventional open technique or subfascial ligation performed via an endoscope, assuming the deep system is patent.

Surgery involves disconnecting the great saphenous vein from the femoral vein; the terminal branches of the great saphenous vein are individually ligated and divided. This may be combined with stripping of the great saphenous vein from groin to knee. If there are other incompetent communications (perforators), these need to be individually ligated or avulsed. Small varicose venules can be avulsed via a small skin incision.

Recurrence of varicose veins after operation is due either to a failure in the original diagnosis (e.g. underlying deep vein incompetence or arteriovenous fistula) or to a defect in operative technique, particularly a failure to divide and excise all the groin tributaries of the saphenous vein. If this error is made, these tributaries will dilate and form new varices. Recurrence may also be due to the development of further varices *de novo*, despite an adequate operation.

Endovenous laser treatment is replacing conventional surgery and sclerotherapy. Laser fibre is passed along the vein under ultrasound guidance. When in position the laser is fired and produces heat within the vein which ablates the endothelium, causing the vein to thrombose. The fibre is gradually withdrawn until all of the vein has been treated. A compression bandage or stockings are applied for 2 weeks.

Complications of varicose veins

Haemorrhage

This is usually due to minor trauma to a dilated vein. The bleeding is profuse owing to the high pressure within the incompetent vein. The treatment is very simple; the patient is laid recumbent with the leg elevated, and a pressure bandage is applied. Subsequent to the emergency, the varicose veins should be treated by operation.

Phlebitis

This may occur spontaneously or may be secondary to trauma to the leg or the sclerosing fluid used in the injection treatment of varicose veins. The varicose vein becomes extremely tender and hard and the overlying skin may be inflamed. The patient may have a constitutional disturbance with pyrexia and malaise. Secondary bacterial infection may occasionally complicate the thrombosis.

Treatment

Bed rest with the foot of the bed elevated and a pressure bandage on the leg, which compresses the superficial veins and increases the speed of flow of blood in the deep veins. If infection is present, antibiotics may be necessary, but this is unusual. In severe cases, systemic anticoagulation may alleviate pain and prevent spread of the condition. Non-steroidal anti-inflammatory drugs may give relief of symptoms but they can cause peptic ulceration.

Deep venous insufficiency

Varicose veins appear when superficial veins are dilated by blood entering via incompetent perforating veins or incompetent superficial valves. Deep venous insufficiency (also known as chronic venous insufficiency, post-thrombotic limb and postphlebitic limb) is the term given to the situation in which the valves of the deep venous system are incompetent. In the normal patient, there is a pressure in the veins at the ankle of around $100\,cmH_2O$, equivalent to the height of the column of blood from the right atrium to the ankle. Upon walking, this pressure drops to around $20\,cmH_2O$ as the calf pump drives the blood upwards. In the presence of incompetent valves, blood is no longer pumped back efficiently, and the venous pressure remains at the high resting state. This raised hydrostatic pressure causes an increase in fluid transudation across the capillaries following Starling's forces.[4]

Aetiology

Primary

- Congenital syndromes where valves are absent.

Secondary

- Venous hypertension. Deep vein thrombosis is the major cause of deep venous insufficiency, where the previous thrombosis has recanalized but left the valves incompetent.
- Arteriovenous fistula.

Features of venous hypertension in the leg

- *Swelling*, particularly of the lower leg, is due to transudation of fluid across capillaries causing oedema, which takes on a brawny character with time.
- *Superficial varicose veins*, caused by perforator incompetence secondary to the raised venous pressure.

---

[4]Sir Ernest Starling (1866–1927), Professor of Physiology, University College, London, UK.

- *Pigmentation of skin*, particularly the medial gaiter area (just above the medial malleolus). The pigment, which appears brown in colour, is haemosiderin and is the breakdown product of haemoglobin in transuded red blood corpuscles.
- *Eczema*, particularly over the pigmented area, causing pruritus. When the patient succumbs to the temptation to scratch this skin, it is further damaged and predisposed to ulcer formation.
- *Lipodermatosclerosis*. The soft subcutaneous tissue is replaced by thick fibrous tissue, a consequence of inflammation and fibrin exudation. In time, this forms a hard enveloping layer around the lower leg through which the veins pass, forming prominent gutters when the leg is elevated. The appearance of the lower leg has been likened to an inverted champagne bottle, with the narrow ankle below and soft oedematous limb above.
- *Ulceration* occurs as a consequence of the poor skin nutrition. Repeated excoriations due to the irritation of the eczema and the impaired nutrition of the fibrotic subcutaneous tissue lead to epithelial damage and ulceration.

Special investigations

- *Venography* to detect perforators that may be treated, and identify occlusions that may explain the aetiology of the condition.
- *Duplex sonography*, in the hands of an experienced operator, will demonstrate deep venous reflux as well as detecting occlusions.

Treatment

There is no successful way to repair or replace the valves of the deep veins. If there is incompetence in the superficial veins they may be removed, and incompetent perforators ligated.

Venous ulceration

As described above, ulceration due to venous hypertension is generally due to incompetence of the deep veins, although superficial vein incompetence may be present. All patients with such an ulcer (also called varicose or gravitational ulcers) should be questioned for any previous history of venous thrombosis, suggested by painful swelling of the leg after an operation, childbirth or immobilization in bed for any reason.

Why the ulcer occurs around the malleoli and not in the foot itself is not fully explained. It is probable that in this area the subcutaneous tissue is less well supported than in the foot. The pressure of the column of blood and the consequent oedema and pericapillary fibrin cuffs result in ischaemia and very poor nutrition to this area so that the skin may break down either spontaneously or more commonly after minor trauma.

Venous ulcers either have an edge which is ragged or, where the ulcer is healing, the margins will be shelving with a faint blue rim of advancing epithelium. Previous scarring appears as a white rim around the ulcer, known as atrophie blanche. Rarely, a squamous carcinoma can develop in the edge of a long-standing ulcer (Marjolin's ulcer[5]).

Treatment

If the patient is confined to bed with the foot of the bed elevated, so that the high venous pressure is abolished, venous ulcers will heal fairly quickly, provided they are kept clean by careful toilet. Antibiotics should be administrated only in the unusual circumstances of the ulcer being grossly infected with a surrounding cellulitis. The antibiotics used will depend on the sensitivity of the bacteria cultured from the ulcer. Topical antibiotic therapy should be avoided; the incidence of sensitivity reaction is high.

Unfortunately, this simple treatment is often not a practical one. The patients are mostly elderly, and prolonged recumbency is obviously of some danger in these cases. Younger patients, from the economic point of view, do not wish to spend several weeks in hospital, in bed.

In such cases, healing can be obtained either by tight elastic bandaging of the leg or by using proprietary paste bandages over which elastoplast is applied. This firm pressure empties the dilated superficial veins and enables the calf muscle pump to act more efficiently. Oxygenated blood is therefore able to reach the previously ischaemic tissues. A split-skin graft may be useful in indolent cases, but grafting must only supplement the other treatment modalities.

[5]Jean Nicholas Marjolin (1780–1850), Surgeon, Hôpital Sainte-Eugènie, Paris, France.

Box 13.1 Differential diagnosis of leg ulcers

- *Venous ulcer complicating venous insufficiency*

- *Ischaemic ulcer*, due to impaired arterial blood supply; the peripheral pulses must always be examined and ankle brachial pressure indexes checked

- *Neuropathic ulcer*: particularly common in diabetics where they are often compounded by ischaemia due to diabetic microangiopathy

- *Malignant ulcer*: a squamous carcinoma, often arising in a pre-existing chronic ulcer, or an ulcerated malignant melanoma

- *Ulcer complicating systemic disease*, e.g. acholuric jaundice, ulcerative colitis and rheumatoid arthritis

- *Arteriovenous fistula-associated ulcer*

- *Repetitive self-inflicted injury*

- *Gummatous ulcer of syphilis*: usually affects the upper one-third of the leg

Once the ulcer has healed, the patient is fitted with a firm elastic graduated compression stocking or advised to continue with the elastic bandage. Incompetent perforating veins are ligated. Unless the incompetent veins are treated thus, either by support or by operation, recurrence is inevitable.

Venous ulcers account for approximately 90% of all ulcers of the legs, but other, rarer, causes should always be considered (Box 13.1). Venous ulcers may be complicated by a poor arterial supply, so the ankle brachial pressure index should be checked (Chapter 12, p. 87).

Deep vein thrombosis

Spontaneous deep vein thrombosis generally presents to, and is managed by, general physicians. To surgeons, it is usually a postoperative complication, which is where it is discussed in full (Chapter 4, p. 15).

14

The brain and meninges

Learning objective

✓ To know the manifestations and causes of raised intracranial pressure, with particular reference to intracranial tumours and pituitary adenomas.

Space-occupying intracranial lesions

Space-occupying lesions within the skull may be caused by the following:

1 Haemorrhage:
   a extradural;
   b subdural – acute or chronic (Chapter 15, p. 123);
   c intracerebral.
2 Tumour.
3 Hydrocephalus.
4 Brain swelling (oedema), e.g. head injury, encephalitis.
5 Cerebral abscess.

Other causes are rare and include hydatid cyst, tuberculoma and gumma.

Clinical features

A space-occupying lesion manifests itself by the general features of raised intracranial pressure and by localizing signs.

Raised intracranial pressure

A space-occupying lesion within the skull produces raised intracranial pressure not only by its actual volume within the closed box of the cranium but also by provoking oedema, and sometimes by

Lecture Notes: General Surgery, 12th edition. © Harold Ellis, Sir Roy Y. Calne and Christopher J. E. Watson. Published 2011 by Blackwell Publishing Ltd.

impeding the circulation or absorption of cerebrospinal fluid (CSF) causing hydrocephalus (see p. 112). For example, a tumour in the posterior fossa may present rapidly with severe symptoms of raised intracranial pressure secondary to hydrocephalus.

A slowly progressive rise in intracranial pressure may lead to the following presenting features:

- *Headache*: may be severe, often present when the patient wakes and is aggravated by straining or coughing.
- *Vomiting*: often without preceding nausea.
- *Papilloedema*: which may be accompanied by blurring of vision and may progress to permanent blindness.
- *Depressed conscious level.*
- *Neck stiffness*: particularly if the lesion is in the posterior fossa.
- *Diplopia, ataxia.*
- *Enlargement of the head*; in children before the sutures have fused.

A rapid rise in intracranial pressure results in a clinical picture of intense headache with rapid progression into coma.

Localizing signs

Having diagnosed the presence of raised intracranial pressure, an attempt must be made to localize the lesion on the basis of the clinical findings, although in some cases this is not possible. There may be upper motor neurone weakness, indicating a lesion of the pyramidal pathway; there may be cranial nerve signs, e.g. a bitemporal hemianopia indicating pressure on the optic chiasma. A lesion of the post-central cortex may produce loss of fine discrimination and of stereognosis. Cerebellar lesions may produce coarse ataxia, muscular hypotonia, incoordination and often nystagmus. A focal fit may provide valuable localizing data. Motor aphasia (the patient knows what he or she wishes to say but cannot do so) suggests a lesion in Broca's area[1] on the dominant side of the lower frontal cortex of the cerebrum. Pupillary dilatation is a late sign, and is caused by the uncus of the temporal lobe being displaced through the tentorial hiatus where it compresses the oculomotor nerve.

Special investigations

The following investigations are required in the study of a suspected space-occupying lesion:

- *Computed tomography (CT)*, with intravenous contrast enhancement, is a non-invasive and extremely accurate investigation for all cerebral tumours and other space-occupying lesions.
- *Magnetic resonance (MR) imaging* gives superb anatomical localization of intracerebral space-occupying lesions.
- *Positron emission tomography (PET)* further complements MR.
- *Chest X-ray* should always be performed if tumour is suspected to exclude a symptomless primary bronchogenic carcinoma; in the case of a cerebral abscess, it may reveal the source of infection.
- *Burr-hole biopsy* may be appropriate to establish a tissue diagnosis.
- *Skull X-ray* has been largely superseded in the diagnosis of space-occupying lesions by cross-sectional imaging (CT and MR). Ten per cent of tumours show calcification, most commonly craniopharyngiomas and oligodendrogliomas. It is occasionally found in astrocytomas, meningiomas and vascular malformations.

The pineal gland may be calcified (30% of 30 year olds, 70% of 70 year olds). Close inspection of the skull X-ray may show a shift of the pineal to one side, indicating a space-occupying lesion on the other.

The sella turcica should be examined; decalcification is evidence of raised intracranial pressure, and expansion of the sella with erosion of the clinoid processes suggests the presence of a pituitary tumour. In children, widening of the coronal sutures and increased convolutional markings may be seen (the 'beaten brass' appearance).

Intracranial tumours

Intracranial tumours can be divided into intrinsic tumours of the brain, arising usually from the supporting (glial) cells, and extracerebral tumours, which originate from the numerous structures surrounding the brain. In addition, 15% of patients with cerebral tumours presenting to neurosurgical units have tumours that are metastatic from distant sites, but many patients dying of widespread metastases have cerebral deposits and do not come under specialist care. The overall incidence of central nervous system (CNS) tumours is around 5 per 100 000 population. The only identified predisposing factor is previous cranial irradiation.

Intracranial tumours cause generalized and focal symptoms. Generalized symptoms reflect a progressive increase in intracranial pressure and include headache (particularly in the early morning), nausea and vomiting. Mental state changes and hemiparesis may also occur. Focal symptoms depend on the tumour location within the brain. Cerebellar tumours therefore lead to ataxia; occipital lobe tumours result in visual field disturbance; and tumours in the posterior aspect of the frontal lobe affecting the motor cortex will result in weakness. Seizures are common and may be focal; post-ictal neurological impairment may help localization. Investigation is outlined above.

Classification

Common tumours include the following.

Intracerebral

- Gliomas (45%), including astrocytoma, oligodendroglioma, ependymoma, medulloblastoma.
- Lymphoma.
- Pineal gland tumour.
- Metastases (15%).

Extracerebral

- Meningioma (15%).
- Neuroma, e.g. acoustic neuroma (5%).
- Pituitary tumours (5%), including pituitary adenomas and craniopharyngioma.

---

[1]Pierre Broca (1826–1880), Professor of Clinical Surgery, Paris, France.

Gliomas

Gliomas arise from the glial supporting cells and are usually supratentorial. They are classified according to the principal cell component. The four important subgroups are as follows.

Astrocytomas (80%)

These are graded according to their mitotic activity, nuclear pleomorphism endothelial proliferation and necrosis. Grade 1 (pilocytic astrocytoma) and grade 2 (diffuse astrocytoma) are less aggressive and are often cystic and slow growing, although they may change over the years into less differentiated and more invasive tumours. Grade 3 (anaplastic astrocytoma) and grade 4 (glioblastoma multiforme) gliomas are more aggressive; about half of all astrocytomas are the highly anaplastic glioblastoma multiforme, the median survival with which is 3 months. Often, a glioma may have cells of different grades of differentiation in different areas of the tumour. It is interesting that the glioblastoma tends to occur in the adult and in the cerebrum, whereas the well-differentiated cystic glioma (juvenile pilocytic astrocytoma) occurs frequently in children and usually arises in the cerebellum.

Medulloblastomas (10%)

These are rapidly growing small-cell tumours generally affecting the cerebellum in children, usually boys. They may block the fourth ventricle, producing an obstructive hydrocephalus, and may spread via the CSF to seed over the surface of the spinal cord. The cells appear to be embryonal in origin with elements of ependymomas and medulloblastoma in varying proportions, and are now more commonly called primitive neuroectodermal tumours (PNETs).

Ependymomas (5%)

These arise from the lining cells of the ventricles, the central canal of the spinal cord or the choroid plexus. They usually occur in children and young adults.

Oligodendrogliomas (5%)

Most are relatively slow growing and are usually found in the cerebrum in adults.

Treatment

Gross surgical removal may prolong survival and improve neurological deficit. This may be followed by radiotherapy to the tumour site. Small tumours less than 3 cm may be suitable for stereotactic radiosurgery (the Gamma Knife). Chemotherapy may confer additional benefit for certain tumours, such as oligodendrogliomas.

Cerebral lymphoma

Primary cerebral lymphoma is uncommon but is increasing in incidence. It occurs in two settings: immunosuppressed patients, whether through disease (e.g. AIDS) or for organ transplantation, have a markedly increased risk of cerebral lymphoma; in non-immunosuppressed patients, the incidence peaks in the sixth and seventh decade, and is often multifocal. Diagnosis is by stereotactic biopsy and the treatment is chemotherapy.

Meningioma

Meningiomas arise from arachnoid cells in the dura mater, to which they are almost invariably attached, and typically are found in middle-aged patients. Special sites are one or both sides of the superior sagittal sinus, the lesser wing of the sphenoid, the olfactory groove, the parasellar region and within the spinal canal. The majority are slow growing and do not invade the brain tissue but involve it only by expansion and pressure, so they may become buried in the brain. The tumour may, however, invade the skull, producing a hyperostosis, which may occasionally be enormous. Most are benign, 5% atypical and 2% frankly malignant.

Treatment

Most meningiomas are surgically removable.

Acoustic neuroma

Neuromas are benign tumours that arise from the Schwann[2] cells of a cranial nerve. The great majority arise from the eighth cranial nerve at the internal auditory meatus (acoustic neuroma). They are usually found in adult patients between the ages of 30 and 60 years and are occasionally associated

---

[2]Theodore Schwann (1810–1882), German physiologist; one of the first to establish the cellular nature of all tissues.

with neurofibromatosis type II, when they may be bilateral.

Neurofibromatosis has three forms (Chapter 9, p. 58). Type II is characterized by neurofibromas on cranial nerves, mental retardation and a tendency to form gliomas and meningiomas.

As the acoustic tumour slowly enlarges, it stretches the adjacent cranial nerves, VII and V anteriorly and IX, X and XII over its lower surface. It also presses on the cerebellum and the brain stem, producing the 'cerebellopontine angle syndrome' with the following features:

- unilateral nerve deafness often associated with tinnitus and giddiness (VIII) is the first symptom;
- facial numbness and weakness of the masticatory muscles (V);
- dysphagia, hoarseness and dysarthria (IX, X and XII);
- cerebellar hemisphere signs and, later, pyramidal tract involvement;
- eventually features of raised intracranial pressure;
- facial weakness with unilateral taste loss (VII) is very uncommon (<5%).

Treatment

Acoustic neuromas can be removed completely but with some risk to the facial nerve. Alternatively, stereotactic radiosurgery is now being used to treat some smaller tumours.

Pituitary tumours

Pituitary tumours have three special features.

1 Local mass effects:
   a *Visual field disturbance* (bitemporal hemianopia) due to compression of the optic chiasm.
   b *Headache*, due to expansion of the pituitary fossa with dural stretching, erosion into the paranasal air sinus, and/or haemorrhage within the tumour (pituitary apoplexy).
2 Hormone defici*ency* (hypopituitarism): as the tumour grows, it compresses the normal pituitary around the tumour, resulting in reduced production of anterior pituitary hormones. Deficiency tends to first suppress luteinizing and growth hormone production, followed in sequence by loss of thyroid-stimulating hormone (TSH),

adrenocorticotrophic hormone (ACTH) and follicle-stimulating hormone (FSH). The posterior pituitary hormones are rarely affected.

3 Hormone excess: hormone-secreting adenomas may present with symptoms from the hormone, for example Cushing's disease[3] from ACTH excess.

They are named according to their staining on light microscopy.

Chromophobe adenoma (80%)

This is the commonest pituitary tumour, which, as it enlarges, compresses the optic chiasm, producing a bitemporal hemianopia. Half are non-secretory tumours, which gradually destroy the normally functioning pituitary, producing hypopituitarism with secondary hypogonadism, hypothyroidism and hypoadrenalism. In childhood there is arrest of growth together with infantilism. Half produce prolactin, which causes infertility, amenorrhoea and galactorrhoea (discharge of milk from the nipple) in females. These tumours rarely extend to involve the hypothalamus, producing diabetes insipidus and obesity.

Eosinophil (acidophil) adenoma (15%)

These are slow-growing tumours, which secrete growth hormone. If they occur before puberty, which is unusual, they induce gigantism. After puberty, acromegaly results.

Basophil adenoma (5%)

These are small tumours that produce no pressure effects and may be associated with Cushing's syndrome (adrenocorticotrophic hormone production, Chapter 40, p. 331).

Special investigations

- *Magnetic resonance (MR) imaging* demonstrates the pituitary fossa, encroachment on the optic chiasm superiorly and laterally into the cavernous sinus.
- *Visual field mapping* looking for evidence of bitemporal hemianopia.

[3]Harvey Cushing (1869–1939), Professor of Surgery, Harvard Medical School, Boston, MA, USA. He was one of the founders of neurosurgery.

- *Hormone assessment*, with basal assays of each pituitary hormone and change in hormone concentrations after stress created by insulin-induced hypoglycaemia.

Treatment

Pituitary tumours which are producing pressure symptoms on the optic chiasm are treated by intracapsular removal through a trans-sphenoidal (or occasionally transcranial) route. Prolactin-secreting tumours (prolactinomas) usually respond to treatment with a dopamine agonist (e.g. cabergoline) to suppress prolactin secretion and reduce tumour size.

Craniopharyngioma

Craniopharyngioma (suprasellar cyst, or cyst of Rathke's pouch[4]) is a benign but locally invasive tumour, usually cystic, which arises in the remnant of the craniopharyngeal duct (the precursor of the anterior pituitary). It presents in childhood or early adult life and lies above and/or within the sella turcica.

The tumour produces hypopituitarism, raised intracranial pressure and optic chiasmal involvement. Craniopharyngiomas may be very difficult to remove completely because of their close relationship to the hypothalamus, so treatment often involves subtotal removal with postoperative radiotherapy.

Secondary tumours

These account for about 15% of intracranial tumours seen on a neurosurgical unit but are more common on the general wards. Common primary tumours are lung, breast, kidney and melanoma, the last occasionally presenting with intracranial haemorrhage.

Intracranial abscess

Aetiology

Intracranial abscesses may be intracerebral, subdural or extradural. There are three common causes for them:

[4]Martin Heinrich Rathke (1793–1860), Professor of Anatomy, Konigsberg, Germany. Gave an early description of the pituitary gland in 1838.

1 *Penetrating wound* of the skull usually with a staphylococcal secondary infection. Such wounds usually cause extradural abscesses.
2 *Direct spread* – the cause in 75% of cases
   a an infected middle ear or mastoid; initially causes a subdural abscess that subsequently spreads to either the temporal lobe or the cerebellum;
   b an infected frontal or ethmoid sinus, spreading to the frontal lobe.
3 *Blood-borne spread.* A septic embolus, especially from a focus of infection in a lung such as bronchiectasis or lung abscess, or occasionally from the systemic circulation in the presence of congenital cyanotic heart disease in which there is a right-to-left shunt. Such abscesses commonly occur in the middle cerebral artery territory.

Clinical features

The clinical features are those of the following:

- the underlying cause (e.g. chronic mastoiditis);
- evidence of the development of an intracerebral space-occupying lesion (raised intracranial pressure);
- localizing features (e.g. epilepsy or a focal neurological defect);
- toxaemia, fever, meningism and a leucocytosis, particularly if there is rapidly spreading cerebral infection. Often, the abscess is walled off by a relatively thick capsule so that the general manifestations of infection (fever and toxaemia) are not evident.

Special investigations

- *Skull X-ray* may show evidence of frontal sinus or mastoid infection.
- *Chest X-ray* may show a primary focus in the lung.
- *CT and MR imaging* provide accurate diagnosis and localization of the abscess, typically appearing as a ring-enhancing lesion with extensive oedema; sinus views may reveal the source.

Treatment

In the first instance, the abscess is aspirated through a burr hole by means of a brain needle. Antibiotics are instilled into the abscess cavity and resolution is followed by serial CT scans. The

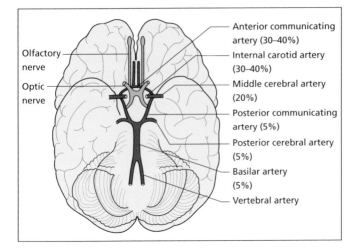

Anterior communicating
artery (30–40%)

Olfactory
nerve

Internal carotid artery
(30–40%)

Optic
nerve

Middle cerebral artery
(20%)

Posterior communicating
artery (5%)

Posterior cerebral artery
(5%)

Basilar artery
(5%)

Vertebral artery

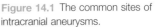

Figure 14.1 The common sites of intracranial aneurysms.

aspirations may require to be repeated and high-dose systemic antibiotics are given, depending on the bacteriology report on the pus. Occasionally, the abscess fails to respond to aspiration and its capsule must be excised.

Epilepsy develops in one-third of patients and anticonvulsant therapy is therefore given prophylactically.

Intracranial vascular lesions

Intracranial vascular lesions may present as either subarachnoid or intracerebral haemorrhage, or a combination of the two. There are two primary lesions: an aneurysm of a cerebral artery or an arteriovenous malformation.

Intracranial aneurysms

Pathology

Intracranial (berry) aneurysms are primary aneurysms of the cerebral arteries. They are saccular, generally arise near the bifurcation of an artery and are probably due to aplasia or hypoplasia of the tunica media. Eighty-five per cent occur in the anterior half of the circle of Willis,[5] with equal distribution between the anterior communicating

artery, internal carotid artery and middle cerebral artery (Figure 14.1). The internal carotid artery aneurysms occur at its terminal bifurcation, origin of the posterior communicating artery and occasionally in the cavernous sinus or at the origin of the ophthalmic artery. Fifteen per cent occur on the basilar or vertebral arteries. About 20% are multiple. Men and women are equally affected, and they may be familial. They are associated with hypertension and cigarette smoking, and also occasionally with polycystic kidney disease, coarctation of the aorta and collagen disorders such as the Ehlers–Danlos syndrome.[6] They are rarely due to arteriosclerosis, trauma or infection (mycotic aneurysms).

Clinical features

These can be divided into two groups.

1 *Subarachnoid haemorrhage:* bleeding into the CSF from a ruptured intracranial aneurysm is the commonest cause of spontaneous subarachnoid haemorrhage. Between 6% and 8% of all strokes are due to subarachnoid haemorrhage. Rupture most commonly occurs at times of stress or exercise, and presents with the following:
   a severe headache of sudden onset ('as if I was hit across the back of my head');
   b vomiting;

[5]Thomas Willis (1621–1675), Physician and Anatomist, first in Oxford then in London, UK.

[6]Edvard Lauritz Ehlers (1863–1937), Professor of Clinical Dermatology, Copenhagen, Denmark. Henri-Alexandre Danlos (1844–1912), Dermatologist, Paris, France.

c photophobia;

d irritability;

e neck stiffness and a positive Kernig's sign[7] (flexion of the hip with extension of the leg causes pain when meningeal irritation present);

f impairment of consciousness;

g focal neurological signs or generalized seizures.

Prior to the haemorrhage, there is often a history of severe headache within the previous 2 weeks, an event that might be due to a small bleed. Aneurysm rupture may also cause intracerebral or subdural bleeding with neurological signs depending on the site of the haematoma. Most cases occur after the age of 40 years, when increasing atheromatous degenerative changes in the arteries and hypertension are probably precipitating factors. The clinical diagnosis is confirmed by CT or, if CT is negative, lumbar puncture will reveal xanthochromia – yellow-stained CSF.

2 *Pressure symptoms due to the aneurysm:* especially third-nerve palsy from an aneurysm of the posterior communicating artery.

Haemorrhage from a ruptured aneurysm is serious and one-quarter of patients die without recovering consciousness. Further deterioration results from the intense spasm that follows several days after the haemorrhage, and from further bleeding. About 50% will bleed again within 6 weeks of the initial haemorrhage and the mortality of such bleeds is high.

Treatment

If the patient is in coma or has significant neurological deficit, but does not have hydrocephalus or a significant intracerebral bleed, conservative management is adopted. This involves flat bed rest, adequate fluid replacement and analgesia, and nimodipine to reduce the risk of development of delayed cerebral ischaemia from vasospasm.

If the patient recovers from the initial bleed, cerebral angiography is performed to locate the site of the aneurysm. If the aneurysm is demonstrated, treatment comprises craniotomy with the direct application of a clip across the base of the aneurysm. Endovascular approaches using platinum

coils to thrombose the aneurysm are increasingly used, and are preferred to surgical clipping in patients with posterior circulation aneurysms (because of the difficult surgical approach) and those with significant comorbidity. Clipping is also associated with a low incidence of recanalization and hence rebleeding. The results of clipping are good in 80% of patients, with a 2–8% mortality.

About 15% of the angiograms are negative and probably indicate that thrombosis has taken place in a microaneurysm. Such patients are treated conservatively and the prognosis is good.

Arteriovenous malformations

Developmental vascular malformations may occur in any part of the CNS, particularly over the surface of the cerebral hemispheres in the distribution of the middle cerebral artery. They comprise a tangle of abnormal vessels, ranging from telangiectasia to cavernous and venous malformations often with arteriovenous fistulae.

They may produce focal epilepsy, headaches or slowly progressive paralysis, and 50% present with subarachnoid or intracerebral bleeding. The subarachnoid haemorrhage is less catastrophic than in rupture of an aneurysm, but accounts for about 10% of all cases of spontaneous subarachnoid bleeding. Half of the cases have a bruit, which may be heard over the eye, the skull vault or the carotid arteries in the neck. Exact diagnosis and localization is made by cerebral angiography.

The haemorrhage rate is around 4% per year. Accessible malformations in non-eloquent parts of the brain (i.e. those not involved in speech production) might be treated by surgery, although stereotactic radiosurgery (known as the Gamma Knife) is now employed for the majority of patients, inducing endarteritis obliterans in the nidus of the lesion. Stereotactic radiosurgery involves focusing multiple beams of low-dose gamma radiation such that only the lesion receives a significant radiation dose. Both surgery and stereotactic radiosurgery may be facilitated by prior embolization.

Sturge–Weber syndrome[8] is an association between a port-wine stain localized to one or more segments of the cutaneous distribution of the trigeminal nerve with a corresponding

[7]Vladimir Kernig (1840–1917), German Physician and Neurologist, St Petersburg, Russia.

[8]William Allen Sturge (1850–1919), Physician, Royal Free Hospital, London, UK. Frederick Parkes Weber (1863–1962), Physician, London, UK, with a life-long interest in rare diseases.

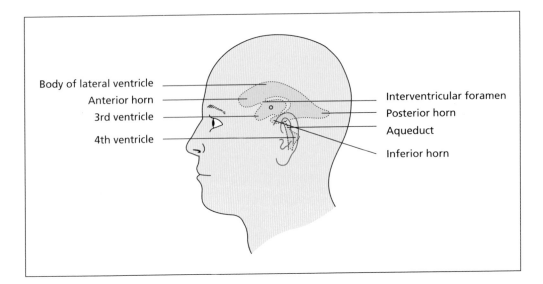

Body of lateral ventricle
Anterior horn
3rd ventricle
4th ventricle

Interventricular foramen
Posterior horn
Aqueduct
Inferior horn

Figure 14.2 The ventricular system. (Reproduced from Ellis H, Mahadevan V. (2010) *Clinical Anatomy*, 12th edn. Oxford: Wiley-Blackwell.)

extensive venous angioma (which may cause contralateral focal fits).

Hydrocephalus

The circulation of CSF

CSF is produced by the choroid plexuses of the lateral, third and fourth ventricles (Figure 14.2). It escapes from the fourth ventricle through the median foramen of Magendie[9] and the lateral foramina of Luschka[10] into the cerebral subarachnoid space. About 80% of the fluid is reabsorbed via the cranial arachnoid villi. The remaining 20% of the CSF is absorbed by the spinal arachnoid villi or escapes along the nerve sheaths into the lymphatics.

Obstruction along the CSF pathway produces a rise in pressure and dilatation within the system proximal to the block. Hydrocephalus may be classified according to whether the block occurs within the ventricular system or outside it.

Non-communicating or obstructive hydrocephalus

CSF cannot escape from within the brain to the basal cisterns. This may be due to congenital narrowing of the aqueduct of Sylvius[11] or the Arnold–Chiari malformation,[12] which is a congenital downward protrusion of the cerebellum into the foramen magnum (with consequent occlusion of the foramina of the fourth ventricle) frequently associated with spina bifida. It may also be acquired as a result of cerebral abscess or tumour, either within or adjacent to a ventricle.

Communicating hydrocephalus

CSF can escape from within the brain but absorption via the villi is prevented as a result of the obliteration of subarachnoid channels. It may be congenital as a result of failure of development of the arachnoid villi, or it may be secondary to meningitis or bleeding into the subarachnoid space (head injury, aneurysm rupture, arteriovenous malformation).

[9]François Magendie (1783–1855), Physician, Hôtel Dieu, Paris, France.
[10]Hubert von Lushka (1820–75), Professor of Anatomy, Tubingen, Germany.

[11]François Sylvius (1614–1672), Professor of Medicine, Leiden, The Netherlands.
[12]Julius Arnold (1835–1915), Professor of Pathology, Heidelberg, Germany. Hans Chiari (1851–1916), Viennese Pathologist, successively Professor at Strasbourg, France, and Prague, Czech Republic.

Clinical features

Clinically, hydrocephalus may be divided into two important groups. The first is the acquired variety, which presents with features of raised intracranial pressure described on p. 105. The second comprises patients with congenital hydrocephalus, who show the characteristic picture of enlargement of the skull (comparison should be made with the size of an infant's skull of the same age obtained from standard charts) over which the scalp is stretched with dilated cutaneous veins. The fontanelles are enlarged and tense and fail to close at the normal times. Typical of this condition is the downward displacement of the eyes ('sun setting') and there may be an associated squint and nystagmus. Papilloedema is not present in these cases. There may be late epilepsy, and mental impairment may be considerable when there is extensive thinning of the cerebral cortex. There may be associated congenital deformities, especially spina bifida.

In some infants with congenital hydrocephalus, natural arrest occurs, presumably as a result of recanalization of the subarachnoid spaces. In the remainder, there is steady progression with inevitable mental deterioration and high mortality unless adequate treatment is instituted.

Special investigations

- *CT scan* confirms ventricular enlargement.
- *Cranial ultrasound* through the fontanelle is useful in the child.

Treatment

The goal of treatment is to divert the CSF around the blockage by means of a shunt. For non-communicating (obstructive) hydrocephalus, direct removal of the occluding mass lesion is desirable.

Decompression of the hydrocephalus can be achieved by diverting CSF into the peritoneum (ventriculoperitoneal shunt) or right atrium via the internal jugular vein (ventriculoatrial shunt). The shunts comprise silicone catheters with a regulator valve mechanism in the middle to permit CSF flow at a certain ventricular pressure without overdrainage of the CSF.

In non-communicating (obstructive) hydrocephalus, an artificial outlet may be created through the floor of the third ventricle into the basal cisterns (endoscopic third ventriculostomy).

15

Head injury

Learning objectives

✓ To know the common causes of coma.

✓ To be able to recognize the severity of a head injury and understand the principles of management.

Head injury is a major cause of death in children and young adults. Many survivors of head injury are catastrophically disabled. Recognizing a severe head injury and administering prompt and appropriate care is important for all medical practitioners who, if not receiving patients with such injuries under their care, may nevertheless be bystanders witnessing such an injury. If presented with a patient in 'coma' (Box 15.1) other causes of unresponsiveness should be considered.

Head injuries are generally classified as closed (concussional) or open (penetrating).

Types of injury

Injuries are usefully classified according to the structures involved (scalp, skull and underlying brain) together with the mechanism of the injury, be it penetrating or blunt, and whether an acceleration/deceleration and/or a rotational brain injury occurred. In reality, isolated injuries are uncommon, and patients more typically experience blunt injury fracturing the skull in which acceleration/deceleration of the brain also occurs.

Scalp injuries

Most scalp injuries are simple penetrating injuries, which are readily managed by debridement and suture. When the skull is also penetrated, the

Lecture Notes: General Surgery, 12th edition. © Harold Ellis, Sir Roy Y. Calne and Christopher J. E. Watson. Published 2011 by Blackwell Publishing Ltd.

brain may be lacerated. However, if the injury occurred when the head was stationary, in the absence of acceleration and deceleration, consciousness may not be lost and neither the patient nor the doctor may appreciate the true extent of the injury.

Skull injuries

Injuries to the skull are a result of crushing or some other severe force. The skull fractures along its weakest plane, which varies according to the position of the injuring force. Typically, this is a linear fracture of the skull vault, but may extend into the skull base. A simple crush injury to a stationary head may leave the scalp intact and not disturb consciousness in the absence of acceleration and deceleration forces, although the subsequent skull X-ray may show extensive fractures.

A skull fracture is most important as an indicator of the force of the injury, and the risk of intracranial haemorrhage. There are several other facets of a skull fracture that are important to note (Box 15.2).

Fractures involving paranasal air sinuses: cerebrospinal fluid rhinorrhoea

Fractures extending through any of the paranasal air sinuses (frontal, ethmoid or sphenoid) communicate with the outside and are therefore compound (open) fractures, as the overlying dura is usually breached. This external communication may manifest as a runny nose, the clear

---

Box 15.1 Causes of coma

The casualty officer is often called upon to make a diagnosis of a patient in coma. The following are the common causes to be considered, the first three groups accounting for the great majority of cases.

- Central nervous system
  - trauma
  - disease (e.g. cerebrovascular accident (the commonest), epilepsy, subarachnoid haemorrhage, cerebral tumour, abscess, meningitis)
- Drugs/toxins
  - alcohol
  - carbon monoxide
  - barbiturates, aspirin, opiates, etc.
- Diabetes
  - hyperglycaemia
  - hypoglycaemia
- Uraemia
- Hepatic failure
- Hypertensive encephalopathy
- Profound toxaemia
- Hysteria

It is usually easy enough to determine that unconsciousness is due to trauma, but it is important to remember that a drunk or epileptic person, for example, may have struck his or her head in falling so that the condition is complicated by a head injury.

Box 15.2 Physical signs of skull fractures

Anterior fossa

- Nasal bleeding
- Orbital haematoma (see text)
- Cerebrospinal fluid rhinorrhoea
- Cranial nerve injuries, nerves I–VI

Middle fossa

- Orbital haematoma
- Bleeding from the ear
- Cerebrospinal fluid otorrhoea (rare)
- Cranial nerve injuries, nerves VII and VIII

Posterior fossa

- Bruising over the suboccipital region, which develops after a day or two (Battle's sign[1])
- Cranial nerve injuries – nerves IX, X and XI (rare)

Fractures of the petrous temporal bone: CSF otorrhoea or rhinorrhoea

Fractures through the petrous temporal bone may result in CSF otorrhoea, as CSF passes through into the external auditory meatus either directly or via the mastoid air cells or middle ear in the presence of a ruptured tympanic membrane. If the tympanic membrane is intact, CSF rhinorrhoea occurs via the eustachian tube. Involvement of the inner ear will result in deafness. Spontaneous resolution of the leak is usual.

Fractures through the temporal bone: middle meningeal vessels

A fracture through the temporal bone may disrupt the middle meningeal artery and/or vein as they traverse the bone, and result in an extradural haemorrhage, which may not manifest immediately (see p. 122).

cerebrospinal fluid (CSF) being rich in glucose and low in mucin content (and positive for tau protein), compared with the normal nasal secretion, which contains no sugar and is rich in mucin. Such a connection may also be indicated by intracranial air (aerocele) or fluid in one of the sinuses on a computed tomography (CT) scan or skull X-ray. Anosmia may occur if the fracture crosses the cribriform plate. Such patients are at risk of meningitis. Some CSF leaks heal spontaneously, particularly those involving the temporal bone, but a persistent leak will require craniotomy and dural repair.

---

[1]William Henry Battle (1855–1936), Surgeon, St Thomas's Hospital, London, UK.

Depressed fractures

A localized blow drives a fragment of bone below the level of the surrounding skull vault. Such fractures are often compound, as the overlying scalp is torn. The depressed bone may be left if it is not deeply depressed (less than the skull thickness) and not otherwise troublesome. Indications for elevation include the debridement of a contaminated wound, depression greater than the bone thickness, associated intracranial haematoma or epileptic focus.

Orbital haematoma

Fractures of the anterior and middle cranial fossae are very frequently associated with orbital haematoma; blood tracks forward into the orbital tissues, into the eyelids and behind the conjunctiva. It may be difficult to differentiate this from a 'black eye', which is a superficial haematoma of the eyelid and surrounding soft tissues produced by direct injury.

An orbital haematoma is suggested by the following features:

- *a subconjunctival haemorrhage*, the posterior limit of which cannot be seen;
- *absence of grazing of the surrounding skin*;
- *confined to the margin of the orbit* (owing to its fascial attachments), whereas a black eye frequently extends onto the surrounding cheek;
- *mild exophthalmos and a degree of ophthalmoplegia*;
- *bilateral haematoma*.

There may also be some confusion in making a diagnosis between a subconjunctival and conjunctival haemorrhage. The subconjunctival haemorrhage extends from the orbit, forwards and deep to the conjunctiva; there is therefore no posterior limit to the haemorrhage. A conjunctival haemorrhage results from a direct blow on the eye and produces a small haematoma clearly delimited on the conjunctiva itself.

Brain injuries

Brain injury can be divided into primary and secondary.

Primary brain injuries are the direct result of trauma, and may have several components which, apart from direct penetrating injuries, are the result of the brain being relatively mobile within the skull and it being violently forced into sudden acceleration and deceleration. These result in both diffuse and local effects.

Secondary brain injuries occur after the initial event and are the result of hypoxia, hypercapnia, hypotension (ischaemia), intracranial haemorrhage or meningitis. These are the main causes of in-hospital mortality after head injury.

Diffuse brain injury

Diffuse neuronal injury occurs as a result of shearing movements, the worst being rotational shearing, as occurs when a blow is delivered off centre. The result is axon damage and rupture of the small vessels, particularly serious in the brain stem. A severe rotational shearing force may be transmitted down along the axis of the brain, and such forces shearing through the brain stem are usually fatal.

Localized brain injury

Local brain damage occurs as the brain impacts against the skull.

Coup and contre-coup (Figure 15.1)

The direct impact of the brain on the skull at the site of injury and the contre-coup injury as it rebounds against the opposite wall of the skull result in oedema and bruising at the sites of impact. Common sites of impaction are the frontal lobes in the anterior fossa and temporal lobes within the middle fossa, with contre-coup to the occipital lobes.

Laceration within the skull

The brain may impinge on sharp bony edges within the skull, such as the sphenoid ridge, and sustain a laceration.

Cerebral perfusion

Understanding the mechanisms underlying the regulation of cerebral perfusion, and how these may be affected in trauma, is important in the management of head injury victims. The main regulatory factors are described below.

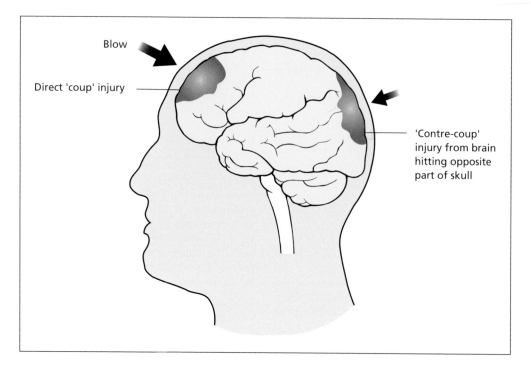

Figure 15.1 Coup and contre-coup injuries – mechanism.

Systemic arterial pressure

Cerebral perfusion is normally autoregulated by the vasoactive cerebral arterioles to maintain constant cerebral blood flow over a wide range of systemic blood pressures. If systemic arterial pressure falls, cerebral vasodilatation occurs to compensate; a further fall may exceed the arterioles' ability to compensate, and cerebral ischaemia occurs.

Intracranial pressure

Since the skull is a closed compartment, a rise in intracranial pressure (ICP) will reduce the cerebral perfusion pressure.

Cerebral perfusion pressure = BP – ICP

where BP is blood pressure. The flow of blood to the brain is autoregulated until the perfusion pressure is around 40 mmHg. A rise in ICP coupled with hypotension in trauma victims with head injuries reduces cerebral blood flow, and the resultant ischaemia affecting the cardiorespiratory centres in the floor of the fourth ventricle leads to reflex increase in systemic pressure and bradycardia – the Cushing reflex.[2] Hence, hypotension in head injury victims is seldom due to the head injury.

Cerebrovascular resistance

The cerebral arterioles can compensate for alterations in systemic blood pressure by altering vascular tone. The arterioles are sensitive to the presence of vasoactive mediators, the most important being pH, and its proxy, $P\text{CO}_2$. An increase in arterial $P\text{CO}_2$ (hypercapnia) causes cerebral vasodilatation. If a reduction in cerebral blood volume is required therapeutically, e.g. in the treatment of post-traumatic cerebral oedema, elective hyperventilation with its resultant hypocapnia is often performed.

Conversely, hypercapnia in the presence of oedema may further raise intracranial pressure and result in exacerbation of the brain injury, one of the causative factors in secondary brain injury.

[2]Harvey Cushing (1869–1939), Professor of Surgery, Harvard Medical School, Boston, MA, USA. He was one of the founders of neurosurgery.

Management of the patient with a head injury

The management of a patient with a head injury can be divided into the following:

- initial assessment;
- immediate management;
- delayed management.

In practice, the initial assessment and immediate management frequently overlap according to clinical priorities.

Initial assessment

The initial assessment is an active process and not just a period of history taking. However, the history is most important, in particular the account of a witness, as most victims of major head injuries are unable to give an accurate history.

History

Important points to note in the history are as follows.

- *The mechanism of the injury*. This may enable some prediction as to the likely injuries, both visible and within the cranium. The nature of the injurious force and its direction relative to the recipient are important.
- *The immediate condition of the injured person*. What was the patient like immediately after the injury? In particular, note the level of consciousness in terms of an accepted scale such as the Glasgow coma scale (see p. 119), as well as other vital signs (pulse, respiration, blood pressure), the size and reaction of the pupils and recorded limb movements (was the patient moving his or her arms and legs after the accident?).
- *Any change in the condition of the injured person*. As well as establishing the patient's condition when first seen after the injury, it is also important to establish whether the condition has changed at all. For example, if the patient was talking and moving all limbs and is now comatose, it suggests that an intracranial mass lesion such as an intracranial haemorrhage is developing.
- *The prior condition of the injured person*. As much history about the injured as possible

should be obtained from relatives and friends. Was the patient drunk at the time? Is the patient diabetic and so could the coma be hypoglycaemic? Does the patient have a glass eye or is he or she on treatment for chronic glaucoma to account for the absence of pupillary responses?

Examination

Your examination should reassess the patient's conscious level to decide whether the condition has worsened or improved, and look for associated injuries, in particular major occult injuries such as a tension pneumothorax or fractured spine. In patients with major injuries, the priorities for examination are usually quoted in terms of the ABC of resuscitation, to which may be added an additional C.

- *Airway*. Is the airway clear without obstruction such as vomitus or blood? If the patient is not maintaining the airway, intubation with an endotracheal tube should be performed. Occasionally, this may not be possible and a tracheostomy may be required.
- *Breathing*. Is the patient breathing spontaneously, or should ventilation be instituted? Controlled hyperventilation may be desirable to reduce intracranial pressure (Chapter 14, p. 106). An arterial blood sample for estimation of oxygen carriage should be taken as soon as convenient, and the patient should be monitored by pulse oximeter to ensure adequate haemoglobin saturation.
- *Circulation*. The patient's pulse and blood pressure should be taken and monitored. Raised intracranial pressure results in bradycardia and hypertension (Cushing reflex, see p. 117). Hypotension is rarely due to head injury and an alternative cause should be sought (a ruptured spleen, a haemothorax or a fractured pelvis for example). Occasionally, extensive scalp bleeding may result in hypotension, as may a head injury in a child.
- *Cervical spine*. Every patient who sustains a head injury should be considered to have a cervical spine injury as well until proved otherwise by good quality radiography or CT scan. The neck should therefore be immobilized in a hard collar.

Following the initial ABC, a full central nervous system (CNS) examination should be performed

---

Box 15.3 The Glasgow coma scale (GCS)

Eye opening

4 Spontaneously

3 To speech/command

2 To pain

1 None

Best verbal response

5 Orientated – knows who he or she is and where he or she is

4 Confused conversation – disorientated; gives confused answers to questions

3 Inappropriate words – random words; no conversation

2 Incomprehensible sounds

1 None

Best motor response

6 Obeys commands

5 Localizes pain

4 Flexes to pain – flexion withdrawal of limb to painful stimulus

3 Abnormal (decorticate) flexion – upper limb adducts, flexes and internally rotates so that it lies across chest; lower limbs extend (Figure 15.2)

2 Extends to pain (decerebrate) – painful stimulus causes extension of all limbs

1 None

When assessing the GCS, it is very important that an adequate stimulus is applied.

Box 15.4 Indications for CT scan

- Impaired conscious level, GCS < 13 on initial assessment or GCS < 15 at 2 hours after the injury

- Suspected open or depressed skull fracture or suspected penetrating injury

- Basal fracture of skull (possibly indicated by cerebrospinal fluid rhinorrhoea or otorrhoea, periorbital haematoma (Battle's sign))

- Focal neurological signs, fits or any other neurological symptoms

- Deteriorating conscious level

- More than one episode of vomiting

- Amnesia for 30 minutes before impact

- Coagulopathy/anticoagulation in patients with a history of significant trauma or impaired consciousness

---

as well as complete examination of the chest, abdomen and limbs. Particular attention should be paid to the parts that are usually forgotten, including examining the back for evidence of trauma and integrity of the spine, and a rectal examination with particular attention to anal tone (or its absence in spinal injury) and the position of the prostate in the male (a ruptured urethra results in a displaced prostate).

The conscious level: the Glasgow coma scale

Vague terms such as comatose, semicomatose, unconscious, stuporose and so on should be avoided; they may be of value to a psychiatrist but not to a surgeon. Instead, the conscious level is charted according to the patient's motor, verbal and eye-opening responses to stimuli; these are very much the reactions of a patient recovering from deep anaesthesia. The most commonly used scale is the Glasgow coma scale (GCS) (Box 15.3), in which the responses within each group are allotted a score, the normal being 15. A mild head injury may score 13–15, a severe injury 8 or less.

Special investigations

With respect to head injury, there are three immediate investigations that may be indicated.

1 *Skull X-ray* used to be the initial investigation but has been replaced owing to the ready availability of CT. It may have a role in children as part of a skeletal survey in suspected non-accidental injury.

2 *CT scan* should be performed on all patients with significant head injuries (Box 15.4) as indicated by impaired conscious level (GCS <15), history of penetrating injury or suspected fracture, signs of a basal skull fracture (e.g. CSF rhinorrhoea or otorrhoea, bilateral orbital haematoma (Battle's sign)), post-traumatic seizure, focal neurological deficit or recurrent (>1) vomiting or amnesia for more than 30 minutes prior to impact. Other indications

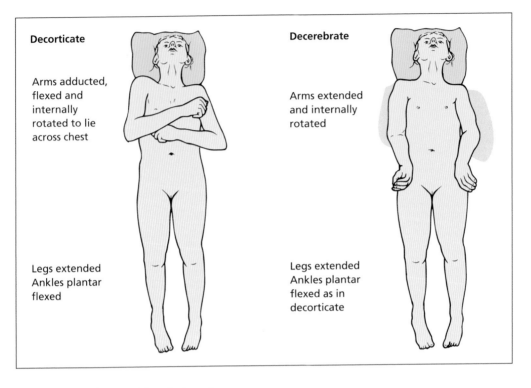

Decorticate

Arms adducted, flexed and internally rotated to lie across chest

Legs extended
Ankles plantar flexed

Decerebrate

Arms extended and internally rotated

Legs extended
Ankles plantar flexed as in decorticate

Figure 15.2 Decerebrate and decorticate postures.

include a history of loss of consciousness or amnesia and a history of significant trauma, coagulopathy (e.g. patient on anticoagulation), or age over 65 years. The resulting images may then be viewed locally or transmitted to a regional neurosurgical centre for specialist opinion.

3 *Cervical spine X-ray* is necessary in all unconscious patients following head injury, unless included in the CT scan. Other indications include neck pain and/or tenderness with a history of possible neck trauma, or where exclusion of neck trauma is necessary prior to intubation for other surgery.

Immediate management

Admission to hospital (Box 15.5), CT scanning (Box 15.3) and neurosurgical referral should all be considered. Consultation with a neurosurgeon is indicated for persistent coma (GCS ≤8), persistent unexplained confusion lasting more than 4 hours, deterioration in GCS and progressive focal neurological signs as well as those in whom neurosurgery is indicated (see below). Transfer should only occur after initial resuscitation and stabilization of the patient.

The immediate management of complicated cases will include correcting any problems identified in the initial assessment, such as draining a pneumothorax, instituting ventilation if the patient is unable to maintain the airway or to breathe, and performing a laparotomy and/or orthopaedic procedures when appropriate.

Following the initial brain injury, further deterioration may be due to the following factors:

- increasing cerebral oedema as the brain swells consequent upon the damage it sustained;
- intracranial haemorrhage – extradural, subdural or intracerebral;
- hypoxia, due to impaired ventilation or ischaemia;
- infection, secondary to compound fractures including fractures involving the paranasal sinuses or petrous temporal bone;
- hydrocephalus, either communicating or non-communicating.

Delayed management

With respect to the head injury, there follows a period of observation, with attention paid to the following:

- conscious level – according to the Glasgow coma scale;
- pupil size and responses – dilatation of a pupil, loss of response to light or asymmetry are late signs of increasing intracranial pressure;
- vital signs – pulse, blood pressure, temperature, oxygen saturation;
- intracranial pressure monitoring – done with a catheter placed within the ventricles, which will help direct treatment and facilitate drainage of ICF to lower pressure.

Pupil size and responses

If a cerebral hemisphere is pressed upon by an enlarging blood clot, the third cranial nerve on that side becomes compressed by descent of the uncus over the edge of the tentorium cerebelli. Paralysis of the third nerve (which transmits parasympathetic pupilloconstrictor fibres) results in dilatation of the corresponding pupil (owing to the intact unopposed sympathetic supply) and failure of the pupil to respond to light. An important sign of cerebral compression is, therefore, dilatation and loss of light reaction of the pupil on the affected side, although, occasionally, pupillary dilatation will be a false localizing sign and will be on the side opposite the mass lesion. Because the optic nerve pathway is intact, a light shone into this unreacting pupil produces constriction in the opposite pupil (consensual reaction to light). As compression continues, the contralateral third nerve becomes compressed, and the opposite pupil in turn dilates and becomes fixed to light. Bilateral fixed dilated pupils in a patient with head injury indicates very great cerebral compression from which the patient rarely recovers. Occasionally, local trauma to the nerves from extensive skull-base fractures may produce the same findings.

Pulse, respiration and blood pressure

With increasing intracranial pressure, the pulse slows and the blood pressure rises (Cushing reflex, see p. 117), the respirations become stertorious and eventually Cheyne–Stokes[3] in nature.

Nursing care of the unconscious patient

The airway

The most important single factor in the care of the deeply unconscious patient, whatever the cause, who has lost the cough reflex is the maintenance of the airway. The patient is transported and nursed in the recovery position, i.e. on one side with the body tilted head downwards, which allows the tongue to fall forward and bronchial secretions or vomit to drain from the mouth rather than be inhaled. Suction may be required to remove excessive secretions or vomit from the pharynx.

An endotracheal tube may be necessary if the airway is not satisfactory and, if after some days it

[3]John Cheyne (1777–1836), an Edinburgh-trained physician who migrated to Ireland. William Stokes (1804–1878), Physician, Meath Hospital, Dublin, Ireland.

is still difficult to maintain an adequate airway, tracheostomy may be required.

Restlessness

Opiates, particularly morphine, are generally contraindicated, as they will depress respiration and disguise the level of consciousness and will also produce constricted pupils, which may mask a valuable physical sign. Paracetamol, barbiturates or codeine preparations may be necessary but, often, all that is required is to protect the patient from self-injury by judicious restraint and padding.

A cause of restlessness may be a distended bladder; often, if the retention is relieved, the patient will then calm down.

Feeding

Many patients with head injury died in the past owing to dehydration and starvation. Orogastric feeding is instituted if the patient remains unable to swallow. A nasogastric tube is contraindicated in patients with craniofacial injuries because of the danger of intracranial penetration.

Skin care

A deeply unconscious patient is liable to bed sores. Careful nursing care and the use of an intermittently inflatable mattress are required for their prevention.

Sphincters

The unconscious patient may be incontinent, and the resultant excoriation of the skin makes the patient still more liable to pressure sores. The use of Paul's tubing[4] on the penis or of an indwelling catheter in female patients will help in the nursing care. Retention of urine may require catheter relief.

Indications for surgery in head injuries

Early

- The excision and suture of scalp lacerations.
- Surgical toilet of a compound fracture.
- Cerebral decompression and evacuation of the haematoma for intracranial bleeding.

[4]Frank Thomas Paul (1851–1941), Surgeon, Liverpool Royal Infirmary, Liverpool, UK.

Delayed

- Repair of a dural tear with CSF rhinorrhoea.
- Late repair of skull defects.
- Late plastic surgery for deforming facial injuries.

Traumatic intracranial bleeding

Classification

Haemorrhage within the skull following injury may be classified as follows.

1 Extradural.
2 Subdural:
   a acute;
   b chronic.
3 Subarachnoid.
4 Intracerebral.
5 Intraventricular.

Extradural haemorrhage

This is sometimes wrongly named 'middle meningeal haemorrhage'. It may indeed arise from a tear of the middle meningeal artery, but an extradural collection of blood may also develop from a laceration of one of the other meningeal vessels, from the torn sagittal sinus or as a result of oozing from the diploë, bone and stripped dura mater on each side of any associated fracture (Figure 15.3a).

Clinical features

The classic story is of a relatively minor head injury producing temporary concussion, recovery ('the lucid period') then, some hours later, the development of headache and progressively deeper coma due to cerebral compression by the extradural clot. This picture may give rise to the tragedies of the drunk who is put into the cells for the night and is found dead in the morning, or the cricketer who goes home to bed after being mildly concussed by a cricket ball and perishes during the evening. It is important to note that this classic picture is not as common as is thought. Often, there is no lucid period; the patient progressively passes into deeper coma from the time of the initial injury.

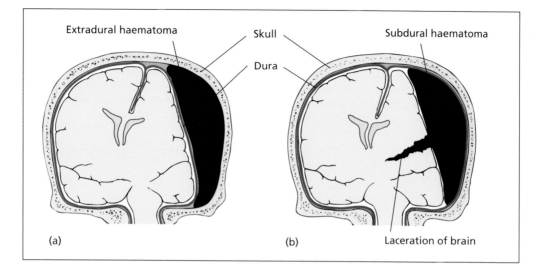

Figure 15.3 (a) Extradural haematoma and (b) acute subdural haematoma. The latter is usually associated with a severe brain injury.

The physical signs are those of rapidly increasing intracranial pressure, which have already been discussed (Chapter 14, p. 105).

In addition, there are certain localizing signs that may help the surgeon decide on which side to explore the skull. These are as follows:

- *The pupils*: a good neurosurgical aphorism is 'explore the side of the dilated pupil' (see p. 121). In 10% of patients, the dilated pupil will be a false localizing sign.
- *Hemiparesis or hemiplegia* (common) or focal fits (uncommon) usually indicate contralateral compression.
- A boggy *scalp haematoma* usually overlies the extradural clot.

Special investigations

- *CT scan* is diagnostic and allows accurate localization of the position and size of the clot.
- *Skull X-ray* may be entirely normal. However, the clot tends to be on the side of the fracture, if one is visible. A calcified pineal gland may be seen to be pushed over from the midline in a good anteroposterior film.

Treatment

An extradural haemorrhage is one of the few surgical emergencies where minutes really can matter. If a neurosurgeon is available, a bone flap will be turned over the clot. Alternatively, a burr-hole is made over the suspected site of the clot, the opening enlarged with nibbling forceps and the clot evacuated. The major bleeding point on the dura is controlled either with diathermy or silver clips or by under-running. Bleeding from the bone edges is plugged by means of bone wax.

Subdural haematoma (Figure 15.3b)

Acute

This results from bleeding into the subdural space from lacerated brain or torn vessels. It is usually part of a severe head injury. The patient is frequently in deep coma from the moment of injury but the condition deteriorates still further.

Treatment
Release of the subdural clot through a craniotomy may give some improvement in the neurological state, but the outcome may be poor because of the severity of the underlying brain trauma.

Chronic subdural haematoma or hygroma

This follows a trivial (often forgotten) injury, usually in an elderly patient, sustained weeks or months before. There is a small tear in a cerebral vein as it traverses the subdural space. Whenever the patient coughs, strains or bends over, a little blood extravasates. The resulting haematoma becomes encapsulated; as the clot breaks down, smaller molecules are formed with a rise in the osmotic pressure within the haematoma. Consequent absorption of tissue fluid produces gradual enlargement of the local collection, which may comprise liquid blood, clot or clear yellow fluid (hygroma).

Clinical features

Clinical features are those of a developing intracranial mass lesion. There is mental deterioration, headaches, vomiting and drowsiness, which progresses to coma. Moderate papilloedema is seen in about half the cases. The condition is indeed often confused with an intracerebral tumour but contrast-enhanced CT scanning will demonstrate the outline of the clot.

Treatment

Treatment comprises the evacuation of the clot or fluid collection through burr-holes.

Subarachnoid haemorrhage

Clinical features

Blood in the CSF after head injury is incidental to most severe head injuries and gives the clinical picture of meningeal irritability with headache, neck stiffness and a positive Kernig's sign.[5] There may be a mild pyrexia.

Treatment

Analgesics and bed rest are required until the severe headache has subsided; rapid rehabilitation follows.

Intracerebral haemorrhage

Scattered small haemorrhages throughout the brain substance are a common post-mortem finding in severe head injuries and may be demonstrated at CT scanning in extensive cerebral injury. At other times, a clot may develop within the brain substance, often in the frontal or temporal lobes. If it is exerting a mass effect and the intracranial pressure is high, the haematoma is evacuated and the injured lobe may have to be removed.

---

[5]Vladimir Kernig (1840–1917), Neurologist, St Petersburg, Russia. He described neck stiffness in meningitis, which at the time was commonly tuberculous in origin.

Intraventricular haemorrhage

Haemorrhage into a ventricle may occur from tearing of the choroid plexus at the time of injury or rupture of an intracerebral clot into the ventricle. It occurs particularly in childhood and is usually part of an overwhelming head injury.

Other complications

Meningitis

Infection of the meninges may complicate a fracture of the skull that is compound, either directly to the exterior or via a dural tear into the nasal or aural cavities (see p. 114).

Confirmation of the diagnosis of meningitis is the only positive indication for performing a lumbar puncture on a patient with a head injury.

Treatment

The treatment of established meningitis is antibiotic therapy. Infection via the nasal route is probably due to *Pneumococcus*; here, penicillin should be the first drug of choice. For infection complicating a compound fracture, or in patients with long inpatient stays or previous antibiotic exposure, *Staphylococcus aureus* or Gram-negative bacilli may be responsible and a broad-spectrum antibiotic which can cross the blood–brain barrier is indicated. The antibiotic may have to be changed when the sensitivity of the organism obtained on lumbar puncture becomes known.

Hyperpyrexia

The temperature of a patient with severe brainstem injury may soar to 40°C (105°F) or more as a result of injury to the heat-regulating centre. This is a serious complication and must be treated vigorously by means of cooling blankets.

Late complications

Post-concussional syndrome

Neurosis following a head injury is not uncommon. Unless reassured and rapidly rehabilitated, the patient who has had concussion is easily led to believe that the brain has been damaged and that he or she will never be fit to lead a normal life again.

Amnesia

Some idea of the severity of the injury is given by the period of amnesia, both the retrograde amnesia up to the time of the accident and the post-traumatic amnesia following injury. Interestingly, the retrograde amnesia is always considerably shorter than the post-traumatic amnesia. If the period of amnesia amounts to a few minutes or hours, the ultimate prognosis is good; amnesia of several days or even weeks indicates a severe injury and poor prognosis for return of full mental function.

Epilepsy

Persistent epilepsy may complicate penetrating compound wounds with resultant cortical scarring. In such cases, anticonvulsant therapy, e.g. phenytoin, is given for at least 6 months following injury. Established post-traumatic epilepsy is treated medically by means of anticonvulsants. Occasionally, success may follow excision of a cortical scar.

Brain death

The medical and nursing care of patients with severe brain damage due to trauma, haemorrhage or intracranial tumour is now so good that the doctors and nurses are often faced with the sad case of a patient whose brain is completely and irreversibly destroyed, but whose heart and circulation are intact, provided the lungs are mechanically ventilated. This state of affairs may persist for some weeks with severe distress to the patient's relatives and to the ward staff.

The diagnosis of brain death depends on the demonstration of permanent and irreversible destruction of brain-stem function. The tests must be performed by two people with experience in the diagnosis of brain-stem death. *All brain-stem reflexes should be absent.* The following should first be excluded before tests for brain-stem death can be performed:

- hypothermia;
- intoxication;
- sedative drugs;

- neuromuscular blocking drugs;
- severe electrolyte and acid–base abnormalities.

In addition, there must be a clearly identified cause of death, which is usually obvious in the presence of head injury but may be less clear in other circumstances. The specific features of brain-stem death are as follows:

- The patient is in a coma and on a ventilator.
- The pupils are dilated and do not respond to direct or consensual light.
- There is no corneal reflex.
- Vestibulo-ocular (doll's eye) reflexes are absent, such that when the head is passively turned, the eyes remained fixed relative to the head.
- Caloric reflexes are absent. These are tested by slow injection of 20 mL of ice-cold water into each external auditory meatus in turn, clear access to the tympanic membrane having been established by direct inspection. If no eye movement occurs during or after the test, it is considered positive.
- No motor responses within the cranial nerve distribution can be elicited by adequate stimulation of any somatic area.
- There is no gag reflex response to bronchial stimulation by a suction catheter passed down the trachea.
- No respiratory movements occur when the patient is disconnected from the mechanical ventilator for long enough to ensure that the arterial P_{CO_2} rises above the threshold for stimulating respiration, i.e. the P_{CO_2} must be above 6.65 kPa (50 mmHg).

If this situation persists over a period of observation and is confirmed by a second practitioner, death can be certified. The period of observation depends upon the age of the patient (child or adult) and the cause of the coma.

The decision to stop mechanical ventilation rests on the above factors. Once this decision has been made, the possibility of the patient becoming an organ donor for transplantation should be considered. This should be discussed fully and sympathetically with available relatives so that their informed consent is obtained for the removal of organs.

16

The spine

Learning objectives
✓ To know the types of spinal injury, their clinical signs and how to manage them.

✓ To know the degenerative diseases of the spine, how they manifest and how they are managed.

Spina bifida

The neural tube develops by an infolding of the neural ectoderm to become the spinal cord. The surrounding meninges and vertebral column derive from mesodermal tissue. Failure of embryonic fusion may result in the following anomalies:

- *Spina bifida occulta*: failure of the vertebral arch fusion only; meninges and nervous tissue normal. It occurs in 10% of the population.
- *Meningocele*: a cystic protrusion of the meninges through a posterior vertebral defect without nervous tissue involvement.
- *Myelomeningocele*: neural tissue (the cord or spinal roots) protrudes into, and may be adherent to, the meningeal sac.
- *Myelocele (rachischisis)*: failure of fusion of the neural tube; an open spinal plate occupies the defect as a red, granular area weeping cerebrospinal fluid (CSF) from its centre.

Antenatal screening (presence of high levels of α-fetoprotein in the amniotic fluid and ultrasound) enables a high degree of accuracy in intrauterine diagnosis of neural tube defects, and gives the opportunity for termination of the pregnancy. The number of infants born with severe spinal abnormalities has, in consequence, greatly

declined. The incidence of open spina bifida (meningocele, myelomeningocele and myelocele) is 1 in 1000 births.

Clinical features

These defects are particularly common in the lumbosacral area, although any part of the spine may be involved. There may be an associated overlying lipoma, tuft of hair or skin dimple, which may be an important clue to the astute clinician of the underlying defect. When nervous tissue is involved, there may be paraparesis, paraplegia, sensory disturbances in the limbs and loss of sphincter control.

Hydrocephalus nearly always coexists with the myelomeningocele owing to the *Arnold–Chiari malformation*,[1] in which the cerebellar tonsils descend below the foramen magnum with consequent obstruction of the CSF pathway.

As with any other congenital deformity, there may be multiple developmental anomalies, e.g. congenital dislocation of the hip, talipes equinovarus, cleft lip or palate, cardiac lesions or supernumerary digits.

Spina bifida occulta is usually an incidental finding noted on X-ray. When overlying skin changes (dimple, hair tuft, lipoma, sinus) are present, the cord beneath may be tethered to the skin by a fibrous band, and, as the child grows,

Lecture Notes: General Surgery, 12th edition. © Harold Ellis, Sir Roy Y. Calne and Christopher J. E. Watson. Published 2011 by Blackwell Publishing Ltd.

[1]Julius Arnold (1835–1915), Professor of Pathology, Heidelberg, Germany. Hans Chiari (1851–1916), Viennese Pathologist, successively Professor at Strasbourg, France, and Prague, Czech Republic.

weakness in the legs may occur with sensory loss, pes cavus or difficulty with bladder and bowel sphincters – 'the tethered cord syndrome'.

Treatment

Dietary supplementation with folic acid before pregnancy and in the first trimester reduces the occurrence of neural tube defects. In the USA, folic acid has been added to grain in an effort to ensure that adequate dietary supplementation is achieved.

Minor degrees of spina bifida are left alone unless there is a risk of tethering or infection. Skin-covered lesions require only cosmetic surgery. All cases with an exposed neural plate should be repaired within a few hours of birth to prevent meningitis. Associated hydrocephalus should be drained within the next 2 weeks provided there is no ascending meningitis. Surgery to improve bladder function and to correct orthopaedic limb problems arising as a result of spasticity or paralysis is often required as the child grows.

Spinal injuries

Spinal injuries have two components – the bony injury and the neurological injury – both of which must be considered in all patients with spinal trauma.

The bony injury

The bony injury may comprise either a fracture or a dislocation or a combination of both (fracture dislocation). The most important consideration is the stability of the fracture. A stable fracture is one that is unlikely to undergo further displacement or neurological damage; an unstable fracture may undergo further displacement with the risk of further neurological damage.

Assessing stability

The assessment of stability is fundamental to the initial management of the patient. It depends upon the integrity of the structures that make up the normal spinal column, namely the vertebrae, intervertebral discs and ligaments. While it is relatively easy to determine stability in upper cervical fractures, it is less easy in lower fractures such as those in the thoracolumbar region. To overcome

this, the concept of the three-column spine is useful (Figure 16.1).

The three columns are made up as follows.

- *The anterior column* comprises the anterior longitudinal ligament, the anterior annulus fibrosus and the anterior part of the vertebral body.
- *The middle column* comprises the posterior longitudinal ligament, the posterior annulus fibrosus and the posterior part of the vertebral body and the facet joints.
- *The posterior column* comprises the posterior arch and the intervening ligament complex, itself comprising supraspinous ligaments, interspinous ligaments and ligamentum flavum.

Disruption of two or all of these columns results in spinal instability. Disruption of a single column, such as in a wedge fracture affecting the anterior half of the vertebral body, is a stable injury without risk of further displacement or further neurological damage.

Types of fracture

Most fractures are caused by a sudden hyperextension or hyperflexion, often combined with compression or distraction. The results of such forces may be considered in terms of five distinct levels in the spine.

1 *Upper cervical spine (C1, C2).* In the upper cervical spine, flexion/extension injuries may result in fracture of the dens (odontoid process) at its base, atlantoaxial dislocation or fracture of the atlas or axis (hangman's fracture). The spinal canal is wide in the upper cervical region and immediate spinal cord damage may be minor, although, in more severe injuries, fatal damage to the cord may occur.

2 *Lower cervical spine (C3–C7).*

   a *Hyperflexion injuries* may result in anterior dislocation of facet joints, with consequent narrowing of the spinal canal and neurological injury. A corresponding step may be seen on a lateral cervical spine X-ray. Either one or both facet joints may be involved. Because of the much closer fit of the cervical cord within the vertebral canal compared with the wider lumbar region, the incidence of cord damage in these injuries is extremely high, with resultant tetraplegia or

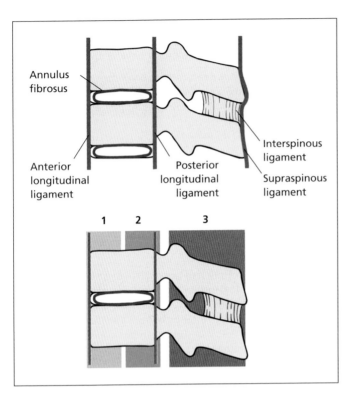

Annulus
fibrosus

Anterior
longitudinal
ligament

Posterior
longitudinal
ligament

Interspinous
ligament

Supraspinous
ligament

1   2   3

Figure 16.1 The three-column spine concept.

paraplegia. If the facet joints do not lock, there may be spontaneous reduction and little to see on a lateral X-ray, although complete transection of the cord may have occurred.

  b *Hyperextension* may result in rupture of the anterior longitudinal ligament and disc with backward displacement of the vertebral body to narrow the spinal canal and impinge on the cord, before springing back.

  c *Compression, combined with flexion,* may result in a wedge-shaped fracture of the vertebral body. Severe compression injuries may result in a comminuted fracture with fragments encroaching on the spinal canal.

3 *Thoracic.* The thoracic spine is relatively stable owing to the splinting afforded by the rib cage and sternum. Pathological fractures, commonly a result of osteoporosis or secondary tumour, are more common in this region.

4 *Thoracolumbar.* The thoracolumbar junction is relatively unsupported, and liable to injuries caused by flexion, rotation and compression. Such injuries may follow a fall from a height

landing on the feet or the buttocks, or forward flexion of the spine in a decelerating car crash, or a heavy weight falling on the shoulders.

5 *Lumbar.*

  a *Compression* injuries may cause wedge-shaped fractures where the body of the vertebra collapses.

  b *Burst fractures* with comminution of the vertebral body and hence disruption of anterior and middle columns may occur following axial compression and result in an unstable fracture, often with cord or cauda equina damage if bone fragments encroach into the canal. Such fractures are often associated with crushing of the intervertebral disc.

In practice, the commonest fractures are those in the cervical and thoracolumbar regions.

Clinical features

There is the typical history of injury followed by localized pain, bruising, tenderness and often a kyphus. Careful neurological examination is imperative (Box 16.1).

Box 16.1 Examining neurological injury

The examination of nerve injuries requires testing for sensation, power and reflexes. The components of sensation include light touch, vibration and joint position sense (dorsal columns), and temperature and pain (spinothalamic tract). Abnormalities should be noted in relation to both dermatome and, in the case of peripheral nerve injuries, innervation.

Motor responses should be examined in relation to spinal level or peripheral nerve according to injury.

Movement	Muscle responsible	Innervation
Arm abduction	Deltoid	C5,6
Elbow flexion	Biceps	C5,6
Wrist extension	Forearm extensors	C6,7
Elbow extension	Triceps	C7,8
Finger abduction	Intrinsic muscles of hand	C8,T1
Hip flexion	Iliopsoas	L2,3
Knee extension	Quadriceps femoris	L2,3,4
Foot dorsiflexion	Tibialis anterior, extensor hallucis longus, extensor digitorum longus	L4,5
Knee flexion	Hamstrings	L5,S1
Hallux extension	Extensor hallucis longus	L5,S1
Foot plantar flexion	Gastrocnemius, soleus, tibialis posterior, flexor hallucis longus, flexor digitorum longus	S1,2
Anal tone	Anal sphincter	S2,3,4

Motor responses should be graded according to the Medical Research Council (MRC) scale:

0 Total paralysis

1 Flicker of movement

2 Active movement with gravity eliminated

3 Normal movement against gravity but not against additional resistance

4 Movement against both gravity and resistance, but still overcome

5 Normal power

The reflexes are innervated as follows:

Biceps jerk	C5,6
Triceps jerk	C7,8
Knee jerk	L3,4
Ankle jerk	S1,2

- *Plantar reflex.* Extension is abnormal and indicates an upper motor neurone lesion.

Two other reflexes are useful in the assessment of patients with spinal cord injuries, the presence of which suggests an incomplete cord lesion:

- *Bulbocavernosus reflex.* Contraction of the anal sphincter in response to pinching of the penile shaft.
- *Anal reflex.* Contraction of the anus in response to stroking of the perianal skin.

It is obligatory to examine every person with a head injury for suspected spinal fracture, as this is easily overlooked in the unconscious patient. Unskilled handling of such a case may produce an irreparable spinal injury.

Special investigations

- *Spine X-ray.* The exact type of fracture is usually shown. Lateral films are the most important. Cervical spine films should show all seven cervical vertebra and T1. Additional views, such as a swimmer's view (a front-crawl position) or an oblique view to visualize the lower cervical spine, and an open-mouth view to show the dens, may be necessary.
- *Computed tomography (CT)* to confirm a fracture and demonstrate the extent of comminution.
- *Magnetic resonance (MR)* imaging to assess injury to the spinal cord or intervertebral disc.

The neurological injury

Mechanism of cord injury

Cord compression

The cord may be compressed by bone, intervertebral disc or haematoma. This is particularly common when a previous abnormality exists, such as congenital spinal stenosis or cervical spondylosis. Facet joint dislocation, in which the cord is trapped in the narrow canal at the level of the dislocation, is another common example.

Direct injury

Open injuries, or shards of fractured bone may penetrate the neural canal and lacerate the cord.

Ischaemia

A vascular insult to the spinal vessels may result in cord damage, and may be delayed and exacerbated by cord oedema and haematoma.

Types of neurological injury

Spinal concussion

Nervous continuity is not lost, paraplegia is only partial and recovery commences within a few hours. Full return of function can be anticipated.

> **Box 16.2 Components of neurological injury**
>
> The neurological injury following spinal cord damage can be divided into three components:
>
> **Sensory loss**
>
> - Somatic and visceral sensations are lost below the level of section. Hyperaesthesia may be present at the level of section
>
> **Motor loss**
>
> - Spinal cord injuries result in an upper motor neurone spastic paralysis with hyperreflexia. Cauda equina injuries, being injuries of nerve roots, produce a lower motor neurone paralysis characterized by reduced tone and areflexia
>
> **Autonomic loss**
>
> - Loss of sympathetic outflow injuries below T5 results in hypotension as a result of loss of vasomotor tone. Thermoregulation, which also depends on vasomotor activity, is also impaired. Sphincter control is also autonomic. With injuries above the level of the sacral outflow the spinal reflex arc triggering micturition remains intact so the bladder empties automatically. Injuries below this level interrupt the reflex and an atonic bladder results

Cord transection

Loss of function owing to anatomical division of the cord is irrecoverable, as the axons within the cord have no power of regeneration. There is an initial period of spinal shock with complete flaccid paralysis below the line of cord section, loss of tendon reflexes, atonicity of the bladder (which becomes distended), faecal retention and priapism. This phase generally lasts for a few days. The cord below the line of transection then recovers reflex function so that the paralysis becomes spastic with muscle spasms, the plantar responses become extensor, and bladder and bowel begin to empty by reflex (Box 16.2).

Cauda equina injury

This may complicate fractures below the level of termination of the spinal cord at the lower border of the first lumbar vertebra. There is saddle anaesthesia (over the buttocks, anus and perineum),

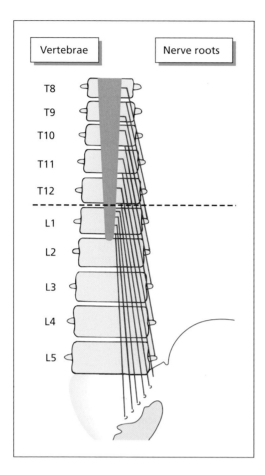

Vertebrae	Nerve roots
T8	
T9	
T10	
T11	
T12	
L1	
L2	
L3	
L4	
L5	

Figure 16.2 The relationship of the spinal cord and nerve roots to the vertebrae. Because of the disparity between the two, a fracture dislocation at the dorsolumbar junction, shown here by the dotted line, will miss the lumbar cord but may transect the sacral segments of the cord together with injury to the lumbar nerve roots.

weakness of the lower leg muscles, absent ankle reflexes and urinary retention. The cauda equina are the roots of peripheral nerves and therefore possess the power of regeneration provided continuity of the nerve trunk is not lost. However, recovery is rarely complete if compression occurs for more than a few hours.

Combined cord and cauda equina injury

As many spinal injuries take place at the thoracolumbar junction, there is usually a combination of spinal cord and nerve-root injury. For example, a fracture dislocation at the T12/L1 junction will divide the cord at the first sacral segment but clinical examination may reveal paralysis being due to damage to the spinal roots as they pass the site of the fracture dislocation (Figure 16.2). In this instance, the roots may recover with return of knee and hip movement, although the sacral paralysis will be permanent.

Brown-Séquard syndrome[2]

A penetrating injury of the spinal cord, which is unilateral and results in spastic paralysis on the affected side (involvement of the ipsilateral pyramidal tract), loss of position and vibration sense also on the affected side (posterior column involvement) and loss of pain and temperature sensation on the opposite side to the lesion (involvement of the spinothalamic tract). Such an injury is often partial, and rarely occurs after a closed injury.

Treatment of spinal injuries

The treatment of spinal injuries depends whether or not there has been neurological injury, and also upon the stability of the fracture.

Immediate management

Spinal injury should be suspected in anyone following severe trauma or who is unconscious following trauma. In addition, any patient with sensory or motor symptoms following minor trauma should be treated as possessing a spinal injury until proved otherwise. Before such a patient is moved, the neck should be immobilized in a hard collar and the patient log rolled or 'scooped' onto a stretcher for transfer.

Airway management is the immediate consideration. The principles are the same as those following head injury. In addition, following spinal cord injury, loss of sympathetic tone may lead to vasodilatation and hypotension, on top of any blood loss which may result from trauma, and so replacing circulating volume is important to prevent ischaemia.

[2]Charles Edward Brown-Séquard (1817–1894), born in Mauritius, trained in Paris, France. Neurologist at The National Hospital for Nervous Diseases, Queen's Square, London, UK, and later Professor of Medicine at Harvard, Boston, MA, USA, and then the Collège de France in Paris, France.

Treatment with no neurological injury

Stable fractures of the spine are treated by bed rest for 2–3 weeks, to allow the associated soft-tissue injury to subside, followed by early exercise and active mobilization. There is no need to reduce the fracture by hyperextension and prolonged fixation; often this results in permanent residual pain.

Unstable fractures require immobilization in order to secure bony stability and thus to protect the cord from later damage. Gross instability in the presence of an incomplete neurological injury is an indication for urgent operative stabilization.

Unstable cervical fractures are immobilized by traction using tongs applied to the skull for 6 weeks, or are fixed by open reduction and plating. This is followed by a cervical collar for a further month. Traction may also be used to try to reduce facet joint dislocation, although open reduction may be necessary.

Unstable thoracolumbar fractures may be treated by operative reduction and internal fixation.

Treatment with paraplegia or tetraplegia

The patient is transported in a neutral position (so that flexion and extension are not possible), to a spinal or neurosurgical centre, the spine being supported by suitably arranged pillows and the patient being moved frequently from side to side to prevent bed sore formation. The distended bladder is best left alone until catheterization can be carried out under full aseptic precautions to prevent infection. High-dose methyl prednisolone given as early as possible and continued for 24 hours has been shown to improve recovery of motor function.

The following are the main principles of treatment.

- *The management of the fracture.* Two techniques of management may be employed. The conservative approach, favoured in most centres in the UK, comprises nursing the patient on a circo-electric bed or a Stryker frame.[3] This allows regular turning of the paraplegic (thus avoiding pressure sores), while keeping the fracture immobilized. This is

[3]Homer Stryker (1894–1980), Orthopaedic Surgeon, Stryker Corporation, Kalamazoo, MI, USA.

continued for 6 weeks. Plaster casts or beds are avoided, as pressure sores are almost inevitable. Once the fracture has become stable, the patient can progress to the rehabilitation stage of treatment. The surgical approach, more often used on the continent and in the USA, consists of open reduction and internal rod fixation of the unstable fracture.

- *Care of the skin.* Pressure sores may develop with extraordinary rapidity in the first weeks because of the combination of anaesthesia and immobilization. Two-hourly turning, aided by use of the circo-electric bed or a Stryker frame, and meticulous skin care are required.
- *The bladder.* In the initial phase of complete bladder paralysis, acute urinary retention is common and continuous catheter drainage by means of a fine Silastic urethral or suprapubic catheter is instituted. With recovery from spinal shock, the patient may develop an automatic (reflex) bladder so that stroking the side of the thigh or abdominal compression may evoke reflex bladder emptying.
- *The bowels.* Acute spinal injury results in paralytic ileus. Following recovery of motility, constipation is common and is best managed by regular enemas. Faecal impaction must be watched for and treated by digital evacuation.
- *Peptic ulceration prophylaxis.* Prophylaxis with antacids, H_2-receptor antagonists, proton pump inhibitors or sucralfate should be initiated since acute peptic ulceration is common in the early days following spinal cord injury.
- *Pulmonary embolism prophylaxis.* Patients with paralysis of the legs following spinal cord injury are at risk of venous thrombosis and pulmonary emboli. Prophylaxis with subcutaneous low-molecular-weight heparin should be instituted and continued until normal mobility is restored.
- *Rehabilitation.* Active development of muscles with an intact or partial innervation by expert physiotherapy can restore mobility in 80% of paraplegic patients. However, these patients require callipers and crutches so that they can swing their paralysed legs by the use of abdominal, flank and shoulder muscles. Of these, latissimus dorsi is the most important. At the same time, vocational training can be commenced and a large percentage of these unfortunate patients can be restored to useful activity.

Degenerative spinal disorders

Degenerative spinal disorders may arise from degenerative changes in the vertebral body, the intervertebral joints or the intervertebral discs. The resulting symptoms may arise from a combination of effects, so apophyseal joint degeneration may result in local back pain (lumbago), together with a radiculopathy attributable to encroachment of osteophyte into the intervertebral foramen.

Neurological sequelae of spinal degeneration

- *Local pain* arises from osteoarthritis of the intervertebral joints. Backache (lumbago) in the lumbar spine, neck ache in the cervical spine.
- *Radiculopathy*, causing lower motor neurone symptoms, arises from compression and irritation of the nerve roots as they exit the intervertebral foramen. This may be due to disc or osteophyte encroachment into the intervertebral canal, and is compounded by loss of intervertebral joint space.
- *Myelopathy* causes upper motor neurone symptoms, results from compression of the spinal cord within the canal, arises from prolapse of an intervertebral disc or osteophyte encroachment into the spinal canal and is exacerbated in the presence of a congenital narrowing of the spinal canal.
- *Claudication of the cauda equina* may arise as a result of lumbar canal stenosis. Symptoms are similar to those resulting from peripheral vascular disease with cramp-like calf pains, but are often associated with paraesthesiae, are worse when standing erect or walking downhill, may be bilateral and are relieved by sitting rather than standing. Contrast claudication from vascular disease, which is usually unilateral, worsens walking uphill and is relieved on standing.

Prolapsed intervertebral disc

Disc herniation comprises a protrusion of the nucleus pulposus posteriorly, or more commonly posterolaterally, through a defect in the annulus fibrosus. It is probable that most ruptures are initiated by trauma, which may be severe but which is more often mild or repetitive. It is probably for this reason that the great majority of prolapsing discs occur in the active adult male.

By far the commonest sites are between the L4 and L5 vertebrae, and between L5 and the sacrum. Cervical disc protrusion most commonly occurs between C5 and C6 or between C6 and C7. The cervical lesion is often associated with degenerative changes in the spine and is therefore usually found more than the lumbar disc prolapse in older patients.

Lumbar disc herniation

Clinical features

There is often lumbar pain early in the history, with exacerbations as a result of straining or heavy lifting. The majority of patients complain of sciatica, their pain being usually unilateral and radiating from the buttock along the back of the thigh and knee and then down the lateral side of the leg to the foot. This pain is aggravated by coughing, sneezing or straining (which raise the intrathecal pressure) or by straight leg raising (which stretches the sciatic nerve). Sometimes there is the complaint of weakness of ankle dorsiflexion (L5) or plantar flexion (S1). There may be paraesthesiae or numbness in the foot. A central prolapse of the lumbar disc is more devastating, producing bilateral sciatic pain, sphincter disturbance and complete or incomplete cauda equina compression.

Examination reveals flattening of the normal lumbar lordosis, scoliosis and limited spinal flexion. The erector spinae muscles are in spasm and straight leg raising is limited and painful. There may be weakness of plantar- or dorsiflexion of the ankle and there may be disuse muscle wasting of the leg on the affected side. Sensory loss on the medial side of the dorsum of the foot and the great toe (L5 innervation) suggest an L4/L5 disc lesion. Sensory loss on the lateral side of the foot (S1 innervation) may occur in L5/S1 disc lesions. The ankle jerk may be diminished in the latter cases.

Special investigations

- *X-rays of the spine* may or may not reveal narrowing of the affected disc space on the lateral view.

- *CT or MR scans* are the investigations of choice and usually demonstrate the disc protrusion.
- *C-reactive protein (CRP)* is normal, and is helpful in the differential diagnosis of tumour or abscess.

Differential diagnosis

This includes the other common spinal lesions: sacroiliac strain, osteoarthritis, spondylolisthesis, spinal tumours and tuberculosis. One should consider, particularly in the elderly patient, an intrapelvic tumour, e.g. of the prostate or rectum, involving the sacral plexus; never omit a rectal examination in any patient with sciatica, both to detect rectal and prostatic tumours and to assess anal tone. Intermittent claudication is readily differentiated by careful history and examination. An abdominal aortic aneurysm may cause low back pain, and upon rupture may cause sciatica.

Treatment

Severe acute pain is treated with analgesia and rest on a firm bed; as soon as the patient can get up, gentle mobilization and physiotherapy should be instituted. Operative removal of the prolapsed disc is indicated if conservative measures fail, if repeated attacks occur, if there are severe neurological disturbances and particularly if a large central protrusion is diagnosed. If bladder sphincter disturbance occurs, surgical decompression must be performed urgently.

Spinal stenosis

Narrowing of the spinal canal may be congenital, but more commonly follows degeneration of the spine with osteophyte formation. It generally extends over several segments, and occurs predominantly in the lumbar spine.

The clinical features have been likened to intermittent claudication (Chapter 12, p. 90), but in spinal claudication the patient presents with pain, numbness and weakness in the legs brought on by standing or walking, and, in contrast to vascular claudication, it is not relieved by standing still but by sitting down or otherwise flexing the spine. Neurological examination of the legs is most revealing after the patient has been walking for a few minutes.

The diagnosis is confirmed by MR (or CT) scan of the spine, which shows evidence of bony and soft-tissue encroachment into the spinal canal.

Treatment is usually conservative, although surgery with decompression and fusion may be required.

Cervical spondylosis

Cervical spondylosis refers to degenerative changes that occur in the neck, with a similar pathological process to that in the lumbar spine. In the cervical spine, coexistent myelopathy and radiculopathy is more common.

Clinical features

Local cervical pain is usually overshadowed by a more severe pain radiating into the arm and accompanied by numbness and tingling in the fingers. Patients with myelopathy also complain of leg stiffness and difficulty in walking. Sensory changes may be present in the legs or arms, and bladder sphincter control may be disturbed. Examination of the arms reveals a lower motor neurone weakness with wasting and decreased tendon reflexes. Sensation is reduced with a nerve-root distribution. Examination of the legs may reveal an upper motor neurone pattern with a spastic paraplegia, increased tone, leg weakness, brisk reflexes and extensor plantars.

Differential diagnosis

There is an extensive differential diagnosis, which includes spinal tumour, multiple sclerosis and motor neurone disease. When the radiculopathy alone is present with unilateral or bilateral arm pain, the differential diagnosis includes cervical rib, carpal tunnel syndrome and angina pectoris.

Treatment

Radiculopathy usually settles with conservative treatment. A severe episode may require a period of neck traction; otherwise, the neck is supported in a plastic collar. Operative removal of the prolapsed cervical disc has the same indications as lumbar disc protrusions.

Extradural spinal abscess

An abscess in the extradural spinal compartment usually represents a metastatic infection as part of a *Staphylococcus aureus* septicaemia. Occasionally, it is secondary to an osteomyelitis of the spine. Diagnosis can be difficult owing to an insidious presentation.

Clinical features

Clinical features are local pain and tenderness, fever, malaise and anorexia, and a rapidly progressive paraplegia. The white blood cell count is raised and the C-reactive protein is elevated.

Treatment

Urgent treatment is required with drainage of the abscess via a laminectomy, and antibiotic therapy is commenced. Provided surgery is performed in the initial stages, the paraplegia recovers but delay carries with it the risk of permanent cord damage.

Spinal tumours

Spinal tumours are conveniently classified, from both the pathological and clinical points of view, into those which occur outside the spinal theca (extradural), those which occur within the theca but outside the cord itself (intradural extramedullary) and those occurring within the cord (intramedullary).

The tumours most commonly encountered are the following.

1 *Extradural.*
  a Secondary deposits in the spine – by far the commonest.
  b Primary vertebral bony tumours (e.g. osteoclastoma, myeloma).
  c Lymphomas (Hodgkin's disease, non-Hodgkin's lymphoma).
2 *Intradural extramedullary.*
  a Meningioma.
  b Neurofibroma.
3 *Intramedullary* (rare).
  a Glioma.
  b Ependymoma.
  c Others, such as haemangioma.

Clinical features

The three groups of spinal tumours listed above each tend to have a fairly distinctive clinical picture.

- *The extradural tumours* are usually fast growing and malignant; they therefore give a picture of rapidly progressive cord compression leading to paraplegia, although symptoms of root irritation (see below) may also be present.
- *The intradural extramedullary tumours* are usually slow growing and benign. Initially, there is irritation of the involved nerve roots; pain occurs in the localized area of nerve distribution, which is often aggravated by recumbency and by factors such as coughing, sneezing or straining, which raise the CSF pressure. There may be hyperalgesia in the affected cutaneous segment. Motor symptoms due to anterior root pressure are not a feature if only one nerve segment is involved, as most major muscle groups are innervated from several segments; however, if more than one segment is affected, there may be localized flaccid paralysis.

  As the tumour increases in size, cord compression takes place. There may be features of the *Brown-Séquard syndrome* (see p. 131). Further compression results in complete paraplegia of the spastic type with increased tendon jerks and extensor plantar response, together with overflow retention of urine and severe constipation.

  Cauda equina tumours produce a lower motor neurone lesion: flaccid paralysis with diminished reflexes and paralysis of the anal and bladder sphincters with incontinence.
- *The intramedullary tumours* may be accompanied by pain, but much more frequently give a picture very similar to that of syringomyelia. Progressive destruction of the cord produces bilateral motor weakness below the lesion and, as the crossed spinothalamic tracts are the first to be involved, there may be dissociation of sensory loss below the lesion, with abolition of pain and temperature but with persistence of vibration and position sense until later on in the progress of the disease.

Differential diagnosis

Spinal tumours are relatively uncommon and are great impersonators of other diseases; indeed, a correct diagnosis made *ab initio* is something of a rarity. The root pain, if it occurs in the thoracic or abdominal segments, is often mistaken for intrathoracic or intra-abdominal disease; if the pains radiate to the leg, they may be at first diagnosed as a prolapsed disc or intermittent claudication. The intramedullary lesions closely simulate syringomyelia and it may be difficult at first to differentiate them from disseminated sclerosis or other intraspinal lesions.

Special investigations

- *MR* has become the definitive investigation and gives almost anatomically perfect imaging of spinal tumours.
- *X-rays of the spine* may show obvious bony deposits within the vertebral bodies. In other cases, pressure erosion from the enlarging tumour may scallop the posterior aspect of the vertebral body, erode one or more vertebral pedicles or enlarge the intervertebral foramen. Occasionally, calcification is seen within a meningioma.
- *Lumbar puncture.* Cytological examination of the CSF, together with its protein content and CSF pressure measurement, may be useful. The protein in the CSF is nearly always raised above the normal 0.4 pg/L and may indeed be grossly elevated with yellow (xanthochromic) fluid, which may actually clot in the container. Queckenstedt's test[4] may show either no rise or else a very slow rise and fall of the CSF pressure on jugular compression, indicating a complete or partial block within the spinal canal.
- *A radiculogram*, in which radio-opaque water-soluble contrast medium is injected into the theca, will confirm the presence of a space-occupying lesion and localize its position accurately.

Treatment

A laminectomy (or vertebral body excision and bone grafting) is required to confirm the pathological nature of the tumour and also to decompress the cord. Wherever possible, the tumour is completely excised; this is usually confined to the benign meningiomas and neurofibroma, in which case complete recovery can be anticipated. In the malignant tumours, radiotherapy is usually the only practical treatment and the prognosis is poor.

[4]Hans Heinrich Queckenstedt (1876–1918), Physician, Leipzig, Germany. He described his test while serving in the German Army; he was killed accidentally 2 days before the Armistice.

17

Peripheral nerve injuries

Learning objectives

✓ To know the different types of nerve injury and their prognosis.
✓ To be able to recognize the patterns of neurological deficit that occur with injury to all the main nerves in the upper and lower limbs.

Although there is no regeneration of divided tracts in the central nervous system (CNS), injured peripheral nerve fibres may recover to a varying extent, depending on the severity of the trauma.

Classification

Nerve injuries are commonly the result of laceration, stretching (traction) or compression (crush) injuries. There are three types of injury:

1 *Neurapraxia.* Damage to the nerve fibres without loss of continuity of the axis cylinder; this is analogous to concussion in the CNS. The conduction along the fibre is interrupted for only a short period of time. Recovery usually commences within a few days and is complete in 6–8 weeks.
2 *Axonotmesis.* This is injury to the axon and myelin sheath without disruption of the continuity of its perineural sheath. The axon distal to the lesion degenerates (Wallerian degeneration[1]) and regrowth of the axon occurs from the node of Ranvier[2] proximal to

the injury. As the sheath is intact, the correct axon will grow into its original nerve ending. The rate of regeneration is approximately 1 mm/day; therefore, the time to recovery depends upon the distance between the injury and end organ.
3 *Neurotmesis.* This is actual physical disruption of the peripheral nerve. Regeneration will take place provided the two nerve ends are not too far apart, but functional recovery will never be complete.

Following the complete disruption of neurotmesis, the distal part of the severed nerve undergoes Wallerian degeneration. The medullary sheath is depleted of myelin and the axon cylinders vanish; the empty endoneural sheaths remain as tubules composed of proliferating neurilemmal cells. The proximal end of the nerve degenerates up to the first uninjured node of Ranvier. New axis cylinders proliferate from this point and grow into the empty neurilemmal tubules. However, there is no selection of tubules for the appropriate axon; the distal growth is governed solely by the position of the nerve fibres. Thus, with most mixed nerves, there is likely to be considerable wastage owing to regenerating fibres growing into endings which will be functionless, i.e. motor nerve fibres growing into sensory nerve endings, and vice versa. Even when a motor nerve grows into a motor nerve ending, it may not supply the original muscle and the patient will have to relearn the affected movement.

---

[1] Augustus Waller (1816–1870), a General Practitioner in London, UK, for 10 years before working as a Physiologist in Bonn, Germany, Paris, France, and Birmingham, UK.
[2] Louis Ranvier (1835–1922), Professor of Histology, Paris, France.

Lecture Notes: General Surgery, 12th edition. © Harold Ellis, Sir Roy Y. Calne and Christopher J. E. Watson. Published 2011 by Blackwell Publishing Ltd.

Because a peripheral nerve contains a large number of individual fibres, it is quite possible in a nerve injury for some fibres to suffer from neurapraxia, others axonotmesis and others neurotmesis. However, a distinction between the first two and the last may be quite clear in that, if the nerve is found to be severed at surgical exploration, neurotmesis must have occurred.

Partial nerve injury may occur as the result of pressure or friction, for instance from a crutch, a tightly applied plaster cast or a tourniquet, as well as from closed injuries or open wounds.

Special investigation

Electromyography (EMG) plays an important part in the diagnosis and assessment of nerve injuries. Serial studies are useful in demonstrating the amount and rate of regeneration. EMG is also useful in the diagnosis of nerve compression syndromes.

Treatment

Neurapraxia and axonotmesis

Those joints whose muscles have been paralysed are splinted in the position of function to avoid contractures. They are put through passive movements several times a day so that, when recovery of the nerve lesion occurs, the joints will be fully mobile.

Neurotmesis

Operative repair using an operating microscope is usually required. If a section of the nerve has been lost such that approximation is not possible, the nerve is freed proximally, or even moved from its original position to a new anatomical plane where more length will be available. For example, the ulnar nerve can be transposed from the posterior to the anterior aspect of the elbow joint to allow compensation for a distal loss of nerve substance.

After nerve suture, recovery cannot be expected to take place until the time for regeneration has been allowed for, at the rate already mentioned of 1 mm/day. Eventual recovery will seldom be full.

Nerve grafts

When important nerves are divided, sometimes useful function can be obtained by grafting sections of non-essential nerves such as the sural nerve to act as conduits for axon regrowth.

Tendon transfers

If restoration of nerve function cannot be achieved after injury, tendon transfers may allow the patient to perform movements that would otherwise be impossible. Thus, wrist drop after a radial nerve lesion may be treated by transposing some of the flexor tendons into the extensor group.

It is beyond the scope of this book to discuss lesions of all the individual nerves, but a few important peripheral nerve injuries will be mentioned.

Brachial plexus injuries

Upper trunk lesions (Erb's paralysis[3])

These are the result of damage to the upper trunk when the head is forced away from the shoulder, a common injury in motor cyclists. It may also occur as an obstetric injury. C5 and C6 are damaged and there is paralysis of the biceps, brachialis, brachioradialis, supinator, supraspinatus, infraspinatus and deltoid. The limb will assume the 'waiter's tip' position, being internally rotated with the forearm pronated (owing to the loss of the powerful supinating action of biceps). The arm hangs vertically (deltoid paralysis) and the elbow cannot be flexed (biceps and brachialis). There will be an area of impaired sensation over the outer side of the upper arm.

T1 injury (Klumpke's paralysis[4])

This may occur with a cervical rib or dislocation or forcible abduction of the shoulder. The small

[3]Wilhelm Erb (1840–1921), Professor of Neurology, Heidelberg, Germany.
[4]Auguste Dejerine-Klumpke (1859–1927), Neurologist, Paris, France; her husband, J. J. Dejerine, was also a distinguished neurologist.

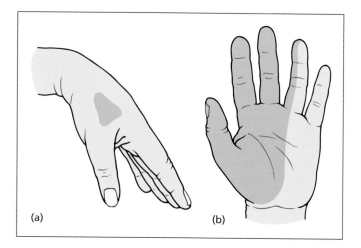

Figure 17.1 (a) Radial nerve injury: wrist drop, together with anaesthesia of a small area of the dorsal aspect of the hand at the base of the thumb and index finger. (b) Median nerve injury: thenar eminence paralysis with anaesthesia of the palmar aspect of the radial three and a half digits and corresponding palm.

muscles of the hand are wasted and there is loss of sensation on the inner side of the forearm. There may also be Horner's syndrome owing to associated damage of sympathetic fibres passing to the inferior cervical ganglion (see p. 142).

Radial nerve injuries (Figure 17.1a)

Usually, the radial nerve is injured by a fracture of the humerus involving the spiral groove where the nerve is closely applied to the posterior aspect of the mid-shaft of the bone. The nerve supply to the triceps comes off the radial nerve before it enters the spiral groove, and the lesions distal to that point will not affect extension of the elbow. However, there will be wrist drop because of paralysis of the wrist extensors and also loss of sensation over a small area on the dorsum of the hand at the base of the thumb and index finger. This surprisingly small sensory loss is due to considerable overlap from the median and ulnar nerves.

Median nerve injuries (Figure 17.1b)

This nerve may be damaged in fractures around the elbow joint or laceration of the forearm or

wrist. In high lesions, the pronators of the forearm and flexors of the wrist and fingers will be involved, with the exception of the flexor carpi ulnaris and the medial half of the flexor digitorum profundus, which are supplied by the ulnar nerve and which produce ulnar deviation of the wrist. When the patient clasps the two hands together, the index finger on the affected side remains extended – the 'pointing sign' of a high median nerve injury. Whether the injury is in the forearm or wrist, there will be paralysis of the small muscles of the thumb so that the thenar eminence is wasted. The patient is unable to abduct the thumb, i.e. lift it at right angles to the plane of the hand. The sensory loss with a median nerve lesion is serious. There is anaesthesia over the palmar aspects of the thumb and the radial two and a half fingers, and the loss extends onto the dorsum of the distal phalanges of these digits. This sensory defect makes it difficult to perform fine and delicate tasks.

Median nerve compression at the wrist (carpal tunnel syndrome)

The median nerve is compressed as it passes through the carpal tunnel formed by the flexor retinaculum stretching from the hook of the hamate and pisiform medially to the trapezium

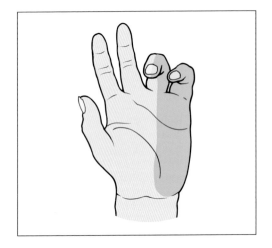

Figure 17.2 Ulnar nerve injury: *main en griffe* with anaesthesia of the ulnar one and a half digits and ulnar border of the hand on both palmar and dorsal aspects.

and scaphoid laterally. This results in wasting of the thenar eminence, diminished sensation and most often unpleasant pain (characteristically at night), paraesthesia (numbness and tingling) in the thumb and radial two fingers and some-times paraesthesia extending up into the arm. The reason for this last symptom is not clear. Women are affected four times more commonly than men, and there is an association with preg-nancy, rheumatoid arthritis, myxoedema and acromegaly. Wrist fractures also predispose to the syndrome.

EMG confirms the diagnosis. Treatment con-sists of dividing the flexor retinaculum at the wrist deep to which the median·nerve is compressed, although conservative management using a wrist splint may also be effective.

Ulnar nerve injuries
(Figure 17.2)

Like the median, this nerve is also injured by frac-tures around the elbow joint and by lacerations of the forearm and, particularly, the wrist.

The ulnar nerve supplies all the intrinsic muscles of the hand apart from the three muscles of the thenar eminence (abductor pollicis brevis, oppo-

nens and flexor pollicis brevis) and the two radial lumbricals, all of which are supplied by the median nerve. The affected intrinsic muscles are the adductor pollicis, the muscles of the hypothenar eminence, the ulnar two lumbricals and the inter-ossei, which are the abductors and adductors of the fingers and which also extend the interphalan-geal joints. In the forearm, the ulnar nerve sup-plies flexor carpi ulnaris and the medial half of flexor digitorum profundus.

Damage to the ulnar nerve produces the typical deformity of clawed hand or *main en griffe*. The clawed appearance results from the unopposed action of the long flexors and extensors of the fingers. The flexor profundus and sublimis, inserted into the bases of the distal and middle phalanges respectively, flex the interphalangeal joints, while the long extensors, inserted into the bases of the proximal phalanges, extend the meta-carpophalangeal joints.

If the nerve is injured at the elbow, flexor digitorum profundus to the fourth and fifth finger is paralysed so that the clawing of these fingers, rather anomalously, is less intense than in injuries at the wrist. Paralysis of flexor carpi ulnaris produces a tendency to radial deviation at the wrist. In late cases, wasting of the intrinsic muscles is readily evident on inspecting the dorsum of the hand and the web space between the thumb and index finger. Sensory loss occurs over the dorsal and palmar aspects of the ulnar one and a half digits and the ulnar border of the hand on both palmar and dorsal aspects. If the ulnar nerve is divided at the level of the wrist, the sensory loss is confined to the palmar surface, as the dorsal branch of the ulnar nerve, supplying the dorsal aspects of the ulnar one and a half fingers, is given off 5 cm above the wrist and thus escapes injury.

Division of the ulnar nerve leaves a surprisingly efficient hand. The long flexors enable a good grip to be taken; the thumb, apart from the loss of adductor pollicis, is intact, and the important sensation over the palm of the hand is largely maintained. Indeed, it may be difficult to be certain clinically that the nerve is injured. A reli-able test is loss of the ability to abduct and adduct the fingers with the hand laid flat, palm down-wards, on a table. This eliminates the trick move-ments of adduction and abduction of the fingers occurring as part of their flexion and extension, respectively.

Differential diagnosis of flexion deformities of the fingers

Ulnar nerve lesion

This has been described above; there is hyperextension of the metacarpophalangeal joints and clawing of the hand, with sensory loss along the ulnar border of the hand and ulnar one and a half fingers.

Dupuytren's contracture[5]

This is a common condition in the elderly, usually male, subject in whom there is fibrosis of the palmar aponeurosis. This produces a flexion deformity of the fingers at the metacarpophalangeal and proximal interphalangeal joints, usually starting at the ring finger and spreading to the little finger and sometimes the middle finger. As the aponeurosis extends distally only to the base of the middle phalanx, the distal interphalangeal joint escapes. The contracture is often bilateral and may occasionally affect the plantar fascia also.

Volkmann's contracture[6] due to ischaemic fibrosis of flexors of the fingers (see Chapter 12, p. 141)

The fingers will be curled up in the hand with metacarpophalangeal and interphalangeal joint flexion. This deformity can to some extent be relieved by flexion of the wrist when the shortened tendons are no longer so taut and the fingers can be partially extended.

Congenital contracture

This usually affects the little finger and produces very little, if any, disability. The proximal interphalangeal joint is typically affected, the condition is usually bilateral and, of course, it dates from birth.

[5]Baron Guillaume Dupuytren (1777–1835), Surgeon, Hôtel Dieu, Paris, France.
[6]Richard von Volkmann (1830–1889), Professor of Surgery, Halle, Germany.

Mallet finger

This follows trauma (common in cricketers) with flexion deformity of the distal interphalangeal joint due to avulsion of the extensor tendon insertion to the base of the distal phalanx.

Trauma

Scar formation following burns, injury or surgery to the fingers or the palm may produce gross flexion deformities wherever a scar crosses a joint line.

Sciatic nerve injuries

This nerve may be wounded in penetrating injuries or torn in posterior dislocation of the hip associated with fracture of the posterior lip of the acetabulum, to which the nerve is closely related. Injury is followed by paralysis of the hamstrings and all the muscles of the leg and foot; there is loss of all movement below the knee joint with foot drop deformity. Sensory loss is complete below the knee, except for an area extending along the medial side of the leg over the medial malleolus to the base of the hallux, which is innervated by the saphenous branch of the femoral nerve, the longest cutaneous nerve in the body.

Common peroneal nerve injuries

The common peroneal nerve is in a particularly vulnerable position as it winds around the neck of the fibula. It may be injured at this site by direct trauma or compression, such as the pressure of a tight plaster cast, or in severe adduction injuries to the knee. Damage is followed by foot drop (due to paralysis of the ankle and foot extensors) and inversion of the foot (due to paralysis of the peroneal muscles with unopposed action of the foot flexors and invertors). There is anaesthesia over the anterior surface of the leg and foot. The medial side of the foot, innervated by the saphenous branch of the femoral nerve, and the lateral side of the foot, supplied by the sural branch of the tibial nerve, both escape.

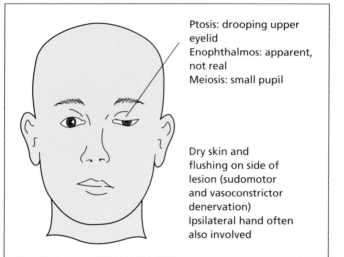

Ptosis: drooping upper eyelid
Enophthalmos: apparent, not real
Meiosis: small pupil

Dry skin and flushing on side of lesion (sudomotor and vasoconstrictor denervation)
Ipsilateral hand often also involved

Figure 17.3 Horner's syndrome.

Lateral cutaneous nerve of the thigh compression: meralgia paraesthetica

The lateral cutaneous nerve of the thigh may be trapped as it emerges beneath the inguinal ligament, a finger's breadth medial to the anterior superior iliac spine. It commonly occurs in overweight middle-aged men and in athletes undergoing physical training. Symptoms comprise painful paraesthesiae over the anterolateral aspect of the thigh, worse on standing and relieved on sitting (hip flexion). Sensation in the distribution of the nerve is diminished.

Cervical sympathetic nerve injuries: Horner's syndrome[7]

If the T1 contribution to the cervical sympathetic chain is damaged, the result is known as Horner's

syndrome (Figure 17.3), in which there are the following characteristics:

- *Meiosis:* paralysis of the dilator pupillae, resulting in constriction of the pupil.
- *Ptosis:* paralysis of the sympathetic muscle fibres transmitted via the oculomotor nerve to the levator palpebrae superioris results in drooping of the upper eyelid.
- *Anhidrosis:* loss of sweating on the affected side of the face and neck.
- *Enophthalmos:* the eye appears sunken within the orbit, an illusion due to the ptosis.

Horner's syndrome may follow operations on, or injuries to, the neck in which the cervical sympathetic trunk is damaged, malignant invasion from lymph nodes or adjacent tumour or spinal cord lesions at the T1 segment (e.g. syringomyelia).

[7]Johann Horner (1831–1886), Professor of Ophthalmology, Zurich, Switzerland.

18

The oral cavity

Learning objectives
✓ To know the common congenital and acquired lesions occurring around the lips and in the oral cavity.
✓ To know the common features of oropharyngeal carcinomas.

It is a useful exercise (and a favourite examination topic) to consider what can be learned by examining a specific anatomical site, such as the fingers, nails or eyes, in making a clinical diagnosis. The mouth and tongue can be conveniently used to illustrate how best to deal with this subject, which can be considered under three headings:

1 *Information about local disease.* Tumours of the mouth and tongue and congenital anomalies are obviously diagnosed by local examination.
2 *Local manifestations of diseases elsewhere.* The smooth tongue of pernicious anaemia, the ulcerated fauces of agranulocytosis or of severe glandular fever, the hemiatrophy of the tongue in hypoglossal nerve palsy, the pigmentation of Addison's disease,[1] the pigmented spots of the Peutz–Jeghers syndrome[2] and the gingivitis, swollen bleeding gums and loosened teeth of vitamin C deficiency are examples of intrabuccal signs of more widespread diseases.
3 *Information given about the general condition and habits of the patient.* The dry tongue of dehydration, the brown dry tongue of uraemia,

[1]Thomas Addison (1773–1860), Physician, Guy's Hospital, London, UK.
[2]Johannes Peutz (1886–1957), Physician, The Hague, The Netherlands. Harold Jeghers (1940–1990), Professor of Medicine, Georgetown University School of Medicine, Washington, DC, and Tufts University Medical School, Boston, MA, USA.

Lecture Notes: General Surgery, 12th edition. © Harold Ellis, Sir Roy Y. Calne and Christopher J. E. Watson. Published 2011 by Blackwell Publishing Ltd.

the coated tongue with foetor oris of acute appendicitis and the typical response of the hypochondriac to the command 'show me your tongue', upon which the patient opens his or her mouth to an extraordinary degree and enables the nethermost recesses of the oral cavity to become exposed.

The lips

Cleft lip and palate

These developmental abnormalities are very common. Cleft lip occurs in 1 in every 750 live births, cleft palate in 1 in every 2000, with half the cases of cleft lip being associated with cleft palate. It is important here, as in all congenital anomalies, to make a careful search for other developmental defects – 10% of patients with clefts have some other malformation.

Embryology

These deformities can only be understood if the embryological development of the face and palate is revised (Figure 18.1).

Around the primitive mouth or stomodaeum the following develop:

• *The frontonasal process*, which projects downwards from the cranium. Two olfactory pits develop in this process, and then rupture into the pharynx to form the nostrils. The frontonasal process forms the nose, the nasal

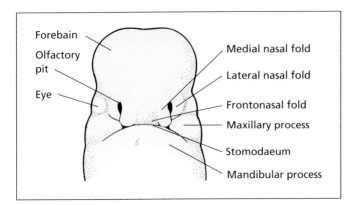

Figure 18.1 The ventral aspect of a fetal head showing the three processes – frontonasal, maxillary and mandibular – from which the face, nose and jaw are derived.

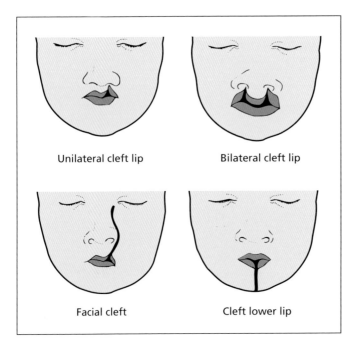

Figure 18.2 Types of cleft lip.

septum, the nostril, the philtrum of the upper lip and the premaxilla; this is the V-shaped anterior portion of the upper jaw, which usually bears the four incisor teeth.
- *The maxillary processes* on either side, which fuse with the frontonasal process to become the cheeks, the upper lip (exclusive of the philtrum), the upper jaw and the palate apart from the premaxilla.
- *The mandibular processes*, which meet in the midline to form the lower jaw.

Cleft lip (Figure 18.2)

This condition was once termed hare lip, but only rarely is the cleft a median one like the upper lip of a hare, although this may occur as a failure of development of the philtrum from the frontonasal process. Much more commonly, the cleft is on one side of the philtrum as a result of failure of fusion of the maxillary and frontonasal process. In 15% of cases, the cleft is bilateral. The cleft may be a small defect in the lip or may extend into the

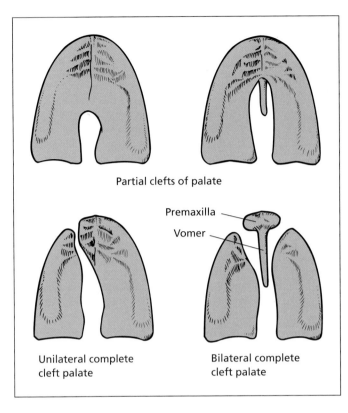

Partial clefts of palate

Premaxilla

Vomer

Unilateral complete
cleft palate

Bilateral complete
cleft palate

Figure 18.3 Types of cleft palate.

nostril, split the alveolus or even extend along the side of the nose as far as the orbit as a very rare anomaly. Associated with the deformity is an invariable flattening and widening of the nostril on the same side.

Cleft of the lower lip occurs very rarely but may be associated with a cleft of the tongue and of the mandible.

Cleft palate

A failure of fusion of the segments of the palate. The following stages may occur (Figure 18.3):

- *Bifid uvula*, which is of no clinical importance.
- *Partial cleft*, which may involve the soft palate alone or the posterior part of the hard palate also.
- *Complete cleft*, which may be unilateral, running the full length of the maxilla and then alongside one face of the premaxilla, or bilateral, in which the palate is cleft with an anterior V which separates the premaxilla completely. The premaxilla floats forward to produce a hideous deformity.

Principles of management

The details of surgical repair belong to the realms of the specialist plastic surgeon, but the principles underlying management are of importance to the paediatrician and the general practitioner.

Cleft lip alone presents no feeding or nursing problems. Repair is required at an early stage so that normal moulding of the bones of the face may occur during growth. Early repair within a few days of birth is now preferred to the previous practice of waiting 3–6 months.

Cleft palate interferes with the normal suckling mechanism. The infant is fed either by using a spoon or by dripping milk into the mouth from a bottle provided with a large hole in the teat. The defect is repaired at between 6 months and 1 year in order to allow normal speech to develop. If delayed beyond this time, the child will develop bad speech, which will require considerable rehabilitation to restore to normal.

Where both defects coexist, the lip is repaired early (before 10 weeks) and the palate then operated upon at a second stage at the age of about 6 months.

Lesions on the lip

Angular stomatitis

Superficial ulceration at the corners of the mouth. Causes range from iron-deficiency anaemia to habitual licking in children.

Retention cyst

A mucous retention cyst represents an obstructed mucous gland. It appears as a blue, domed, translucent swelling of the buccal aspect of the lower lip.

Herpes simplex (cold sores)

Painful ulceration, which starts as a crop of vesicles near the vermilion border and develops into a crusting ulcer before resolving. The cause is a herpes simplex virus (usually type 1), which remains latent in the nerve ganglion and recurs when triggered by viral infection (hence 'cold sores'), trauma, sunburn or endogenous factors such as menstruation. Recurrence starts with a pricking sensation, followed by lip swelling and the appearance of a cluster of vesicles, which break down to produce painful ulcers. Early topical treatment with aciclovir or famciclovir may curtail the infection and reduce symptoms.

Carcinoma

Ulcerating squamous carcinomas are indurated and have characteristic raised edges. Evidence of regional lymph node involvement should be sought (see p. 149).

Less common lesions include Peutz–Jeghers circumoral pigmentation, which is associated with intestinal hamartomatous polyps, and telangiectasia typical of hereditary haemorrhagic telangiectasia (Osler–Rendu–Weber syndrome[3]), which is associated with intestinal telangiectasia and bleeding.

[3]Sir William Osler (1849–1919), Professor of Medicine, successively at McGill University, Montreal, Canada; Johns Hopkins University, Baltimore, MD, USA; and the University of Oxford, Oxford, UK. Henri Rendu (1844–1902), Physician, Necker Hospital, Paris, France. Frederick Parkes Weber (1863–1962), a London physician with an interest in rare disorders.

Ulcers in the mouth

Traumatic

Usually occurs as a result of a sharp edge of a tooth or a denture, and usually present on the tongue. Healing rapidly takes place when the cause is removed. Nowadays, the ulcer produced on the under-aspect of the tongue as this is rubbed against the lower incisor teeth in whooping cough is rarely seen.

Aphthous ulcer

Recurrent, small, round, white, painful ulcers, which may occur singly or in crops anywhere in the mouth but particularly on the edge of the tongue. The ulcers have a sloughy base and a rim of erythema surrounding them. The cause is unknown. They are particularly common around puberty and occasionally they are associated with inflammatory bowel disease. The ulcer will usually heal rapidly if a hydrocortisone tablet is held against it.

Herpes simplex

Can be extensive in the oropharynx, nose, oesophagus and larynx in patients on immuno-suppressive drugs or infected with human immunodeficiency virus (HIV).

Carcinoma

Carcinoma (see p. 148) and lymphoma may cause intraoral ulceration.

Syphilitic ulcers

Now rarely seen, ulcers were features of the first, second and third stages of syphilis: a chancre in the first, a 'snail-track' ulcer in the second and a midline punched-out gumma in the third. In addition, tertiary syphilis may produce leucoplakia or diffuse fibrosis of the tongue. All these conditions are extremely rare now that early syphilis is efficiently treated.

Other causes of ulceration

Rarer causes of oral ulcers include neutropenia

and agranulocytosis, Behçet's syndrome,[4] Reiter's syndrome,[5] Wegener's granulomatosis[6] and tuberculosis. Some drugs, such as sirolimus and everolimus, may also cause mucosal ulceration.

Other lesions within the mouth

Leucoplakia

Leucoplakia refers to thickened white patches of mucosa. In contrast to *Candida* infection, the lesions cannot be rubbed off. This condition may occur anywhere within the mouth, particularly on the tongue. Other sites are the larynx, the anus and the vulva. The affected area may show cracks or fissures.

Microscopically, there is hyperplasia of the squamous epithelium with hyperkeratosis. It is usually found in middle-aged or elderly subjects. Its aetiology may result from chronic irritation, or may relate to smoking, syphilis, sepsis, spices, sore tooth and spirits – the list of S's – but it must be confessed that often no cause at all can be found.

The importance of the condition is that it is often premalignant. Malignant change especially occurs within the fissures and should be suspected if there is local thickening, pain or bleeding or areas of erythema.

Treatment

Remove any underlying irritant cause. Any area suspicious of malignancy should be biopsied. Superficial areas of leucoplakia are usually satisfactorily treated by excision, with skin grafting if the area is large.

Mucous retention cysts

These result from leakage of mucus due to minor trauma of the mucous glands and are better termed extravasation cysts. They are commonly found on the inside of the lips and inner aspects of the cheek. They are blue in appearance and contain glairy mucoid fluid. Their nuisance value is that they tend to be chewed upon by the patient.

Ranula

A large mucous extravasation cyst on one or the other side of the floor of the mouth arising from a sublingual salivary gland. Often, the submandibular duct can be seen passing over the cyst. The word ranula means a small frog and the lesion is so called because it resembles a frog's belly. Small cysts may be excised; larger cysts are marsupialized.

Midline dermoid

This occupies the floor of the mouth and may project below the chin. It represents a congenital seeding of ectoderm during the process of fusion of the two mandibular processes. Similar inclusion dermoid cysts occur at the outer and inner margins of the orbit (external and internal angular dermoids). Treatment is excision.

Epulis

Epulis is a non-specific term applied to a localized swelling of the gum. This may be:

- *Fibrous:* a nodule of dense fibrous tissue covered by epithelium, which arises from the submucosa of the gum.
- *Giant cell:* with the histological appearance of an osteoclastoma.
- *Granulomatous:* peculiarly likely to occur in pregnancy and probably arises as a result of minor trauma followed by chronic infection.
- *Denture granuloma:* originates from the persistent irritation of an ill-fitting denture.
- *Dental abscess:* while not a true epulis, it initially presents as an acute inflammatory swelling of the mucosa adjacent to the diseased tooth.

Malignant disease of the mouth and pharynx

General features

In broad principles, the pathology, diagnosis and treatment of malignant disease of the lips, tongue,

---

[4]Hulusi Behçet (1889–1948), Professor of Dermatology, Istanbul, Turkey.
[5]Friederich Wegener (1907–1990), German Pathologist.
[6]Hans C. J. Reiter (1881–1969), German Bacteriologist, who described the syndrome in a fellow officer while serving as a doctor in the Great War.

floor of the mouth, gums, inner aspects of the cheek, hard and soft palate, tonsils, fauces and pharynx can be considered as one. Specific features of each site are given in the next section. Common hiding places for oral tumours include the base of the tongue, sulci lateral to the base of the tongue, tonsillar fossa (is one tonsil bigger than the other?) and nasopharynx.

Pathology

Sex distribution

For the most part, oral tumours are more common in men than in women. However, tumours of the hard palate and posterior one-third of the tongue have an equal sex distribution and post-cricoid tumours affect women more often than men.

Predisposing factors

These can be divided into three groups:

1 *Chronic irritation:* the common causes begin with S: smoking, syphilis, sepsis, spices, sore tooth and spirits. Certainly mouth cancer is seen particularly among old men of poor social class with gross dental caries and heavy smoking habits. Especially at risk is the heavy smoker who is also a heavy drinker. In India, betel nut chewing is associated with a high incidence of mouth cancer.
2 *Leucoplakia:* a definite precancerous condition (see p. 147).
3 *Iron deficiency:* the Plummer–Vinson[7] syndrome with smooth tongue, cracks at the angles of the mouth (cheilosis), koilonychia, dysphagia and an iron-deficiency anaemia is often present in oral and pharyngeal cancer in women.

Macroscopic appearance

Macroscopically, malignant tumours of the mouth present as one of three types:

1 a nodule;
2 an ulcer or fissure which feels hard to the palpating finger;
3 a warty or papilliferous growth.

[7]Henry Plummer (1874–1937) and Porter Paisley Vinson (1890–1959), Physicians, Mayo Clinic, Rochester, MN, USA.

Microscopic appearance

Microscopically, by far the commonest tumours are keratinizing squamous cell carcinomas. In addition, two other types may be seen, particularly in the posterior third of the tongue, the tonsil and the nasopharynx. These are as follows:

1 *transitional cell carcinoma,* made up of undifferentiated epithelial cells, which simulate the transitional carcinomas of the urinary tract;
2 *lymphoepithelioma,* comprising sheets of rather anaplastic epithelial cells pervaded with a diffuse lymphocytic infiltration.

It is probable that these variations are merely examples of undifferentiated squamous cell tumours. Tumours may also arise in the minor salivary glands, which are abundantly distributed over the mucous membrane of the mouth.

Spread

They occur by local infiltration, which often transgresses nearby anatomical boundaries. Thus, a carcinoma of the tongue may invade the floor of the mouth, the gum and the fauces. Cervical lymph node involvement is common and is often the presenting feature. Thirty per cent of patients have cervical node involvement at the time of diagnosis. Distant blood-borne spread (e.g. to the lung and liver) is late and relatively uncommon.

Causes of death

Tumours of the mouth and pharynx are particularly horrible in their late stages. The patient becomes cachectic because of difficulty in swallowing and anorexic as a result of the infected, foul-smelling, fungating ulcer within the mouth. As a result of this sepsis, inhalation bronchopneumonia is a common cause of death. Fatal haemorrhage may occur, either from the primary ulcerating growth or from invasion of tumour from cervical lymph nodes into the internal jugular vein or carotid artery.

Special investigations

- *Endoscopy* and examination under anaesthetic to look at the larynx and exclude second primaries, or diagnose the primary in patients presenting with cervical lymphadenopathy.

- *Orthopantomogram (OPG)* may demonstrate bone invasion in tumours arising close to the mandible.
- *Chest X-ray* to exclude the rare pulmonary secondary spread.
- *Computed tomography (CT)* may demonstrate local disease including bone invasion and involvement of the maxillary sinus, and may demonstrate cervical nodal involvement.
- *Magnetic resonance (MR) imaging* has a slightly better resolution than CT.

Principles of treatment

The diagnosis is first confirmed by biopsy. The search for predisposing factors includes syphilis serology and haemoglobin estimation. In every case, treatment must be considered with respect to (1) the primary tumour and (2) the regional lymph nodes.

Management of the primary tumour

The treatment of choice is radiotherapy. When the tumour is readily accessible, e.g. the lip, the anterior part of the tongue and the buccal mucosa, this is conveniently carried out by implantation of radioactive needles. More posteriorly placed tumours are treated by external beam radiotherapy.

With conventional radiotherapy, invasion of the mandible or maxilla by the tumour was a contraindication to treatment because bone necrosis almost invariably took place. In such circumstances, only radical surgery could be offered. Fortunately, modern external beam radiotherapy only infrequently causes radionecrosis so that jaw involvement is no longer a bar to treatment.

Irradiation is abandoned under two circumstances: first, if the tumour proves to be radioresistant, and, second, if recurrence takes place subsequent to satisfactory regression. In these circumstances, it may be necessary to consider radical surgical excision, e.g. a hemiglossectomy or mandibulectomy and block dissection of the cervical nodes in continuity.

Management of the regional lymph nodes

If the lymph nodes are not enlarged, the patient is kept under close regular observation.

If the lymph nodes are enlarged but mobile and obviously operable, block dissection is performed providing the primary tumour is controllable; clearly there is little point in carrying out a radical block dissection of the neck in the presence of a hopelessly inoperable malignant mass within the mouth.

If the lymph nodes are enlarged but are fixed and clinically irremovable, palliative irradiation is given and may be combined with cytotoxic chemotherapy.

Prognosis

The prognosis becomes increasingly worse the further backwards into the mouth the tumour occurs; the outlook is best in tumours of the lip, then of the anterior two-thirds of the tongue, but it is usually grave in tumours of the pharynx and tonsil. As with tumours elsewhere, the prognosis also depends on the degree of differentiation of the tumour on histological examination and on the extent of spread, particularly whether or not the lymph nodes are involved.

Specific features

The local pathological and clinical features at specific sites can now be considered. In every case, the management of the tumour and the regional lymph nodes are as described in the above scheme.

Carcinoma of the lip

Clinical features

This disease commonly affects men (90%), nearly always elderly, and those exposed to a weather-beaten outdoor life associated with sunlight exposure. The lower lip is by far the commonest site, accounting for 93% of the tumours. Five per cent occur on the upper lip and 2% at the angle of the mouth – these last have a particularly bad prognosis. The lesion appears as a fissure, as a typical malignant ulcer or as a warty papilliferous tumour. The majority are slow growing, and spread to the regional lymph nodes is comparatively late: first to the submental, then the submandibular and finally the internal jugular chain of nodes. Distant metastasis is rare.

Differential diagnosis

The differential diagnosis of carcinoma of the lip conveniently sums up the other swellings that may be found in this situation. They are as follows:

- simple papilliferous wart, which may itself be premalignant;
- keratoacanthoma (molluscum sebaceum; see Chapter 9, p. 48);
- haemangioma;
- lymphangioma;
- herpes simplex;
- mucous cyst – this is probably the commonest swelling to be found upon the lip (see p. 147);
- chancre – the lip is the commonest extragenital site for a chancre. Usually, the upper lip is affected; it is accompanied by considerable local oedema and exuberant enlargement of the regional lymph nodes.

Carcinoma of the tongue

Carcinoma of the tongue occurs more commonly in men than in women, affecting older men who drink and smoke excessively. The tumours are conveniently divided into those of the anterior two-thirds and those of the posterior one-third of the tongue.

Clinical features

The tumour itself tends to occur on the lateral border of the tongue, and rarely affects the dorsum.

Anterior tumours commence as a nodule, fissure or ulcer, although occasionally a widely infiltrating type of tumour is seen. At first the lesion is painless but becomes painful as it invades and becomes grossly septic. The pain often radiates to the ear, being referred from the lingual branch of the trigeminal nerve, supplying the tongue, along its auriculotemporal branch. Ulceration is accompanied by bleeding. The typical picture of late disease is an old man sitting in the outpatient department spitting blood into his handkerchief, with a plug of cotton wool in his ear. As the tumour extends onto the floor of the mouth and the alveo-

lus, speech and swallowing become difficult because of fixation of the tongue (ankyloglossia). Palpation is especially valuable. Malignant ulcers in the mouth, as in the rectum, feel hard with surrounding induration.

Lymphatic spread occurs to the submental, submandibular and deep cervical nodes. Unless the primary tumour is situated far laterally on the margin of the tongue, this lymphatic spread may be bilateral.

Posterior third tumours of the tongue are rapidly growing and are of the lymphoepitheliomatous type with early spread bilaterally to the cervical nodes.

Any nodule or chronic ulcer of the tongue must be regarded with great suspicion of malignant disease, particularly if there is any predisposing factor such as leucoplakia.

Differential diagnosis

This is to be made from the other ulcers of the tongue discussed on p. 146, from the comparatively rare benign tumours of the tongue (papilloma, haemangioma, lymphangioma and fibroma) and from the still rarer lingual thyroid which occurs as a midline nodule. More commonly, the nervous patient may suddenly notice a circumvallate papilla on the tongue viewed in the mirror, and may present to the surgeon having decided it is a cancer of the tongue.

Carcinoma of the soft palate and fauces

These tumours usually resemble those of the posterior third of the tongue in their behaviour.

Carcinoma of the hard palate

Tumours in this region are usually warty, spread over the palate and later invade the bone. Differential diagnosis must be made from secondary involvement of the palate from an antral tumour and from mixed salivary tumours, which arise from the small accessory salivary glands scattered over the hard palate.

Carcinoma of the floor of the mouth, alveolus and cheek

Here the tumour is commonly an ulcerating carcinoma, which often involves more than one of these structures; thus, an ulcer is often found wedged in the floor of the mouth extending upwards onto the gum and backwards to involve the root of the tongue. There is early spread to the regional nodes.

In addition, adenomas or adenocarcinomas occasionally arise in the mucous and salivary accessory glands of this region.

Carcinoma of the tonsil

About 85% of the tumours of the tonsil are squamous carcinomas, about 10% are lymphomas arising from the lymphoid tissue of the tonsil and 5% are lymphoepitheliomas, which show rapid lymph node spread.

Carcinoma of the nasopharynx

As elsewhere, the predominant tumour is a squamous carcinoma. In addition, a rapidly growing lymphoepithelioma occurs in younger subjects and for some unexplained reason is particularly common among the Chinese, with a high incidence of raised antibody titres to the Epstein–Barr virus;[8] indeed, in this race, it is second in frequency only to uterine cancer. Rarely, a fibrosarcoma of the nasopharynx arises from the periosteum of the basiocciput.

These tumours may present with nasal obstruction and bleeding, eustachian tube blockage with deafness, involvement of one or more of the cranial nerves and severe deeply situated head-

[8]Michael Anthony Epstein (b. 1921), Professor of Pathology, University of Bristol, Bristol, UK. Yvonne Barr (b. 1932), Epstein's assistant, Middlesex Hospital, London, UK.

ache. Tumours at this site are notoriously difficult to locate even on careful inspection and palpation under anaesthesia. One-third present first as a cervical node mass.

Carcinoma of the oro- and laryngopharynx

Carcinomas at these sites present first with discomfort in the throat, excessive salivation and expectoration of blood-stained mucus, which then becomes foetid. Later, there may be alteration of the voice progressing to hoarseness and then dysphagia. Often, however, these tumours present with enlarged cervical lymph nodes.

The hypopharyngeal tumours (post-cricoid carcinoma) are almost always confined to women, many of whom present features of the Plummer–Vinson syndrome (see Chapter 20, p. 162). Diagnosis is confirmed by oesophagoscopic examination and biopsy.

Tumours of the jaw

Tumours of the jaw are of extremely wide pathological variety because they may arise from the bone of the jaw itself, from the tissues over the surface of the jaw or, in the case of the maxilla, from the mucosa lining the maxillary antrum.

Tumours of the bone

These may originate from any of the histological structures forming the bone, e.g. osteoma or osteogenic sarcoma from the bone itself, chondroma and chondrosarcoma from the cartilage, osteoclastoma from the osteoclasts, myeloma from the marrow cells, haemangioma from the blood vessels and fibrosarcoma from the periosteum. In addition to this, the jaw is the occasional site for secondary deposits, the common sources of which are lung, breast, prostate, thyroid and kidney.

Ameloblastoma (adamantinoma)

This is an interesting benign tumour, which is derived from the epithelial cells of the enamel organ. Its histological appearance resembles these cells arranged in clumps within a fibrous stroma. Gradual destruction of the jaw takes place but the tumour metastasizes only rarely. It is multilocular, and usually involves the lower jaw towards its angle. Any age may be affected, but the majority present in the second and third decades with equal sex distribution.

Surface tumours

Carcinoma, mixed salivary tumour or rarely melanoma of the palate, gum, cheek or floor of the mouth may invade the underlying bone.

Antral tumours

Probably the commonest tumour of the upper jaw is the squamous carcinoma arising from the mucous membrane of the maxillary antrum.

The antral carcinoma occurs in middle-aged and elderly subjects with equal sex distribution.

Clinical features

Symptoms and signs are late in manifesting themselves; indeed, the tumour must burst through the bony walls of the antrum before it becomes obvious. Presentation then depends on the direction of growth of the tumour and can be deduced by the application of some knowledge of the anatomy of the region.

Medial extension

Blockage of the ostium of the maxillary antrum with consequent infection of the sinus, or with nasal obstruction and epistaxis.

Lateral extension

Swelling of the face, which often has an inflammatory appearance and may well be mistaken for an acute infection.

Upward extension

Orbital invasion with proptosis, diplopia and lacrimation due to blockage of the tear duct. Anaesthesia of the cheek may result from invasion of the maxillary branch of the trigeminal nerve.

Inferior extension

Bulging and ulceration into the palate. Metastases to the upper jugular lymph nodes occur at a relatively late stage.

Special investigations

- *Skull X-rays* usually reveal decalcification and erosion of the maxilla. There may be opacification of the normally translucent maxillary antrum.
- *CT and MR imaging* are valuable in indicating the exact spread of the tumours.

Treatment

- *Benign tumours* are treated by local excision; in the case of the lower jaw, this may require bone graft to the resected portion of the mandible.
- *Malignant tumours* of the mandible and of the maxillary antrum are treated initially by radiotherapy, followed by hemi-mandibulectomy or maxillectomy.

19

The salivary glands

Learning objective
✓ To know the common inflammatory and malignant conditions of the salivary glands and their treatment.

The salivary glands comprise three paired glands – the parotid, submandibular and sublingual – together with tiny accessory salivary glands scattered over the walls of the buccal cavity. The parotid gland secretes a serous saliva, in contrast to the mucus product of the sublingual glands. The submandibular saliva is seromucus, and represents 75% of the total saliva produced. The parotid and submandibular glands drain into the mouth via long ducts, the parotid (Stensen's[1]) duct opening adjacent to the second upper molar tooth, while the submandibular (Wharton's[2]) duct opens on the floor of the mouth through a papilla at the base of the frenulum of the tongue. Their orifices are easily visible in your own mouth and saliva will be seen to flow if you press on the glands themselves. The sublingual gland's mucus secretion drains by a series of very short ducts into the floor of the mouth.

The two principal surgical conditions of the salivary glands are inflammation, with or without calculus, and neoplasm. The nature of the glandular cells determines the saliva's composition, explaining the different incidence of these conditions in each of the salivary glands.

[1]Niels Stensen (1638–1686), Professor of Anatomy, University of Copenhagen, Denmark. Gave up his Chair in 1669 to become a Bishop.
[2]Thomas Wharton (1614–1673), Physician, St Thomas's Hospital, London, UK.

Lecture Notes: General Surgery, 12th edition. © Harold Ellis, Sir Roy Y. Calne and Christopher J. E. Watson. Published 2011 by Blackwell Publishing Ltd.

Inflammation

Aetiology

- *Calculus*, usually affecting the submandibular gland (see below).
- *Mumps*, usually affects the parotid, rarely the submandibular gland.
- *Acute bacterial infection* usually occurs postoperatively and involves the parotid.
- *Chronic recurrent sialadenitis*, usually occurs in the parotid.
- *Mikulicz's syndrome*: involving all the salivary and the lacrimal glands.

Mumps

A viral infection (incubation period 17–21 days), which is common in children and affects the parotid glands; it is usually bilateral. Rarely the submandibular or sublingual glands may be involved. Most children are now immunized against mumps before starting school.

Mumps may present to the surgeon in the following ways:

- *Acute parotitis:* usual in childhood but may occasionally occur as a painful parotid swelling in an adult (Boxes 19.1 and 19.2).
- *Mumps orchitis:* usually presents in adolescents or young adults, and rare before puberty. Pain and swelling in the testicle occur 7–10 days after the onset of the parotitis and may lead to testicular atrophy. If bilateral orchitis occurs, there may be sterility or

eunuchoidism. Very rarely the orchitis occurs without prodromal parotitis.
- *Pancreatitis, mastitis, thyroiditis or oöphoritis* are also rarely caused by mumps.

Acute bacterial parotitis

Ascending infection of the parotid gland via its duct may occur after major surgical procedures. Aetiological factors include dental sepsis, dehydration, prolonged presence of a nasogastric tube and poor oral hygiene. This complication may also occur in any severe debilitating illness and in uraemia. The infection is usually streptococcal (*Streptococcus viridans* or *S. pneumoniae*) and occasionally staphylococcal.

Clinical features

Clinically, there is swelling and intense pain in one or both parotid glands, which are hard, enlarged and tender, often with associated trismus (masseter spasm). There may be a purulent discharge from the duct. Abscess formation occasionally occurs.

Treatment

Prophylaxis is important. Adequate hydration with elimination of the above aetiological factors has rendered this complication rare nowadays. In the established case, the patient must be kept fully hydrated and the flow of saliva encouraged by sucking sweets or chewing gum. Parenteral antibiotic therapy is commenced. Occasionally, surgical drainage is required.

Chronic recurrent parotid sialadenitis

Repeated episodes of pain and swelling in one or both parotids is not uncommon and is caused by a combination of obstruction and infection of the gland. There may be an associated dilatation of the duct system and alveoli of the gland, termed sialectasia (which resembles bronchiectasis in the lung), associated with a stricture of the duct or a stone. These changes are best demonstrated by performing a *sialogram*.

Treatment

An associated stricture is treated by dilatation or surgical enlargement, and if stones are present these must be removed. Massage of the gland several times a day, and the use of sialogogues (such as 'acid drops') encourage drainage. Occasionally, in severe and refractory cases, excision of the gland with preservation of the facial nerve is required.

Mikulicz's syndrome[3]

Mikulicz's syndrome is characterized by enlargement of the salivary and lacrimal glands, and is associated with dry eyes, leading to conjunctivokeratitis, and dry mouth (xerostomia). It may occur in the following conditions:

- sarcoid (commonest);
- lymphoma, particularly non-Hodgkin's lymphoma;
- tuberculosis;
- Sjögren's syndrome[4], principally affecting middle-aged women and associated with connective tissue disorders such as rheumatoid arthritis and systemic lupus erythematosus.

Calculi

Stone formation is common in the submandibular gland and its duct, rare in the parotid and unknown in the sublingual. The different composition of the saliva from each gland probably explains this difference. Stasis of the more viscid secretion of the submandibular gland in its long duct, changes in composition of the saliva, trauma to the duct, infection, stricture and several metabolic diseases such as hyperparathyroidism may predispose to stone formation. The stones themselves consist of calcium phosphate and calcium carbonate, and are therefore radio-opaque.

Clinical features

There is painful swelling of the affected gland, aggravated by food (classically by sucking a lemon) and there may be an unpleasant taste in the mouth due to the purulent discharge. On examination, the obstructed gland is enlarged and tender. The submandibular duct, visible in the floor of the mouth, is red and swollen and the calculus may be visible or palpable on bimanual examination of the duct. Gentle pressure on the gland may produce a purulent exudate from the orifice of the duct.

[3]Jan Mikulicz-Radecki (1850–1905), Professor of Surgery successively at Cracow, Konigsberg and Breslau, Poland. One of the first surgeons to use rubber gloves and to wear a face mask.
[4]Henrik Sjögren (1899–1986), Ophthalmologist, Gothenburg, Sweden.

Special investigations

- *X-rays* invariably confirm the presence of the stone.
- A *Sialogram*, in which contrast material is injected into the duct, may be necessary if no stone is visible. This may reveal stenosis of the ostium of the duct, which mimics the symptoms of a stone, or sialectasis.

Treatment

If the stone lies within the submandibular duct, it can be removed from within the mouth, with the duct being marsupialized at the site of extraction. If one or more stones are impacted in the gland substance, excision of the whole gland is required.

Salivary tumours

Classification

Benign

- Pleomorphic adenoma (mixed salivary tumour).
- Adenolymphoma.

Malignant

- *Primary:* carcinoma.
- *Secondary:* direct invasion from skin or from secondarily involved lymph nodes.

Pleomorphic adenoma

Ninety per cent occur in the parotid, although occasionally they are found in the submandibular, sublingual or accessory salivary glands. Ninety per cent present before the age of 50 years, although any age may be affected. Sex distribution is equal.

Pathology

Macroscopic appearance

The tumour is lobulated and lies within a false capsule of compressed salivary tissue. The cut surface is glistening and translucent; the consistency is crumbly.

Microscopic appearance

The tumours vary across a spectrum from a typical adenoma to a frank carcinoma. The majority show glandular acini within a blue-staining stroma, which gives the appearance of a cartilage but which is, in fact, mucus. The appearance of epithelial cells and 'cartilage' gave rise to the older concept of a 'mixed tumour'.

Surgical considerations

If treated by enucleation, at least 25% of the tumours recur, because:

- the capsule surrounding the tumour is a false one, which itself is incomplete and may contain tumour cells;
- serial sections show that the tumour often has 'amoeboid' processes, which may be left behind; and
- implantation of tumour cells may occur into the wound.

Although slow growing, these tumours cannot be considered benign because of the lack of encapsulation, the occasional wide infiltration of surrounding tissues and the tendency to recur. Moreover, the less differentiated tumours, which are extremely difficult to distinguish from frank carcinoma, may metastasize to the regional lymph nodes and distantly via the bloodstream.

Clinical features

The patient presents with a slow-growing swelling anywhere within the parotid gland, but usually in the lower pole and in the region of the angle of the jaw. The lump is well defined, usually firm or hard but sometimes cystic in consistency. It is usually placed in the superficial part of the gland but may occasionally be in its deep prolongation and indeed may project into the pharynx. The facial nerve is never involved, except by frankly malignant tumours. Its integrity should be confirmed.

Treatment

Wide excision of the tumour and the surrounding parotid tissue, with careful preservation of the fibres of the facial nerve (superficial parotidectomy). Where the tumour involves one of the other salivary glands, complete excision of the gland is performed.

Prognosis

Providing the tumour is completely excised, the prognosis is excellent but inadequate surgery is followed by a recurrence in a high percentage of cases.

Adenolymphoma

Adenolymphoma (Warthin's tumour[5]) accounts for about 10% of parotid tumours, and is very rare elsewhere. Adenolymphomas usually occur in men over the age of 50 years, and are occasionally bilateral.

Macroscopically, the tumour is soft and cystic. Microscopically, it consists of columnar cells forming papillary fringes, which project into cystic spaces and which are supported by a lymphoid stroma. These tumours probably arise from the salivary duct epithelium, the lymphoid tissue originating from the lymphoid aggregates that are present in the normal parotid gland. Presence of the lymphoid tissue may lead to confusion with lymphoproliferative disorders. Prognosis is excellent after local removal.

Carcinoma

Clinical features

Again this usually affects the parotid. Sex distribution is equal, and the patients are usually over the age of 50 years. The tumour is hard and infiltrating. Clinically, the diagnosis is based on rapid growth, pain and involvement of the facial nerve and regional lymph nodes. Eventually, surrounding tissues are infiltrated and the overlying skin becomes ulcerated.

Microscopically, most tumours are adenocarcinomas, rapidly progressive with a high incidence of metastasis to regional lymph nodes. A small proportion represent malignant change in slow-growing pleomorphic adenomas.

Treatment

When the tumour lies in the parotid, radical

---

[5]Aldred Scott Warthin (1866–1931), Professor of Pathology, University of Michigan, Ann Arbor, MI, USA.

parotidectomy is performed with sacrifice of the facial nerve. This is combined if necessary with block dissection of the regional lymph nodes if these are involved, and is followed by radiotherapy. When the tumour arises in the other sites of salivary tissue, wide local excision is performed, again with block dissection if this is indicated by the presence of enlarged but mobile lymph nodes.

The prognosis is not good for this tumour, particularly when the submandibular gland is the site of origin.

20

The oesophagus

Learning objectives

✓ To know the common causes of dysphagia.
✓ To know the presentation and management of oesophageal carcinoma.

Dysphagia

Dysphagia is difficulty in swallowing. The causes may be local or general. The local causes of obstruction of any tube in the body can be subdivided into those in the lumen, those in the wall and those outside the wall.

Local causes

In the lumen

- Foreign body.

In the wall

- Congenital atresia.
- Inflammatory stricture, secondary to reflux oesophagitis.
- Caustic stricture.
- Achalasia.
- Plummer–Vinson syndrome with oesophageal web.
- Pharyngeal pouch.
- Schatzki ring.[1]
- Tumour of oesophagus or cardia.
- Systemic sclerosis (scleroderma).

Outside the wall

- Pressure of enlarged lymph nodes (secondary cancer or lymphoma).
- Thoracic aortic aneurysm.
- Bronchial carcinoma.
- Retrosternal goitre.

General causes

- Myasthenia gravis.
- Bulbar palsy.
- Bulbar poliomyelitis.
- Diphtheria.
- Hysteria.

Investigation

History

The subjective site of obstruction is not always exact; the patient often merely points vaguely to behind the sternum. The diagnosis may be given by a history of swallowed caustic in the past. A previous story of reflux oesophagitis suggests peptic stricture. Patients with achalasia tend to be young and the history is often long, usually without loss of weight.

Malignant stricture has a short history, occurs usually in elderly people and is associated with severe weight loss.

Examination

Often this is negative, but search is made for clinical evidence of Plummer–Vinson syndrome (a smooth tongue, anaemia and koilonychia, see

---

[1]Richard Schatzki (1901–1992), Radiologist, Boston, MA, USA. Described a circumferential ring of mucosal tissue in the distal oesophagus.

Lecture Notes: General Surgery, 12th edition. © Harold Ellis, Sir Roy Y. Calne and Christopher J. E. Watson. Published 2011 by Blackwell Publishing Ltd.

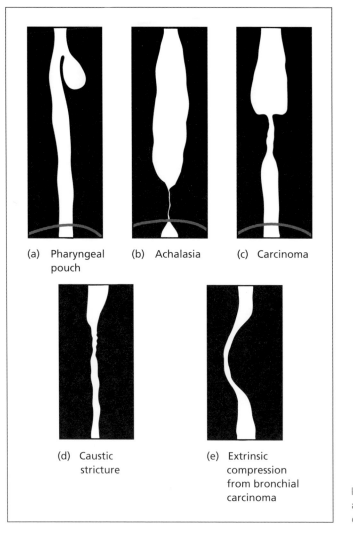

(a) Pharyngeal pouch (b) Achalasia (c) Carcinoma

(d) Caustic stricture (e) Extrinsic compression from bronchial carcinoma

Figure 20.1 (a–e) Barium swallow appearances of common causes of dysphagia.

p. 164), secondary nodes from a carcinoma of the oesophagus which may be felt in the neck and supraclavicular fossae, and the upper abdomen is carefully palpated, as a carcinoma of the cardia is a common cause of dysphagia in elderly patients and indeed is more common in this country than carcinoma of the oesophagus.

Special investigations

- *Fibreoptic oesophagoscopy* enables biopsies to be taken to confirm malignancy, and permits therapeutic dilatation or intubation if indicated.

- *Barium swallow*, with cine-radiography, may demonstrate the characteristic appearances of a cervical web, extrinsic compression and the dilated oesophagus of achalasia (Figure 20.1).

The investigations are complementary and both may be indicated.

Swallowed foreign bodies

Foreign bodies are swallowed either accidentally, usually by children, or deliberately by mentally disturbed people, prison inmates and circus sideshow performers. A recent phenomenon is the 'body-packer', a smuggler who swallows condoms packed with cocaine or heroin. These may present with bowel obstruction, or may rupture producing coma or death from absorption of the drug.

Obstruction of the oropharynx and tracheal opening by a large portion of meat can rapidly become fatal. A sharp blow just below the xiphoid, Heimlich's manoeuvre,[2] causing a sudden rise in intra-abdominal pressure, may dislodge the plug and save the patient's life.

Unless they are sharp or irregular, amazingly large foreign bodies will pass into the stomach. If a smooth object such as a bolus of food impacts in the oesophagus, one must suspect the presence of a stricture. Occasionally a carcinoma of the oesophagus presents as an acute dysphagia when a morsel of food lodges above it. Absolute dysphagia, with failure to swallow even saliva, is then characteristic.

The presenting feature is painful dysphagia. The danger depends on the nature of the foreign body. Perforation may occur with resultant mediastinitis; rarely, perforation of the aorta occurs with fatal haematemesis. The diagnosis may be confirmed by a plain X-ray if the foreign body is radio-opaque; otherwise, it may be shown up on a barium swallow.

Treatment

Oesophagoscopic removal is indicated when the foreign body is stuck in the oesophagus. Occasionally, oesophagotomy is required. The great majority of foreign bodies, once they have passed into the stomach, proceed uneventfully along the alimentary canal and are passed per rectum. Occasionally, a sharp foreign body penetrates the wall of the bowel (there is a particular tendency for it to lodge in, and pierce, a Meckel's diverticulum; see Chapter 23, p. 194).

The treatment of a foreign body that has passed the cardia is initially conservative. The patient is watched and serial X-rays taken to observe the object's progress if it is radio-opaque. Operation is performed if a sharp object fails to progress or if abdominal pain or tenderness develop.

If the foreign body is potentially toxic when ingested, emetics or laxatives may be indicated.

[2]Henry J. Heimlich (b. 1920), Thoracic Surgeon, Xavier University, Cincinnati, OH, USA.

Perforations of the oesophagus

Classification

From within

- Swallowed foreign body – may occur anywhere in the oesophagus.
- Rupture at oesophagoscopy – usually at the level of cricopharyngeus or above a stricture.
- Rupture during dilatation or biopsy – usually at the lower end of the oesophagus and especially likely in the presence of oesophageal disease (carcinoma or stricture).
- Rupture during oesophageal echocardiography – again usually at the lower end, often in the presence of a hitherto unknown stricture.

From without

- Perforating wounds (rare).

Spontaneous

- Lower thoracic oesophagus (Boerhaave's syndrome[3]).

Clinical features

After instrumentation, perforation is suspected if the patient complains of pain in the neck, chest or upper abdomen, together with dysphagia and pyrexia. Diagnosis is certain if subcutaneous emphysema is felt in the supraclavicular area.

Spontaneous rupture of the oesophagus occurs rarely and is associated with vomiting after a large meal (Boerhaave's syndrome). There is severe pain in the chest, the dorsal region of the spine or the upper abdomen (acute mediastinitis). The patient is collapsed and cyanosed. The abdomen may be rigid and often a false diagnosis of perforated peptic ulcer or myocardial infarction is made. Surgical emphysema (subcutaneous crepitation) is usually palpable in the neck owing to gas escaping into the mediastinum.

[3]Hermann Boerhaave (1668–1738), Physician, Leiden, The Netherlands. Diagnosed spontaneous rupture of the oesophagus at post-mortem on the Grand Admiral of the Dutch Fleet.

Special investigations

- *Chest X-ray* shows gas in the neck and mediastinum and there may be fluid and gas in the pleural cavity.
- *Thoracoabdominal computed tomography (CT)*, combined with oral gastrograffin (a water-soluble contrast fluid), will confirm the perforation and define its position.

Treatment

Cervical perforation is managed conservatively with parenteral antibiotics, nil by mouth and intravenous drip. Abscess formation in the superior mediastinum requires drainage via a supraclavicular incision.

Thoracic rupture is treated by immediate suture (or resection if a carcinoma is instrumentally perforated). The prognosis from spontaneous rupture is inversely related to the time to surgery, and after 12 hours is very poor.

Caustic stricture of the oesophagus

This follows accidental or suicidal ingestion of strong acids or alkalis (particularly caustic soda and ammonia). It often occurs in children.

In the acute phase, there are associated burns of the mouth and pharynx. The mid- and lower oesophagus are usually affected, as these are the sites of temporary hold-up of the caustic material where the oesophagus is crossed by the aortic arch and at the cardiac sphincter.

Treatment

In the acute phase treatment aims to neutralize the cause, so alkali ingestion with vinegar and acid with bicarbonate of soda. The damaged oesophagus is rested by instituting feeding via a gastrostomy, nil being given by mouth. Systemic steroids are given to reduce scar formation. If a stricture develops, gentle dilatation with bougies is commenced after 3 or 4 weeks. An established, impassable stricture is treated by a bypass operation, a loop of colon or small bowel being brought up on its vascular pedicle between the stomach below and the upper oesophagus above.

Achalasia of the cardia

This is a neuromuscular failure of relaxation at the lower end of the oesophagus with progressive dilatation, tortuosity, incoordination of peristalsis and often hypertrophy of the oesophagus above.

Clinical features

Achalasia may occur at any age but particularly in the third decade. The ratio of women to men is 3:2. It is indistinguishable from Chagas' disease,[4] which occurs in South America secondary to *Trypanosoma cruzi* infection. The parasite destroys the intermuscular ganglion cells of the oesophagus.

There is progressive dysphagia over months to years, sometimes associated with a spasm-like chest pain. Regurgitation of fluids from the dilated oesophageal sac may be followed by an aspiration pneumonia. Occasionally, malignant change occurs in the dilated oesophagus.

Special investigations

- *Chest X-ray* may reveal the dilated oesophagus as a mediastinal mass, with an air–fluid level, and pneumonitis from aspiration of oesophageal contents. (Note that there are three other 'pseudotumours': scoliosis, tuberculous paravertebral abscess and thoracic aortic aneurysm, all of which may simulate a mediastinal tumour on a chest X-ray – Chapter 10, p. 67.)
- *Barium swallow* shows gross dilatation and tortuosity of the oesophagus leading to an unrelaxing narrowed segment at the lower end (said to resemble a bird's beak) (Figure 20.1).
- *Oesophagoscopy* demonstrates an enormous sac of oesophagus containing a pond of stagnant food and fluid.
- *Oesophageal manometry* confirms increased lower oesophageal sphincter pressure.

Treatment

Satisfactory results are obtained by Heller's operation,[5] which is a cardiomyotomy dividing the muscle of the lower end of the oesophagus and the

[4]Carlos Chagas (1879–1934), Professor of Tropical Medicine, Rio de Janeiro, Brazil.
[5]Ernst Heller (1877–1964), Surgeon, Leipzig, Germany.

upper stomach down to the mucosa in a similar manner to Ramstedt's operation (see Chapter 21, p. 168) for congenital pyloric hypertrophy. This procedure is best performed laparoscopically, thus reducing morbidity.

The same effect may be achieved by forcible dilatation of the oesophagogastric junction by means of an endoscopic balloon that is inflated under fluoroscopic (X-ray) control. Although this avoids open operation, it is accompanied by the risk of rupture of the oesophagus. A newer alternative involves endoscopic injection of botulinum toxin (Botox) to paralyse the lower oesophageal sphincter, a treatment that gives relief in many patients and which may last for a year.

Plummer–Vinson syndrome[6]

A syndrome actually described by Paterson and Kelly before Plummer and Vinson, and which sometimes rejoices in all four names, comprising dysphagia and iron-deficiency anaemia (with its associated smooth tongue and koilonychia – spoon-shaped nails) usually in middle-aged or elderly women.

The dysphagia is associated with hyperkeratinization of the oesophagus and often with the formation of a web in the upper part of the oesophagus. The condition is premalignant and is associated with the development of a carcinoma in the cricopharyngeal region.

Treatment

The dysphagia responds to treatment with iron, although the web may require dilatation through an oesophagoscope.

Oesophageal diverticula

The only common diverticulum of the gullet is the pharyngeal pouch.

Pharyngeal pouch

This is a mucosal protrusion between the two parts of the inferior pharyngeal constrictor – the thyropharyngeus and cricopharyngeus (Figure 20.2). The weak area between these portions of the muscle is situated posteriorly (Killian's dehiscence[7]). The pouch is believed to originate above the cricopharyngeus muscle which is in spasm; it develops first posteriorly but cannot then expand in this direction and protrudes to one or the other side, usually the left. As the pouch enlarges, it displaces the oesophagus laterally. It is an example of a pulsion diverticulum, forming as a result of increased intraluminal pressure.

Clinical features

It occurs more often in men and usually in the elderly. There is dysphagia, regurgitation of the food that has collected in the pouch, and often a palpable swelling in the neck, which gurgles. Food retained in the pouch leads to a foetor, and late regurgitation may lead to aspiration pneumonia and lung abscess. Diagnosis is confirmed by a barium swallow.

Treatment

Traditional surgery involved a cervical incision with excision of the pouch combined with a posterior myotomy of the cricopharyngeus. Alternatively, the pouch can be treated by division of the wall between pouch and oesophagus using an endoscopic stapling device (endoscopic diverticulotomy), leaving the pouch *in situ* and avoiding the risk of fistula formation and leaks associated with the open operation.

Other oesophageal diverticula

Other oesophageal diverticula are very rare.

- *Traction diverticula* may occur in association with fixation to tuberculous nodes or to pleural adhesions.
- *Pulsion diverticula* may be associated with cardiospasm and occur at the lower end of the oesophagus.

[6]Henry Strong Plummer (1874–1937), Physician, Mayo Clinic, Rochester, MN, USA. Porter Paisley Vinson (1890–1959), Physician, Mayo Clinic, Rochester, MN, USA. Donald Ross Paterson (1863–1939), ENT Surgeon, Royal Infirmary, Cardiff, UK. Adam Brown-Kelly (1865–1914), ENT Surgeon, Victoria Infirmary, Glasgow, UK.

[7]Gustav Killian (1860–1921), Professor of Otorhinolaryngology, Freiburg and Berlin, Germany.

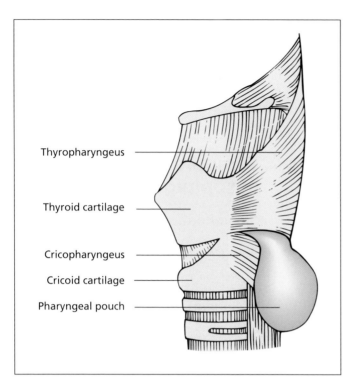

Thyropharyngeus

Thyroid cartilage

Cricopharyngeus

Cricoid cartilage

Pharyngeal pouch

Figure 20.2 A pharyngeal pouch emerging between the two components of the inferior constrictor muscle.

- *Congenital diverticula* are occasionally found. These are usually X-ray findings only, although they may occasionally produce dysphagia.

Reflux oesophagitis

This is produced by the reflux of peptic juice through the incompetent cardiac sphincter into the lower oesophagus, resulting in ulceration and inflammation and eventually in stricture formation. The exact mechanism of the cardio-oesophageal sphincter is not understood; it is sufficient to prevent regurgitation into the oesophagus when standing on one's head or in forced inspiration, when there is a pressure difference of some 80 mmHg between the intragastric and intraoesophageal pressure, yet it can relax readily to allow vomiting or belching to occur. The mechanism is probably a complex affair comprising the following:

- positive intra-abdominal pressure acting on the lower (intra-abdominal) oesophagus, maintaining a high-pressure zone at the cardia;

- physiological muscle sphincter at the lower end of the oesophagus;
- valve-like effect of the obliquity of the oesophagogastric angle;
- pinch-cock effect on the lower oesophagus of the diaphragmatic sling when the diaphragm contracts in full inspiration;
- plug-like action of the mucosal folds at the cardia.

The diaphragm is an important but not essential part of the cardiac sphincter mechanism, as sliding hiatus hernias are not necessarily accompanied by regurgitation. Similarly, free regurgitation occurs in some subjects with a normal oesophageal hiatus, presumably because of some defect in the function of the physiological sphincter.

Reflux oesophagitis may also occur in association with the following:

- repeated vomiting, especially in the presence of a duodenal ulcer with high acid content of gastric juice;
- long-standing nasogastric intubation;
- resections of the cardia with gastro-oesophageal anastomosis;

- the presence of ectopic acid-secreting gastric mucosa within the oesophagus ('Barrett's oesophagus', see p. 166).

Special investigations

- *Fibreoptic oesophagoscopy* demonstrates the presence of oesophagitis, and facilitates biopsy to exclude carcinoma, or the presence of gastric-type epithelium.
- *24 hour oesophageal pH studies*: a probe in the oesophagus will demonstrate reflux of gastric acid and its temporal relation to pain.
- *Barium swallow*: this will demonstrate the outline of a hernia and the presence of any associated stricture. Tilting the patient head down will demonstrate reflux, but does not necessarily confirm that the pain is due to reflux.

Differential diagnosis

The pain of oesophagitis may be confused with cholecystitis, peptic ulcer or angina pectoris; indeed, these conditions often coexist.

The obstructive symptoms of an associated stricture must be differentiated from carcinoma of the oesophagus or of the cardia.

Treatment

Medical treatment comprises weight loss, stopping smoking and dietary manipulation. Regurgitation is discouraged by avoiding stooping or lying and by sleeping propped up in bed. Alginate antacids (e.g. Gaviscon) taken after meals neutralize the acidity as well as line the gullet. H$_2$-receptor antagonist drugs (e.g. cimetidine or ranitidine) and proton pump inhibitors (e.g. omeprazole) provide more complete reduction in gastric acidity. Prokinetic drugs to increase gastric emptying, such as metoclopramide, may also be useful. Many patients with mild symptoms obtain considerable relief from such regimens.

Laparoscopic repair of the hernia is undertaken when medical treatment fails. This may be supplemented by fundoplication in which the fundus of the stomach is sutured around the lower oesophagus in an inkwell fashion in order to produce an anti-reflux valve.

In the presence of *stricture*, surgical treatment is indicated. In a mild case, continuous acid reduction treatment with a proton pump inhibitor (e.g. omeprazole) and endoscopic balloon dilata-tion will provide good palliation, with repeat dilatation every year or so. Anti-reflux surgery to repair the hernia in younger patients combined with preoperative dilatation may also give good long-term palliation. In the advanced case, where frequent dilatation is required or is unsuccessful, resection of the stricture may be necessary.

Tumours of the oesophagus

Classification

Benign

- Leiomyoma.

Malignant

- Primary:
  - carcinoma;
  - leiomyosarcoma.
- Secondary: direct invasion from lung or stomach.

Carcinoma

Post-cricoid carcinoma usually occurs in women and is associated with the Plummer–Vinson syndrome (see p. 162). The remaining oesophageal growths occur more often in men, usually elderly men. The commonest site has changed in recent years, with distal tumours becoming more common than tumours of the mid-third, with upper oesophageal tumours being least common.

Risk factors for oesophageal carcinoma include tobacco and alcohol, with squamous carcinoma also being linked to achalasia and coeliac disease; adenocarcinoma may occur in association with Barrett's oesophagus as a consequence of metaplastic change at the gastro-oesophageal junction.

Carcinoma of the oesophagus is a relatively common tumour in the UK (12 per 100000 incidence), but is 20 times more common in China, and twice as common in France. The incidence is rising in the Western world. The overall prognosis is less than 10% survival at 3 years.

Pathology

The tumour commences as a nodule, which then develops into an ulcer, a papilliferous mass or an annular constriction.

Microscopically, the majority are now adeno-carcinomas arising at the lower end of the oesophagus, either in gastric metaplasia (Barrett's oesophagus) or as a result of an invasion of the oesophagus from a tumour developing at the cardiac end of the stomach. Tumours of the upper two-thirds are usually squamous carcinomas.

Spread

- *Local:* into the mediastinal structures – the trachea, aorta, mediastinal pleura and lung.
- *Lymphatic:* to para-oesophageal, tracheobronchial, supraclavicular and subdiaphragmatic nodes.
- *Bloodstream:* to liver and lungs (relatively late).

Clinical features

Carcinoma of the oesophagus may present because of the following:

- *local symptoms* – dysphagia;
- *secondary deposits* – enlarged neck nodes, occasionally jaundice and/or hepatomegaly;
- *general manifestations of malignant disease* – loss of weight, anorexia, anaemia.

Dysphagia in an elderly male with a short history is almost invariably due to carcinoma of the oesophagus or the upper end of the stomach. Progression is from dysphagia for solids to dys-phagia for liquids. Hoarseness and a bovine cough suggest invasion of the left recurrent laryngeal nerve by an upper oesophageal tumour.

Special investigations

The purpose of these investigations is to confirm the diagnosis and to assess extent (stage) of disease.

- *Oesophagoscopy* enables the tumour to be inspected and a biopsy taken. This may be combined with endoluminal ultrasound to evaluate local invasion.
- *CT* of the thorax and abdomen to assess the primary growth, local invasion and secondary spread to the liver and lymph nodes.
- *Endoscopic ultrasound* enables assessment of the tumour's depth of invasion and detection of local and lymphatic spread; it also facilitates fine needle aspiration of lymph nodes to facilitate preoperative staging.
- *Positron emission tomography (PET),* in conjunction with CT, may also be used to screen for metastatic disease and stage the tumour.
- *Laparoscopy* may be indicated to exclude peritoneal metastases prior to resection.

Differential diagnosis

Other causes of dysphagia (p. 158).

Treatment

The two treatment aims are to cure the cancer when possible, and to palliate the dysphagia. The treatment options are curative resection and pal-liative intubation or laser.

Curative resection

When cure is possible, resection is undertaken fol-lowing a course of chemotherapy. The growth is removed and the defect is usually bridged by mobilizing the stomach up into the chest, with anastomosis to residual oesophagus or to the pharynx in the neck. Even with successful resec-tion, survival is poor.

Palliation

- *Intubation* with a stent may relieve dysphagia if the tumour is inoperable.
- *Endoscopic laser therapy* may vaporize the growth and restore the lumen. Repeated courses may be necessary, but disease progression rapidly overtakes the patient.
- *Radiotherapy,* either external beam or intraluminal, is useful for squamous tumours.
- *Chemotherapy,* particularly with a platinum-based regimen, has shown increasing promise when combined with radiotherapy.

The average expectation of life is in the region of 3 months with a maximum survival of about 1 year, but at least the patient is spared the misery of total dysphagia.

Barrett's oesophagus[8] and adenocarcinoma

This is an increasingly common condition with an estimated prevalence of about 2% of adults in the UK. The normal oesophagus is lined by stratified squamous epithelium. In patients with long-standing reflux of duodenogastric contents, the lower oesophageal epithelium undergoes metaplasia to an intestinal-type columnar epithelium. Continued inflammation may lead to dysplasia and subsequently to malignant change.

Carcinomas in such cases are adenocarcinomas, and most occur in the lower third of the oesophagus or at the gastro-oesophageal junction. They are commonest in male smokers, with a long history (over 10 years) of Barrett's metaplasia and frequent symptoms (more than three times a week) of gastro-oesphageal reflux.

As metaplasia to a Barrett-type oesophagus is premalignant, such patients should undergo regular endoscopic surveillance, with biopsies to look for dysplasia. Severe dysplasia (carcinoma *in situ*) is an indication for endoscopic treatment or resection.

[8]Norman Barrett (1903–79), Thoracic Surgeon, St Thomas's Hospital, London, UK.

The stomach and duodenum

Congenital hypertrophic pyloric stenosis

Aetiology

The aetiology of the pyloric muscle 'tumour' in pyloric obstruction in infants is unknown. It may result from an abnormality of the ganglion cells of the myenteric plexus; failure of the pyloric sphincter to relax may then produce an intense work hypertrophy of the adjacent circular pyloric muscle.

It is a familial condition; 80% of cases occur in male infants; 50% are first-born; and the condition often occurs in siblings.

Clinical features

The child usually presents at 3–4 weeks old, although symptoms may be present, rarely, at or soon after birth. It is extremely uncommon for a previously healthy infant to develop this condition after 12 weeks old.

The presenting symptom is projectile vomiting. The vomit does not contain bile and the child takes food avidly immediately after vomiting, i.e. it is always hungry. There is failure to gain weight and, as a result of dehydration, the baby is constipated (the stools resembling the faecal pellets of a rabbit).

The infant may be dehydrated and visible peristalsis of the dilated stomach may be seen in the epigastrium. Ninety-five per cent of infants have a palpable pyloric tumour, which is felt as a firm 'bobbin' in the right upper abdomen, especially after vomiting a feed.

Differential diagnosis

- *Enteritis:* diarrhoea accompanies this.
- *Neonatal intestinal obstruction* from duodenal atresia, volvulus neonatorum or intestinal atresia: symptoms commence within a day or two of birth and the vomit contains bile.
- *Intracranial birth injury.*
- *Overfeeding:* here there are no other features to suggest pyloric stenosis apart from vomiting.

Special investigations

If the clinical features are characteristic and a pyloric mass is palpable, no further investigations are necessary.

Lecture Notes: General Surgery, 12th edition. © Harold Ellis, Sir Roy Y. Calne and Christopher J. E. Watson. Published 2011 by Blackwell Publishing Ltd.

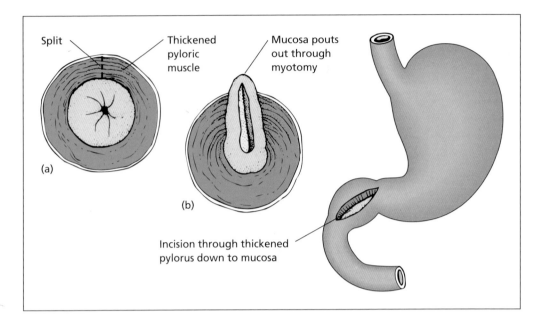

Figure 21.1 Ramstedt's pyloromyotomy. The thickened muscle at the pylorus is split down to the mucosa. (a and b) The pathology and the operative procedure in transverse section.

- *Ultrasound scan* demonstrates the thickened pylorus and large stomach.
- *Abdominal X-ray* reveals a dilated stomach with minimal gas in the bowel, in contrast to dilated coils of bowel in intestinal obstruction.
- *Barium meal* reveals the pyloric obstruction with characteristic shouldering of the pyloric antrum due to the impression made on it by the hypertrophied pyloric muscle. However, this investigation is rarely called for.

Treatment

This is anomalous in that the more seriously ill the child, the less urgent is the operation. With prolonged vomiting, the infant becomes dehydrated with a hypochloraemic metabolic alkalosis. In such cases, a day or two must be spent in gastric lavage and fluid replacement (saline with added potassium chloride), by either the subcutaneous or intravenous route. The otherwise healthy child can be submitted to operation soon after admission.

Surgical treatment

Ramstedt's pyloromyotomy[1]

A longitudinal incision is made through the hypertrophied muscle of the pylorus down to mucosa and the cut edges are separated (Figure 21.1). This is now commonly performed laparoscopically. The infant is given glucose water 3 hours after the operation and this is followed by 3 hourly milk feeds, which are steadily increased in amount.

Results are excellent and the mortality is extremely low.

Duodenal atresia

Duodenal atresia may be partial or complete, and principally affects the second part of the duodenum near the ampulla of Vater. An annular pancreas may be present (Chapter 32, p. 276).

[1]Conrad Ramstedt (1867–1963), Surgeon, Munster, Germany.

Clinical features

Antenatally, the diagnosis is suggested by the presence of polyhydramnios and ultrasound appearances. Vomiting occurs from birth and the stomach may be visibly distended. As the common bile duct usually enters above the obstruction, the vomit usually contains bile.

There is a strong association between duodenal atresia and Down syndrome, with 30% of neonates with duodenal atresia having trisomy 21.

Differential diagnosis

- *Oesophageal atresia:* there is choking rather than vomiting.
- *Pyloric stenosis:* bile is absent from the vomit, there is a palpable pyloric tumour and onset is later.
- *Congenital intestinal obstruction:* there is abdominal distension and X-rays show multiple distended loops of bowel with fluid levels (Chapter 22, p. 185).

Plain X-ray of the abdomen is diagnostic and shows distension of the stomach and proximal duodenum with absence of gas throughout the rest of the bowel (the 'double bubble' sign).

Treatment

Duodenojejunostomy or gastrojejunostomy is performed after rehydration and gastric aspiration.

Peptic ulcer

Pathology

The pathogenesis of peptic ulcer involves a disturbance in the balance between the secretion of acid and pepsin by the stomach on the one hand and the mucosal barrier (a thick layer of mucus) on the other. The normal stomach mucosa is adapted to contain the acid produced by the parietal (oxyntic) cells. Where the mucosal defence is compromised, or non-existent, the acid causes mucosal ulceration. Ulcers also occur where acid attacks mucosa not specialized to deal with it. Hence, typical sites for peptic ulcers are the oesophagus (peptic oesophagitis), stomach, first part of duodenum, at the stoma of a gastrojejunal anastomosis or adjacent to a Meckel's diverticulum[2] when ectopic parietal cells are present.

Aetiology

Historical background

The vast majority of peptic ulcers are caused by infection with *Helicobacter pylori*. Until the publication of the link between this organism and ulcers in 1983, the majority of peptic ulcers were thought to be due to overactivity of the gastric parietal cells. The stimuli to parietal cell function are neural (via the vagus nerve) and humoral (gastrin and histamine). Earlier treatments were therefore directed at reducing acid secretion by surgical denervation of the stomach (vagotomy) or removal of the parietal cells (partial gastrectomy). More recently, pharmacological control has been possible with histamine H_2-receptor antagonists (e.g. cimetidine and ranitidine), and proton pump inhibitors (e.g. omeprazole). With hindsight, we now realize that none of these treatments dealt with the most important cause of the peptic ulceration, *H. pylori*.

Helicobacter pylori

H. pylori (previously called *Campylobacter pyloridis*) is a spiral-shaped, Gram-negative, motile rod that is able to penetrate the viscid mucus layer lining the stomach. Its potent urease activity splits any urea in the vicinity, producing ammonia and thus neutralizing the pH in the local milieu surrounding the organism. Many *H. pylori* strains also produce cytotoxins that possess protease and phospholipase activity, allowing them to attack and damage mucosal membranes. This direct damage, together with the resultant inflammation, impairs the gastric mucosal barrier and allows further damage by gastric acid. Non-cytotoxin-producing strains explain asymptomatic carriage of the organism.

Evidence identifying *H. pylori* as a causative agent in peptic ulceration includes the following observations:

- Ingestion of *H. pylori* results in chronic gastritis (as demonstrated Barry Marshall, who

[2]Johann Frederick Meckel (1781–1833), Professor of Anatomy and Surgery, Halle, Germany. His grandfather and father were both Professor of Anatomy.

with Robin Warren[3] identified the relationship between infection with the organism and peptic ulceration, and proved it by inoculating himself).

- Animal inoculation with *H. pylori* mimics human gastritis.
- Antimicrobial treatment which eradicates *H. pylori* also eliminates gastritis.
- *H. pylori* can be identified in almost all patients with duodenal ulcers, and most patients with gastric ulcers.

Zollinger–Ellison syndrome[4]

This is a syndrome in which a non-insulin-secreting islet cell tumour of the pancreas produces a potent gastrin-like hormone (Chapter 32, p. 284). It is an uncommon cause of peptic ulceration. In this syndrome, the ulcers are often multiple, and ulceration may be more widespread within the small bowel.

Other factors in the aetiology of peptic ulceration

A number of other factors decrease the effectiveness of the mucosal defences against gastric juice. In particular, non-steroidal anti-inflammatory drugs (NSAIDs) inhibit the production of protective prostaglandins in the mucosa. Steroids also predispose to ulceration, as do smoking and stress, which are thought to have an effect on both acid secretion and mucosal defences.

The acute peptic ulcer

This may be single or multiple (multiple erosions), may occur without apparent cause or may be associated with ingestion of alcohol or NSAIDs (aspirin is a common culprit), steroid therapy, acute stress, a major operation, head injury (Cushing's ulcer[5]) or severe burns (Curling's ulcer[6]). It may present with sudden pain, haemorrhage or perforation. A proportion of acute ulcers probably go on to become chronic.

The chronic peptic ulcer

At least 80% of peptic ulcers occur in the duodenum. Duodenal ulcers may occur at any age, but especially in the thirties to forties; about 80% occur in men. Women are relatively immune to duodenal ulceration before menopause and especially during pregnancy.

Gastric ulcers occur predominantly in men, but the sex preponderance is less marked – about 3:1 for men to women. Any age may be affected, but especially the forties to fifties (i.e. a decade later than the peak for duodenal ulceration).

Clinical features

Physical signs in the uncomplicated case are absent or confined to epigastric tenderness. Clinical diagnosis depends on the careful history.

The pain is typically epigastric, occurs in attacks that last for days or weeks and is interspersed with periods of relief. Pain that radiates into the back suggests a posterior penetrating ulcer. Peptic ulcer pain may come on immediately after a meal but more typically commences about 2 hours after, so that the patient says it precedes a meal ('hunger pain'). Characteristically, it wakes the patient in the early morning, so much so that the patient may adopt the habit of taking a glass of milk or an alkali preparation to bed. However, it is a myth to say that one can differentiate between a gastric and a duodenal ulcer merely on the time relationship of the pain. The pain is aggravated by spicy foods and relieved by milk and alkalis, although the relief is lost in deep and penetrating ulcers. There may be associated heartburn, nausea and vomiting. The patient may lose weight because of the pain produced by food but often may gain weight because of the high intake of milk.

[3]Barry Marshall (b. 1951), Gastroenterologist, Royal Perth Hospital, Australia. J. Robin Warren (b. 1937), Pathologist, Royal Perth Hospital, Australia. Won Nobel Prize for their observation in 2005. Spiral-shaped organisms were identified in stomach biopsies in 1875, and their relation to gastritis suggested in 1899 by Walery Jaworski, a Polish physician; the observation was largely overlooked until the work of Marshall and Warren in 1982.
[4]Robert Milton Zollinger (1903–1992), Professor of Surgery, Ohio State University, Columbus, OH, USA. Edwin Homer Ellison (1918–1970), Associate Professor at the same institution.

[5]Harvey Cushing (1869–1939), Professor of Surgery, Harvard Medical School, Boston, MA, USA.
[6]Thomas Blizzard Curling (1811–88), Surgeon, The London Hospital, London, UK.

Special investigations

- *Fibreoptic endoscopy:* enables the oesophagus, stomach and duodenum to be examined. The ulcer can be identified and, particularly in the case of a gastric lesion, biopsy material obtained to enable differentiation between a benign and malignant ulcer.
- H. pylori *detection.*
  - *Endoscopic biopsy.* Histological examination will confirm the presence of the organism and identify mucosal damage. A urease test, in which a biopsy sample is placed in a solution of urea together with a pH indicator, is highly specific and sensitive for the organism. *H. pylori* splits urea, releasing ammonia, which changes the pH of the solution.
  - *^{13}C-labelled urea breath test.* The patient ingests a solution containing ^{13}C-labelled urea (non-radioactive). The urease from the organism cleaves the urea load and bicarbonate (HCO_3^-) is released into the blood and expired as $^{13}CO_2$. Measurement of labelled CO_2 in breath samples taken before and after ingestion of the urea solution confirms the diagnosis, and serial tests can be used to confirm eradication of the organism.
  - *Serological testing.* Infection with *H. pylori* results in generation of antibodies, which may be detected. Antibody titre falls slowly after eradication.
- *Barium meals* are seldom performed nowadays to diagnose ulcers.
- *Faecal occult blood examination* is often positive in the presence of an ulcer.

Treatment

Treatment of a peptic ulcer is medical in the first instance; surgery is indicated when complications supervene. The complications are chronicity, perforation, stenosis, haemorrhage and, in the case of gastric ulcer, malignant change. They are considered in detail later in this chapter.

Principles of medical treatment

The main principles of treatment are to eradicate *H. pylori* and to reduce and neutralize (using alkalis and milk) acid secretion. Failure to eradicate *H. pylori* by giving antacid therapy alone results in high relapse rates.

- H. pylori *eradication.* A 2 week course of antimicrobial therapy combined with acid reduction therapy will eradicate *H. pylori*. Acid reduction is usually afforded by a proton pump inhibitor (e.g. omeprazole, lanzoprazole) and the antimicrobial therapy is based on either clarithromycin or amoxicillin, together with metronidazole. The combination of two antibiotics is recommended because of the high incidence of antibiotic resistance. Such protocols will eradicate *H. pylori* in over 90% of patients.
- *Acid reduction.* Acid reduction with a proton pump inhibitor such as omeprazole (or less commonly a H_2 receptor blocker such as ranitidine) alone results in the majority of ulcers healing within 1–2 months; the ulcers will recur if *H. pylori* has not been eradicated.

Violent gastric acid stimulants such as alcohol should be avoided. Rest, sedation, avoidance of smoking and dealing with underlying anxiety states are helpful. Aspirin and other NSAIDs should be avoided wherever possible.

Principles of surgical treatment

Surgical treatment is now reserved for those patients in whom complications of ulceration occur. In the emergency situation, minimal surgery is practised with the confidence that medical cure of the underlying disease may be effected. The commonest indications for emergency surgery are bleeding or perforation (see below).

- *Gastric ulcers* are treated by removing the ulcer together with the gastrin-secreting zone of the antrum. Traditionally, this was done by the Billroth I gastrectomy[7] (Figure 21.2), but is now more commonly achieved by an antrectomy combined with a Roux-en-Y gastroenterostomy, the latter to limit bile reflux.
- *Duodenal ulcers* will heal providing the high acid production of the stomach is abolished. This can be effected by removing the bulk of the acid-secreting area of the stomach (the body and the lesser curve), and re-establishing gastric drainage via a Roux-en-Y

[7]Theodor Billroth (1829–94), Professor of Surgery, Vienna, Austria. He performed the first successful gastrectomy for cancer at the pyloric end of the stomach in 1881.

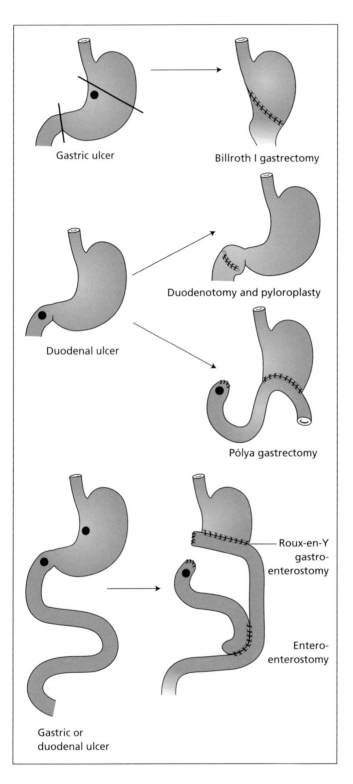

Gastric ulcer

Billroth I gastrectomy

Duodenal ulcer

Duodenotomy and pyloroplasty

Pólya gastrectomy

Gastric or
duodenal ulcer

Roux-en-Y
gastro-
enterostomy

Entero-
enterostomy

Figure 21.2 The principal operations once commonly performed for peptic ulcer. Surgery is still indicated in the presence of haemorrhage from an ulcer, and usually comprises a partial gastrectomy with drainage into a Roux-en-Y loop of jejunum. The more traditional procedures are also shown here: for a gastric ulcer a Billroth I gastrectomy with gastroduodenal anastomosis was performed; for a duodenal ulcer, a simple longitudinal duodenotomy, closed as a pyloroplasty, with under-running of the bleeding vessel was performed, combined with acid suppression with a proton pump inhibitor (instead of the traditional vagotomy); a Pólya gastrectomy with under-running of the vessel was an alternative. Eradication of *Helicobacter pylori* should be undertaken when necessary. For gastric cancer, a gastrectomy with Roux-en-Y drainage is now preferred.

gastroenterostomy. The traditional procedures involved a partial (Pólya[8]) gastrectomy with closure of the duodenum and a gastrojejunostomy, or division of the vagus nerves. As total vagotomy interferes with the mechanism of gastric emptying, this operation must be accompanied by a drainage procedure, either gastrojejunostomy or pyloroplasty. If the branches of the vagus that supply the pyloric sphincter (the nerves of Latarjet[9]) are left intact, the remaining vagal fibres can be divided without the necessity of gastric drainage (highly selective vagotomy), but nevertheless the goal of reduction in the vagal phase of acid secretion is achieved.

- *Postgastrectomy syndromes.* Even though about 85% of patients are well following Pólya partial gastrectomy for peptic ulcer, a large number of unpleasant sequelae may occur. These may be classified into the following:
  - *Small stomach syndrome:* a feeling of fullness after a moderate-sized meal.
  - *Bilious vomiting* due to emptying of the afferent loop of a Pólya gastrectomy into the stomach remnant.
  - *Anaemia* due usually to iron deficiency (HCl is required for adequate iron absorption) or, occasionally, vitamin B12 deficiency owing to loss of intrinsic factor with extensive gastric resection.
  - *Dumping:* comprises attacks of fainting, vertigo and sweating after food, rather like a hypoglycaemic attack. This is probably an osmotic effect due to gastric contents of high osmolarity passing rapidly into the jejunum, absorbing fluid into the gut lumen and producing a temporary reduction in circulating blood volume.
  - *Steatorrhoea.* In the presence of a long afferent loop, food passing into the jejunum traverses the bowel without mixing adequately with pancreatic and biliary secretions. Calcium deficiency and osteomalacia may occur.
  - *Stomal ulceration* complicates about 2% of gastrectomies for duodenal ulcer; it is extremely rare after resection for gastric ulcer. It may be due to inadequate removal

of the acid-secreting area of the stomach or, rarely, because of the Zollinger–Ellison syndrome (Chapter 32, p. 284). A stomal ulcer, like any other peptic ulcer, may perforate, stenose, invade surrounding structures or bleed. It is treated by either vagotomy or higher gastric resection.

- *Postvagotomy syndromes.* The following sequelae may occur after truncal vagotomy:
  - *Steatorrhoea and diarrhoea.* Frequently transient or episodic, they may be severe and persistent in about 2% of patients. The incidence is reduced in patients subjected to highly selective vagotomy without drainage.
  - *Stomal ulceration* may occur if vagotomy is incomplete.

Complications of peptic ulceration

Peptic ulcer at any site may undergo the following complications:

- *perforation* either into the peritoneal cavity or into adjacent structures, e.g. the pancreas, liver or colon;
- *stenosis*;
- *haemorrhage*;
- *chronicity* due to formation of fibrous tissue in the ulcer base;
- *malignant change* which does not occur in duodenal ulcers but may rarely take place in a gastric ulcer; a long history does not necessarily mean that the ulcer was not malignant *de novo*. Both gastric ulcer and gastric carcinoma are common conditions and there may merely be a chance association between the two. It would seem that about 1% of all gastric carcinomas arise in a gastric ulcer.

Perforated peptic ulcer

Pathology

Perforation of a peptic ulcer is a relatively common and important emergency. The incidence of perforation fell steadily from the 1950s (i.e. before the introduction of the H_2-receptor antagonists), but has been relatively constant for the past 10 years. Male preponderance, once very high, is now about 2:1. Until recently, perforation occurred particularly in young adults, but now the shift is towards

---

[8]Eugen Alexander Pólya (1876–1944), Surgeon, St. Stephen's Hospital, Budapest, Hungary.
[9]André Latarjet (1876–1947), Professor of Anatomy, Lyon, France.

the older age groups, especially in patients who are on either steroids or NSAIDs (aspirin, indometacin, etc.).

Gastric carcinomas may occasionally present with perforation.

Clinical features

A previous history of peptic ulceration is obtained in about half the cases, although this may be forgotten by the patient in agony. Typically, the pain is of sudden onset and of extreme severity; indeed, the patient can often recall the exact moment of the onset of the pain. Subphrenic irritation may be indicated by referred pain to one or both shoulders, usually the right. The pain is aggravated by movement and the patient lies rigidly still. There is nausea, but only occasionally vomiting. Sometimes, there is accompanying haematemesis or melaena.

Examination reveals a patient in severe pain, cold and sweating with rapid, shallow respirations. In the early stages (hours), there may be no clinical evidence of true shock: the pulse is steady and the blood pressure normal; the temperature is either normal or a little depressed. The abdomen is rigid and silent, although in some instances an occasional bowel sound may be heard. Liver dullness is diminished in about half the cases owing to escape of gas into the peritoneal cavity. Rectal examination may reveal pelvic tenderness.

In the delayed case, after 12 hours or more, the features of generalized peritonitis with paralytic ileus become manifest; the abdomen is distended, effortless vomiting occurs and the patient is extremely toxic and in oligaemic shock.

Special investigations

- *Chest X-ray*, with the patient erect, shows free gas below the diaphragm in over 70% of cases.
- *Computed tomography (CT)* is more sensitive in the detection of free intraperitoneal gas, and can exclude common differential diagnoses such as pancreatitis when doubt exists.

Differential diagnosis

The four conditions with which perforated ulcer is most commonly confused are the following:

- perforated appendicitis;
- acute cholecystitis;
- acute pancreatitis;
- myocardial infarction.

Treatment

A nasogastric tube is passed to empty the stomach and diminish further leakage. It is an essential preanaesthetic measure. Opiate analgesia is given to relieve pain and an intravenous fluid resuscitation is started. Antibiotics are given to contend with the peritoneal infection, and an intravenous H_2-blocker or proton pump inhibitor commenced. Most surgeons are in favour of immediate operative repair of the perforation.

Surgery involves suturing an omental plug to seal the perforation, together with lavage of the peritoneal cavity. In addition, a gastric ulcer is biopsied at all four quadrants to exclude malignancy. An obviously malignant gastric ulcer is removed by partial gastrectomy (see p. 182). Definitive ulcer treatment at the time of emergency surgery is now uncommon, and medical control of acid secretion together with *H. pylori* eradication is undertaken postoperatively. A definitive procedure may be indicated when medical therapy has failed.

Prognosis

The mortality for perforated peptic ulcer lies between 5% and 10%. Most deaths are in patients incorrectly diagnosed, with consequent delay in correct treatment, or in those who are too ill for operation. The subjects who die are typically either over the age of 70 years or reach hospital 12 hours or more from the time of perforation.

The late prognosis following perforation depends on whether or not the ulcer is chronic, and whether a treatable cause, such *as H. pylori* or NSAIDs, is present. Some patients may come to further surgery.

Pyloric stenosis

This is an inaccurate term when applied to duodenal ulceration, as the obstruction is in the first part of the duodenum.

Pathology

At first, fibrotic scarring is compensated by dilatation and hypertrophy of the stomach muscle.

Eventually, failure of compensation occurs, much like the failure of a hypertrophied ventricle of the heart with valvular stenosis.

Clinical features

During the phase of compensation, there is nothing in the history to suggest stenosis. Once failure occurs, there is characteristic profuse vomiting, which is free from bile. The vomitus may contain food eaten 1–2 days previously and appear and smell faeculent. Because of copious vomiting, there is associated loss of weight, constipation (because of dehydration) and weakness because of electrolyte disturbance.

On examination, the patient may appear dehydrated and wasted. The progressive dilatation and hypertrophy of the stomach can be summed up as 'the stomach you can hear, the stomach you can hear and see, and the stomach you can hear, see and feel'. At first, a gastric splash (*succussion splash*) can be elicited by shaking the patient's abdomen several hours after a meal. As the stomach enlarges, visible peristalsis can also be seen, passing from left to right across the upper abdomen. Finally, the grossly dilated, hypertrophied stomach, full of stale food and fluid, can actually be palpated.

Gastric aspiration yields a morning resting juice of over 100 mL. In advanced cases, it may amount to several litres of foul-smelling gastric contents.

Special investigations

- *Gastroscopy* following decompression of the stomach with a nasogastric tube will identify the cause in most cases.
- *CT scan* will provide further anatomical information about the diagnosis and its aetiology.
- *Arterial blood gases and electrolyte estimation* may show a hypochloraemic alkalosis, with hypokalaemia and uraemia (see below).

Biochemical disturbances

Pyloric obstruction with copious vomiting results in not only dehydration from fluid loss but also alkalosis due to loss of hydrogen ions from the stomach. The alkalotic tendency is compensated by the renal excretion of sodium bicarbonate, which may keep the blood pH within normal limits. During this phase, the dehydration results in diminished volume and increased concentration of urine, the chloride content of which is first diminished and then disappears and the pH of which is alkaline. If vomiting continues, a large sodium deficit becomes manifest. This loss of sodium is partly accounted for by loss in the vomitus but it is mainly the result of urinary excretion consequent upon the bicarbonate lost in the urine as sodium bicarbonate. As the body's sodium reserves become depleted, hydrogen and potassium ions are substituted for sodium as the cations that are excreted with the bicarbonate. This results in the paradox that the patient with advanced alkalosis now excretes an acid urine. The blood urea rises, partly because of dehydration and partly because of renal impairment secondary to the electrolyte disturbances. Eventually, the patient may develop tetany as a result of a shift of the ionized, weakly alkaline calcium phosphate to its unionized state, in attempted compensation for the alkalosis. The concentration of calcium ions in the plasma therefore falls, although the total calcium concentration is not affected.

The metabolic disturbances may be summarized as follows:

- The patient is dehydrated and the haematocrit level is raised.
- The urine is scanty, concentrated, initially alkaline, but later acid; the chloride content of the urine is reduced or absent.
- Serum chloride, sodium and potassium are lowered and the plasma bicarbonate and urea are raised.

Differential diagnosis

- Carcinoma of the pylorus.

Other causes of pyloric obstruction are unusual in the adult:

- scarring associated with a benign gastric ulcer near the pylorus;
- carcinoma of the head of the pancreas infiltrating the duodenum and pylorus;
- chronic pancreatitis;
- invasion of the pylorus by malignant nodes.

The differential diagnosis from a pyloric carcinoma cannot always be established until endoscopy and biopsy, or even laparotomy, but a reasonable attempt can be made on the following points:

- *Length of history:* a history of several years of characteristic peptic ulcer pain is in favour of benign ulcer. Cancer usually has a history of only months and indeed may be painless.
- *Gross dilatation of the stomach* favours a benign lesion, as it may take several years for this to develop.
- *The presence of a mass* at the pylorus indicates malignant disease, although, rarely, a palpable inflammatory mass in association with a large duodenal ulcer can be detected.

Treatment

The treatment of established pyloric obstruction is invariably surgical. Before operation, dehydration and electrolyte depletion are corrected by intravenous replacement of saline together with potassium. Daily gastric lavage is performed to remove the debris from the stomach. In addition, this often restores function to the stomach and allows fluid absorption to take place by mouth. Vitamin C is given, as the patient with a chronic duodenal ulcer is often deficient in ascorbic acid. This may be a direct effect of *H. pylori* or it may be the result of a diet low in fruit and vegetables.

Surgical correction is carried out after a few days of preoperative preparation. Surgery usually involves an antrectomy with a Roux-en-Y gastroenterostomy.

Gastrointestinal haemorrhage

Management

The management of patients presenting with haematemesis and/or melaena is threefold:

1 assessment and resuscitation of the patient;
2 diagnosis of the source of the bleeding;
3 treatment and control of the source of bleeding.

Assessment of the patient

An initial appraisal of the patient's airway and breathing are undertaken; oxygen is administered when necessary. Indicators of severe blood loss are the features of shock, namely pallor, cold, clammy and peripherally shut down, with a tachy-cardia and a systolic blood pressure below 100 mmHg. It should be remembered that patients on beta-blockers tend not to become tachycardic, and if the patient is known to have hypertension a systolic pressure well above 100 mmHg does not rule out shock.

The presence of shock is an indication for immediate fluid replacement with normal saline or compound sodium lactate solution; at the same time, blood should be taken for cross-matching. Additional evidence of significant bleeding is a marked difference between lying and standing blood pressure (postural hypotension) and a low central venous pressure. Every patient presenting with gastrointestinal haemorrhage should have blood taken for grouping and cross-matching.

Direct inspection of the amount of blood vomited and melaena passed will generally under-estimate losses; however, it may help to distinguish old from recent bleeding. The haemoglobin estimation on admission is of only limited value, as it may be more than 24 hours before haemodilution will reduce the haemoglobin level from its normal value.

Once resuscitation is under way, a further history should be taken to establish the possible aetiology of the bleeding.

Aetiology

In considering the aetiology of the bleeding both general and local causes should be borne in mind.

Local causes of bleeding are best considered anatomically, as follows.

1 Oesophagus:
   a reflux oesophagitis (associated with hiatus hernia);
   b oesophageal varices (associated with portal hypertension, Chapter 30, p. 259);
   c peptic ulcer;
   d tumours (benign and malignant).
2 Stomach:
   a gastric ulcer;
   b acute erosions (small ulcers <5 mm; associated with aspirin, other NSAIDs and corticosteroids);
   c gastritis (generalized inflammation, appearing as red dots through the endoscope);
   d Mallory–Weiss syndrome (see below);

e vascular malformation, (e.g. Dieulafoy[10] lesion);

f tumours (benign and malignant).

3 Duodenum:

  a duodenitis;

  b duodenal ulcer;

  c erosion of the duodenum by a pancreatic tumour;

  d aortoduodenal fistula, in patients with previous aortic graft.

4 Small intestine:

  a tumours;

  b Meckel's diverticulum;

  c angiodysplasia;

  d aortoenteric fistula.

5 Large bowel:

  a tumours (benign and malignant, commonly adenocarcinomas);

  b diverticulitis;

  c angiodysplasia;

  d colitis (ulcerative colitis, ischaemic colitis and infective colitis).

General causes of bleeding include haemophilia, leukaemia, anticoagulant therapy and thrombocytopenia. While it is accepted that general bleeding diatheses do not cause bleeding by themselves, they alter the course of bleeding from a local lesion.

Hereditary haemorrhagic telangiectasia is an inherited condition characterized by numerous mucosal arteriovenous malformations, any of which may cause bleeding; the common presentation is, however, with nose bleeds.

About 55% of patients in the UK with upper gastrointestinal bleeding of an acute form have a peptic ulcer or erosion of the stomach or duodenum. About 5% of patients have oesophageal varices, and the remainder are accounted for by the other causes listed above.

Diagnosis is made on history, examination and special investigations.

History

There may be a typical story of peptic ulceration (see p. 170) with epigastric pain and often a history of a previous positive endoscopy. It is important to take a history of drug habits, as many obscure bleeds are found to be due to recent ingestion of aspirin, clopidogrel, anticoagulants, steroids, NSAIDs etc. A story of alcoholism or previous viral hepatitis may suggest cirrhosis, and an alcoholic binge may also have precipitated an acute gastric erosion or gastritis. Repeated violent vomits after a large meal or alcohol followed by a bright red haematemesis is typical of the Mallory–Weiss syndrome,[11] in which a mucosal tear at the gastrooesophageal junction may result in brisk haemorrhage.

Clinical examination

This is usually negative apart from the clinical features that enable assessment of blood loss. It is important to note the following:

- *purpura*, suggesting a bleeding tendency;
- *features of cirrhosis* (enlargement of the liver and spleen, the presence of spider naevi, jaundice and liver palms) suggesting oesophageal varices;
- *circumoral telangiectasia* suggesting hereditary haemorrhagic telangiectasia.

Special investigations

- *Haemoglobin estimation.* Useful as a baseline, it will not reflect acute blood loss until the circulating volume is restored. Until then, the haemoglobin concentration is unchanged.
- *Serum urea.* This is usually raised following upper gastrointestinal bleeding, so it is helpful in distinguishing upper from lower gastrointestinal bleeding.
- *Coagulation screen and platelet count.* An early assessment of any underlying bleeding tendency is essential, and should stimulate treatment if abnormal.
- *Liver function tests* may identify an underlying liver disease.
- *Upper gastrointestinal fibreoptic endoscopy*, viewing the oesophagus, stomach and duodenum, is the most valuable investigation, and should be carried out as an emergency as soon as the patient has been resuscitated and stabilized. It will usually identify the exact site of the bleeding in upper gastrointestinal haemorrhage.

[10]George Kenneth Mallory (1900–1986), Professor of Pathology, Boston University, Boston, MA, USA. Soma Weiss (1898–1942), Professor of Medicine, Harvard University, Boston, MA, USA.

[11]Santiago Ramóny Cajal (1852–1934), Histologist and Professor, successively in Valencia, Barcelona and Madrid, Spain. Awarded the Nobel Prize in 1906 with Golgi for studies of the neurone.

Most actively bleeding peptic ulcers can be treated endoscopically by injection of adrenaline (epinephrine) into and around the vessels in the ulcer bed; dual modality treatment is superior to injection alone, and other modalities include coagulation with a heater probe or placement of a clip directly onto the bleeding vessel. Bleeding oesophageal varices can be treated by band ligation.

If upper gastrointestinal endoscopy fails to detect a source for the blood loss, the following may be considered:

- *Colonoscopy* is performed to identify colonic sources of bleeding, particularly the presence of angiodysplasia in the right colon.
- *Technetium scan*, in a child or young adult, will identify the presence of ectopic gastric mucosa in a Meckel's diverticulum. Gastric mucosa takes up technetium, which is then detected by scintigraphy.
- *Selective visceral angiography* using a catheter inserted via the femoral artery into the mesenteric arteries may localize the source of haemorrhage in an obscure case, but usually only in the presence of significant active bleeding.
- *Red cell scintigraphy* using radiolabelled red cells to identify the site of bleeding. More sensitive than angiography but poorer at localization of the bleeding source.
- *Capsule endoscopy*, which uses a small capsule containing a camera that takes pictures as it traverses the gastrointestinal tract; this is not useful in acute haemorrhage. Its role is in identifying lesions in the small bowel that are not accessible by fibreoptic endoscope.
- *Laparotomy and on-table enteroscopy* is required rarely when bleeding continues and upper and lower gastrointestinal endoscopy are unproductive. An enterotomy is made at laparotomy through which an endoscope is passed and guided throughout the entire small bowel, seeking an obscure cause of bleeding such as an arteriovenous malformation.

Treatment

In the first instance this is on medical lines.

1 The patient is reassured, and reassurance is supplemented with morphine if the patient is in pain.

2 A careful watch is kept on the patient's general condition, pulse and blood pressure, and urine output.

3 Shock, if present, is treated with fluid replacement including blood transfusion. A central venous catheter is placed after the initial resuscitation to measure central venous pressure and assist in fluid replacement; a urinary catheter is passed to monitor urine output.

4 Intravenous proton pump inhibitor therapy may be considered to reduce acid secretion.

5 Treatment of *H. pylori* should be commenced only once infection is proven in patients with duodenal or gastric ulcers.

6 As soon as active bleeding ceases, patients can commence oral fluids and light diet. Oral anti-ulcer therapy is commenced as soon as possible, and the patient is transferred to a semisolid diet.

Indications for surgery

The mortality of gastrointestinal haemorrhage is in the region of 10%. This is almost confined to patients over the age of 45 years, especially the elderly, who continue to bleed, or in whom bleeding recurs, while in hospital on the above regimen.

1 Clinical features suggesting poor prognosis:
   a age over 60 years;
   b chronic history;
   c relapse on full medical treatment;
   d serious coexisting medical conditions;
   e continued melaena or haematemesis;
   f more than four units of blood transfusion required during resuscitation.

2 Endoscopic features suggesting poor prognosis:
   a active bleeding;
   b visible vessel in the ulcer base;
   c clot adherent to the ulcer;
   d blood in the stomach but the source not identifiable.

In most cases therapeutic endoscopy will be able to control the haemorrhage, although it may require more than one treatment. Indications for surgery are:

1 continued bleeding in spite of adequate endoscopic treatment;

2 torrential bleeding preventing adequate views of the bleeding lesion;

3 rebleeding that cannot be treated endoscopically.

At operation, the source of bleeding is found and controlled. For a chronic gastric ulcer, this usually takes the form of a simple ulcer excision or partial gastrectomy; for duodenal ulceration, pyloroplasty and undersewing of the gastroduodenal artery at the base of the ulcer. In other cases, it may be possible to undersew an acute erosion or bleeding ulcer, particularly in the desperately ill patient who is unfit for gastrectomy.

In most cases, preoperative endoscopy will identify the cause of the haemorrhage. If blood is present in the stomach but the source of haemorrhage is not immediately obvious, the stomach is opened by a gastrotomy, the blood clot evacuated and the bleeding point sought by direct inspection of the gastric and duodenal mucosa.

In patients unfit for laparotomy, angiographic embolization of the bleeding vessel, such as the gastroduodenal artery for a duodenal ulcer, may be effective.

In patients who are treated medically and who settle down, careful assessment is made in the convalescent period. If the presence of a chronic duodenal or gastric ulcer is established, in the absence of *H. pylori*, surgery may be advised as an elective procedure; once a chronic ulcer has bled, subsequent haemorrhages are likely to occur. *H. pylori* eradication therapy should be attempted first when it is found. However, it is now rare for surgery to be required.

The management of haemorrhage from oesophageal varices

This is considered in Chapter 30, p. 261.

Tumours of the stomach

Classification

Benign

1 *Epithelial* – adenoma:
  a single;
  b multiple (gastric polyposis).
2 *Connective tissue*: gastrointestinal stromal tumour.
3 *Vascular*: haemangioma.

Malignant

1 *Primary*:
  a adenocarcinoma;
  b gastrointestinal stromal tumour;
  c lymphoma;
  d Hodgkin's disease.
2 *Secondary*: invasion from adjacent tumours (pancreas or colon).

Gastrointestinal stromal tumours

Pathology

These are uncommon tumours, previously thought to arise from the muscular layer or from nerve cells in the gut wall; in fact, they are now believed to arise from the interstitial cells of Cajal[12] (ICCs), the pacemaker cells of the gastrointestinal tract. ICCs are part of the autonomic nervous system, and when the tumour has the appearance of neural tissue it is often called a gastrointestinal autonomic nervous tumour (GANT). Other tumours may have an appearance more like smooth muscle cells; hence, they were previously thought to be leiomyomas. Gastrointestinal stromal tumours (GISTs) may be malignant or benign, and, although they may occur anywhere in the gastrointestinal tract, they are most common in the stomach, but not infrequent in the rest of the small intestine. They appear as small tumours within the muscular wall, or larger tumours growing out from the bowel wall. Large tumours may outstrip their blood supply and become partly cystic; sometimes, the cyst communicates with the bowel lumen. GISTs typically present with either intestinal bleeding or obstruction; some are found during investigation of non-specific abdominal pain.

Aetiology

The aetiology of GISTs is unclear, but they are associated with type 1 neurofibromatosis in some cases. Typically, patients are over 40 and there is no sex difference in incidence. The pathogenesis is a spontaneous mutation in the *c-kit* gene, which

---

[12]Rudolf Ludwig Karl Virchow (1821–1902), Professor of Pathology in Würzburg and later Berlin, Germany.

codes for a transmembrane receptor (*c-kit*/CD117) for a growth factor called stem cell factor. The *c-kit* mutation results in a continuous signal for cell growth which is mediated via a tyrosine kinase in the intracellular domain of the molecule. Some GISTs arise from mutations in platelet-derived growth factor receptor α (PDGFA); occasional cases demonstrate an inherited predisposition.

Special investigations

- *Endoscopy* usually detects the tumour, which appears as a submucosal polyp and which often has an ulcerated surface.
- *CT* may also identify the presence of a tumour.
- *Endoscopic ultrasound (EUS)* can be used to confirm the nature of the polyp and demonstrates clearly the origin of the polyp from the muscular layer of the stomach wall.
- *Positron emission tomography (PET)* is used both for detection and for staging of the tumours.

Once a tumour is found, diagnosis is by biopsy. Owing to the polyp's submucosal origin, mucosal biopsies are frequently non-diagnostic and confirmation of the diagnosis relies on EUS appearances with or without EUS-guided biopsy. Percutaneous biopsies are undertaken in the presence of metastases, but not undertaken otherwise to avoid the risk of seeding tumour cells along the biopsy track. The presence of c-kit protein (CD117) on the cell surface is almost diagnostic. Most small GISTs (<5 cm) have a low mitotic rate and behave like benign tumours; larger GISTs (>5 cm) have a more malignant phenotype and require adjuvant chemotherapy.

Treatment

- *Surgical. Wide excision* is the treatment of choice.
- *Chemotherapy. Molecular targeted chemotherapy* with imatinib mesilate (Glivec), an inhibitor of the *c-kit* tyrosine kinase, is very effective. It can be either given prior to surgery to shrink a large tumour in order to make it operable or given postoperatively to treat metastases or when complete resection was not possible. This is an example of the new generation of chemotherapy relying on unique molecular features of the tumour to target and control.

Carcinoma

Pathology

This is a common (incidence 10 per 100 000 in the UK) and important tumour, although its incidence is falling, in both Europe and the USA. It is the fifth most common cancer killer in the UK, preceded only by lung, colorectal, breast and prostate cancer. Distribution is worldwide, although it is particularly frequent in some races, especially the Japanese. Any age may be involved, but it especially affects the 50–70 year age group.

Risk factors

The risk factors for stomach cancer can be classified into three groups.

1 *Predisposing conditions.*
   a Pernicious anaemia and atrophic gastritis, conditions where achlorhydria is present.
   b Previous gastric resection (two- to threefold increased incidence).
   c Chronic peptic ulcer, believed to give rise to 1% of gastric cancer cases.
2 *Environmental factors.*
   a *H. pylori* infection. Seropositive patients (indicating past or present infection) have a six- to ninefold risk of gastric cancer. However, fewer than 1% of those infected with *H. pylori* will go on to develop gastric cancer.
   b Low socioeconomic status.
   c Smoking.
   d Nationality. Gastric cancer is much more common in Japan, although recent work suggests much of this excess is related to *H. pylori*. The incidence declines in Japanese immigrants to America.
3 *Genetic factors.*
   a Blood group A.
   b Hereditary non-polyposis colon cancer syndrome (HNPCC, Chapter 25, p. 211), associated with an increased incidence of gastric as well as colon cancer.

Macroscopic pathology

One-third diffusely involve the stomach; one-quarter arise in the pyloric region; and the remainder are distributed fairly evenly throughout the rest of the organ.

There are four macroscopic appearances:

1 a *malignant ulcer* with raised, everted edges;
2 a *polypoid tumour* proliferating into the stomach lumen;
3 a *colloid tumour*: a massive, gelatinous growth;
4 the *leather-bottle stomach (linitis plastica)* caused by submucous infiltration of tumour with marked fibrous reaction. This produces a small, thickened, contracted stomach without, or with only superficial, ulceration; hence, occult bleeding is rare in this group.

Microscopic appearances

These tumours are all adenocarcinomas with varying degrees of differentiation. The leather-bottle stomach consists of anaplastic cells arranged in clumps with surrounding fibrosis.

Malignant change in a benign ulcer is suggested when a chronic ulcer, with characteristic complete destruction of the whole muscle coat and its replacement by fibrous tissue and chronic inflammatory cells, has a carcinoma developing in its edge.

Spread

- *Local.* Spread is often well beyond the naked-eye limits of the tumour, and the oesophagus or the first part of the duodenum may be infiltrated. Adjacent organs (pancreas, abdominal wall, liver, transverse mesocolon and transverse colon) may be directly invaded. A gastrocolic fistula may develop.
- *Lymphatic.* Lymph nodes along the lesser and greater curves are commonly involved. Lymph drainage from the cardiac end of the stomach may invade the mediastinal nodes and thence the supraclavicular nodes of Virchow[13] on the left side (Troisier's sign[14]). At the pyloric end, involvement of the subpyloric and hepatic nodes may occur.
- *Bloodstream.* Dissemination occurs via the portal vein to the liver and thence occasionally to the lungs and the skeletal system.

- *Transcoelomic spread.* May produce peritoneal seedlings, ascites and bilateral Krukenberg[15] tumours owing to implantation in both ovaries.

Clinical features

Symptoms may be produced by the local effects of the tumour, by secondary deposits or by the general features of malignant disease.

Local symptoms

These are epigastric pain and discomfort, pain radiating into the back (suggesting pancreatic involvement), vomiting, especially with a pyloric or antral tumour producing pyloric obstruction (see p. 174) and dysphagia in tumours of the cardia. The patient may also report a feeling of fullness after eating little (early satiety). Occasionally, carcinoma of the stomach may present with perforation or haemorrhage (melaena and/or haematemesis).

Symptoms from secondaries

The patient may first report with jaundice owing to liver involvement or abdominal distension with ascites.

General features

Anorexia (an extremely common presenting symptom), loss of weight and anaemia.

Examination may reveal features corresponding to these three headings. Local examination may reveal a mass in the upper abdomen. A search for secondaries may show enlargement of the liver with or without jaundice, ascites, enlarged, hard left supraclavicular nodes, or a palpable mass on pelvic examination due to secondary deposits in the pouch of Douglas. There may be obvious signs of loss of weight or anaemia.

Paraneoplastic syndromes

Haemolytic anaemia, membranous glomerulonephritis and chronic disseminated intravascular

[13]Charles Émile Troisier (1844–1919), Professor of Pathology, Paris.
[14]Friedrich Krukenberg (1871–1946), Pathologist, Halle, Germany.

[15]Armand Trousseau (1801–1867), Physician, Hôpital St. Antoine and Hôpital Dieu, Paris, France. Noted this sign in himself as confirmation of his own gastric cancer. Also described carpopedal spasm in hypocalcaemic tetany.

coagulation leading to vascular thrombosis (Trousseau's sign[16]) are occasionally seen.

Special investigations

- *Gastroscopy* enables direct inspection and multiple biopsies of any lesion. The detection rate is related to the number of biopsies taken.
- *CT* may show nodal and metastatic spread, information that may influence attempts at curative gastric resection.
- *EUS* enables assessment of lymph node spread and local tumour infiltration into pancreas, crura and liver.
- *Staging laparoscopy* allows assessment of the primary tumour, including its mobility and invasion into adjacent organs, and examination of the peritoneal cavity to exclude small metastases (peritoneal or liver) that are not detectable by CT scanning. If ascites is found, this can be sampled for cytology. The presence of even small metastases means the patient has incurable disease.

It is important to note that considerable pain relief and 'healing' may occur when a gastric carcinoma is treated with acid suppression (H$_2$-antagonists or proton pump inhibitors), owing to diminution in the adjacent oedema, and may lead to a false diagnosis of benign ulcer.

Differential diagnosis

There are five common diseases that give a very similar clinical picture, of a patient with slight lemon-yellow tinge, anaemia and loss of weight:

1 carcinoma of the stomach;
2 carcinoma of the caecum;
3 carcinoma of the pancreas;
4 pernicious anaemia;
5 uraemia.

They form an important quintet, and should always be considered together.

The principal differential diagnosis of gastric carcinoma is a benign gastric ulcer. If in doubt, resection should be advised, but it may be difficult, even at operation, to decide between the two, and a perioperative frozen section microscopic examination is then useful in planning treatment.

Treatment

- *Curative*: partial or total gastrectomy, with extensive lymph node clearance, depending on the extent of the tumour. Patients undergoing gastrectomy now commonly receive chemotherapy before and after surgery
- *Palliative*: palliative gastrectomy may be carried out even in the presence of small secondary deposits elsewhere. A gastroenterostomy may be performed for an irremovable obstructive lesion of the pylorus. However, more commonly, stenting of the pylorus is performed for gastric outflow obstruction in unresectable disease. Stenting is also used for carcinoma of the cardiac end that is unresectable and producing dysphagia. Irradiation and cytotoxic drugs are of limited value.

Prognosis

This depends on the extent of spread and degree of differentiation of the tumour. Microscopic spread is much further than apparent at operation, and lymph node spread has a poor prognosis. Early gastric carcinomas confined to the stomach wall (stage 1) have a 72% 5 year survival with resection. Perigastric lymph node involvement (stage 2) reduces survival to 32%, whereas more distant nodal involvement more than 3 cm away from the tumour (stage 3) has a survival rate of only 10% at 5 years. The presence of metastases (stage 4) is associated with death before 5 years.

---

[16]Paul Georges Dieulafoy (1839-1911), Physician, Paris. The lesion is a submucosal artery running abnormally close to the mucosa, typically occurring in the gastric fundus near the oesophagogastric junction and a cause of recurrent bleeding.

Mechanical intestinal obstruction

Learning objective

✓ To know the causes of obstruction in all age groups. In particular, the reader should recognize the four common clinical features, the key points of clinical examination and the management principles.

Mechanical obstruction

Classification

Intestinal obstruction (Box 22.1) is a restriction to the normal passage of intestinal contents. It may be divided into two main groups: paralytic and mechanical. Paralytic obstruction (paralytic or adynamic ileus) is discussed in Chapter 28.

Mechanical intestinal obstruction is further classified according to the following:

- *speed of onset*: acute, chronic, acute on chronic;
- *site*: high or low;
- *nature*: simple versus strangulating;
- *aetiology*.

Speed of onset

The speed of onset determines whether the obstruction is acute, chronic or acute on chronic. In acute obstruction, the onset is rapid and the symptoms severe. In chronic obstruction, the symptoms are insidious and slowly progressive (as, for example, in most cases of carcinoma of the large bowel). A chronic obstruction may develop acute symptoms as the obstruction suddenly

becomes complete, e.g. when a narrowed lumen becomes totally occluded by inspissated bowel contents. This is termed acute-on-chronic obstruction.

Site

The site of the obstruction is classified into high or low, which is roughly synonymous with small or large bowel obstruction.

Nature

The nature of the obstruction is divided into simple or strangulated.

- *Simple obstruction* occurs when the bowel is occluded without damage to its blood supply.
- *Strangulating obstruction* is when the blood supply of the involved segment of intestine is cut off (as may occur, for example, in strangulated hernia, volvulus, intussusception or when a loop of intestine is occluded by a band). Gangrene of the strangulated bowel is inevitable if left untreated.

Aetiology

Whenever one considers obstruction of a tube anywhere in the body, the causes should be classified into the following:

- causes in the lumen;
- causes in the wall;

Lecture Notes: General Surgery, 12th edition. © Harold Ellis, Sir Roy Y. Calne and Christopher J. E. Watson. Published 2011 by Blackwell Publishing Ltd.

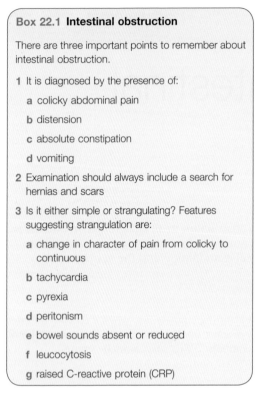

> **Box 22.1 Intestinal obstruction**
>
> There are three important points to remember about intestinal obstruction.
>
> 1 It is diagnosed by the presence of:
>
>   a colicky abdominal pain
>
>   b distension
>
>   c absolute constipation
>
>   d vomiting
>
> 2 Examination should always include a search for hernias and scars
>
> 3 Is it either simple or strangulating? Features suggesting strangulation are:
>
>   a change in character of pain from colicky to continuous
>
>   b tachycardia
>
>   c pyrexia
>
>   d peritonism
>
>   e bowel sounds absent or reduced
>
>   f leucocytosis
>
>   g raised C-reactive protein (CRP)

- causes outside the wall.

This can be applied to intestinal obstruction.

- *In the lumen*: faecal impaction, gallstone 'ileus', food bolus, parasites (e.g. ascaris worms in small bowel), intussusception.
- *In the wall*: congenital atresia, Crohn's disease, tumours, diverticulitis of the colon.
- *Outside the wall*: strangulated hernia (external or internal), volvulus and obstruction due to adhesions or bands.

It is also useful to think of the common intestinal obstructions that may occur in each age group.

- *Neonatal:* congenital atresia and stenosis (e.g. duodenal atresia), imperforate anus, volvulus neonatorum, Hirschsprung's disease and meconium ileus.
- *Infants:* intussusception, Hirschsprung's disease, strangulated hernia and obstruction due to Meckel's diverticulum.
- *Young adults and middle age:* strangulated hernia, adhesions and bands, Crohn's disease.

- *The elderly:* strangulated hernia, carcinoma of the colon, colonic diverticulitis, impacted faeces.

A strangulated hernia is an important cause of intestinal obstruction from infancy to old age. The hernial orifices must therefore be carefully examined in every case.

Pathology

When the bowel is obstructed by a simple occlusion, the intestine distal to the obstruction rapidly empties and becomes collapsed. The bowel above the obstruction becomes dilated, partly with gas (most of which is swallowed air) and partly with fluid poured out by the intestinal wall together with the gastric, biliary and pancreatic secretions. There is increased peristalsis in an attempt to overcome the obstruction, which results in intestinal colic. As the bowel distends, the blood supply to the tensely distended intestinal wall becomes impaired and, in extreme cases, there may be mucosal ulceration and eventually perforation. Perforation may also occur from the pressure of a band or the edge of the hernia neck on the bowel wall, producing local ischaemic necrosis, or from pressure from within the gut lumen, e.g. by a faecal mass (stercoral ulceration).

In strangulating obstruction, the integrity of the mucosal barrier is lost as ischaemia progresses, so bacteria and their toxins can no longer be contained within the lumen. Transudation of organisms into the peritoneal cavity rapidly takes place, with secondary peritonitis. Unrelieved strangulation is followed by gangrene of the ischaemic bowel with perforation.

The lethal effects of intestinal obstruction result from fluid and electrolyte depletion owing to the copious vomiting and loss into the bowel lumen, protein loss into the gut and toxaemia due to migration of toxins and intestinal bacteria into the peritoneal cavity, either through the intact but ischaemic bowel wall or through a perforation.

Clinical features

The four cardinal symptoms of intestinal obstruction are the following:

1 colicky abdominal pain;
2 distension;
3 absolute constipation;
4 vomiting.

It is important to note that not all of these four features need necessarily be present in a case of intestinal obstruction. The sequence of onset of symptoms will help localize the obstruction to the upper or lower intestine.

Pain

This is usually the first symptom of intestinal obstruction and is colicky in nature. In small bowel obstruction, it is periumbilical; in distal colonic obstruction, it may be more suprapubic in location. In postoperative obstruction, the colic may be disguised by the general discomfort of the operation and by opiates that the patient may be receiving.

Distension

This is particularly marked in chronic large bowel obstruction and also in volvulus of the sigmoid colon. In a high intestinal obstruction, there may only be a short segment of bowel proximal to the obstruction, and distension will not then be marked.

Absolute constipation

Absolute constipation is the failure to pass either flatus or faeces. Although it is a usual feature of acute obstruction, a partial or chronic obstruction may be accompanied by the passage of small amounts of flatus. Absolute constipation is an early feature of large bowel obstruction, but a late feature of small bowel obstruction as, even when the obstruction is complete, the patient may pass one or two normal stools as the lower bowel empties after the onset of the obstruction.

Vomiting

This usually occurs early in high obstruction, but is often late or even entirely absent in chronic or in low (large bowel) obstruction. In the late stages of intestinal obstruction, the vomiting becomes faeculent but not faecal. The faeculent vomiting is due to bacterial decomposition of the stagnant contents of the obstructed small intestine and of the altered blood that may transude into the bowel lumen. True vomiting of faeces only occurs in patients with gastrocolic fistula (e.g. because of a carcinoma of the stomach, carcinoma of the colon or ulceration of a stomal ulcer into the colon), or in coprophagists.

Clinical examination

The patient may be obviously dehydrated if vomiting has been copious. He or she is in pain and may be rolling about with colic. The pulse is usually elevated, but the temperature is frequently normal. A raised temperature and a tachycardia suggest strangulation. The abdomen is distended and visible peristalsis may be present. Visible peristalsis itself is not diagnostic of intestinal obstruction, as it may be seen in the normal subject if the abdominal wall is very thin.

During inspection it is important to look carefully for two features: (1) the presence of a strangulated external hernia, which may require a careful search in the case of a small strangulated femoral hernia in a very obese and distended patient, and (2) the presence of an abdominal scar. Intestinal obstruction in the presence of this evidence of a previous operation immediately suggests adhesions or a band as the cause.

Palpation reveals generalized abdominal tenderness. A mass may be present (e.g. in intussusception or carcinoma of the bowel).

Bowel sounds are usually accentuated and tinkling. Rectal examination must, of course, never be omitted. It may reveal an obstructing mass in the pouch of Douglas, the apex of an intussusception or faecal impaction.

Simple obstruction versus strangulating obstruction

Clinically, it is extremely difficult to distinguish with any certainty between simple obstruction and strangulation. The distinction is important, as strangulating obstruction with ensuing peritonitis has a mortality of up to 15%. Features suggesting strangulation include the following:

- toxic appearance, with a rapid pulse and some elevation of temperature;
- colicky pain, becoming continuous as peritonitis develops;
- tenderness and abdominal rigidity more marked;
- bowel sounds becoming reduced or absent, reflecting peritonism;
- raised white cell count, mostly neutrophils, which is usual with infarcted bowel.

Special investigations

- *Abdominal X-rays* (erect and supine) are valuable in diagnosis of intestinal obstruction and in attempting to localize the site of the obstruction. A loop or loops of distended bowel are usually seen, together with fluid levels on an erect film.

- *Small bowel obstruction* is suggested by a ladder pattern of dilated loops, their central position and by striations that pass completely across the width of the distended loop produced by the circular mucosal folds.
- *Distended large bowel* tends to lie peripherally and to show the haustrations of the taenia coli, which do not extend across the whole width of the bowel. A small percentage, perhaps 5%, of intestinal obstructions show no abnormality on plain X-rays. This is because the bowel is completely distended with fluid in a closed loop and without the fluid levels produced by coexistent gas.
- *Computed tomography (CT)*, combined with oral water-soluble contrast (e.g. Gastrografin), is particularly useful; it can localize the site of obstruction, detect obstructing lesions and colonic tumours, and may diagnose unusual hernias (e.g. obturator hernias).
- *Water-soluble contrast study*. An emergency contrast enema may detect a suspected large bowel obstruction due to carcinoma or diverticular disease. Unlike a normal barium enema, no pre-examination laxative is given because of the risk of exacerbating the obstruction, and causing perforation if a closed loop exists.

Treatment

Although the treatment of specific causes of intestinal obstruction is considered under the appropriate headings, certain general principles can be enunciated here.

Chronic large bowel obstruction, slowly progressive and incomplete, can be investigated at some leisure (including sigmoidoscopy, colonoscopy and barium enema) and treated electively.

Acute obstruction, of sudden onset, complete and with risk of strangulation, is invariably an urgent problem requiring emergency surgical intervention.

Preoperative preparation in acute obstruction

This comprises the following:

1 *Gastric aspiration* by means of nasogastric suction. This helps to decompress the bowel and to lessen the risk of inhalation of gastric contents during induction of anaesthesia.
2 *Intravenous fluid replacement.* The large amount of fluid sequestered into the gut, together with losses due to vomiting, means that a lot of fluid may be required. Hartmann's solution or normal saline are given, with potassium if this is low and renal function satisfactory. If the patient is shocked plasma expanders may be required.
3 *Antibiotic therapy* is commenced if intestinal strangulation is likely (or is found at operation).

Operative treatment

The affected bowel is carefully inspected to determine its viability, either at the site of the obstruction (e.g. where a band or the margins of a hernial orifice has pressed against the bowel) or the whole segment of bowel involved in a closed loop obstruction. Non-viability is determined by four signs:

1 loss of peristalsis;
2 loss of normal sheen;
3 colour (greenish or black bowel is non-viable; purple bowel may still recover);
4 loss of arterial pulsation in the supplying mesentery.

Doubtful bowel may recover after relief of the obstruction. It should be reassessed after it has been left for a few minutes wrapped up in a warm wet pack. If extensive areas of bowel are of doubtful viability, it may be worthwhile planning a second-look laparotomy in 48 hours to reassess the necessity for an extensive bowel resection.

The general principle is that small bowel in intestinal obstruction can be resected and primary anastomosis performed with safety because of its excellent blood supply. Large bowel obstruction is treated by resection of the obstructing lesion, with a primary ileocolic anastomosis in the case of obstructing lesions proximal to the splenic flexure. Left-sided lesions are managed by excision of the affected segment and exteriorizing the two ends of colon as a temporary colostomy and mucous fistula (Chapter 25, p. 216). If the distal end will not reach the surface it is closed (Hartmann's procedure[1]). This difference in management of colonic

---

[1]Henri Hartmann (1860–1952), Professor of Surgery, Hôtel Dieu, Paris, France.

obstruction reflects the intraluminal bacterial flora and poorer blood supply of the large bowel; a colonic primary anastomosis is very liable to leak in the presence of obstruction. Where a primary colo-colonic anastomosis is performed, the proximal bowel is first lavaged via a catheter passed through the appendix stump, flushing effluent along the colon and out via a large-bore tube in the proximal end of the colon; a defunctioning loop ileostomy may be performed at the same time to minimize the complications of an anastomotic leak, should one occur.

Conservative treatment

Conservative treatment of obstruction by means of intravenous fluid and nasogastric aspiration ('drip and suck') is indicated only under the following conditions.

- When distinction from postoperative paralytic ileus is uncertain (Chapter 28, p. 236) and when a period of careful observation is indicated.
- When the obstruction is one of repeated episodes due to massive intra-abdominal adhesions, rendering surgery hazardous, and when, once again, a short period of observation with conservative treatment is indicated. An increase in distension, aggravation of pain, an increase in abdominal tenderness or a rising pulse are indications to abandon conservative treatment and to re-explore the abdomen.
- When chronic obstruction of the large bowel has occurred. Here, it is reasonable to attempt to remove the obturating faeces by enema, prepare the bowel and carry out a subsequent elective operation.

Closed loop obstruction

This is a specific form of mechanical obstruction. It is characterized by increasing distension of a loop of bowel due to a combination of complete obstruction distally and a valve-like mechanism proximally allowing the bowel to fill, but preventing reflux back. It is most commonly seen with a left-sided colonic obstruction, in the presence of a competent ileocaecal valve. The caecum, the most distensible part of the large bowel, blows up like a balloon, and perforation of the caecum, with faecal peritonitis, may occur if the obstruction is not rapidly relieved. Diagnosis is made on X-ray showing characteristic dilatation of the caecum. Other examples of closed loop obstruction include volvulus (gastric, caecal, sigmoid) and stomal obstruction of the afferent loop following Pólya[2] partial gastrectomy.

Adhesive obstruction

Intra-abdominal adhesions are an almost invariable consequence of abdominal or pelvic surgery. In most cases these are symptomless, but a small number of patients develop small bowel obstruction as a consequence. This may occur at any time from the immediate postoperative period to many years later. Because abdominal surgery is now so common, adhesions account for about three-quarters of all cases of small bowel obstruction. (Large bowel obstruction from this cause is extremely rare.) Treatment is initially conservative, with nasogastric suction and intravenous fluid replacement. However, clinical features of strangulation, peritonitis or failure to respond to the conservative regimen are indications for urgent laparotomy.

Volvulus

Definition

A twisting of a loop of bowel around its mesenteric axis, which results in a combination of obstruction together with occlusion of the main vessels at the base of the involved mesentery.

Most commonly, it affects the sigmoid colon, caecum and small intestine, but volvulus of the gallbladder and stomach may also occur.

Aetiology

Precipitating factors include the following:

- an abnormally mobile loop of intestine, e.g. congenital failure of rotation of the small intestine, or a particularly long sigmoid loop;
- an abnormally loaded loop – as in the pelvic colon of chronic constipation;

[2]Eugen Alexander Pólya (1876–1944), Surgeon, St. Stephen's Hospital, Budapest, Hungary.

- a loop fixed at its apex by adhesions, around which it rotates;
- a loop of bowel with a narrow mesenteric attachment.

Sigmoid volvulus

This occurs usually in elderly, constipated patients. It is four times more common in men than in women. It is relatively rare in the UK (about 2% of intestinal obstructions) but is much more common in Russia, Scandinavia and central Africa. The loop of sigmoid colon usually twists anticlockwise, from one-half to three turns.

Clinical features

There is a sudden onset of colicky pain with characteristic gross and rapid dilatation of the sigmoid loop.

A plain X-ray of the abdomen shows an enormously dilated oval gas shadow on the left side, which may be looped on itself to give the typical 'bent inner-tube' sign. If left untreated, the strangulated bowel undergoes gangrene, resulting in death from peritonitis. The caecum is usually visible and dilated in the right lower quadrant, distinguishing it radiologically from caecal volvulus.

Treatment

A long, soft rectal tube is passed through a sigmoidoscope and advanced into the sigmoid colon. This often untwists an early volvulus and is accompanied by the passage of vast amounts of flatus and liquid faeces. If this method fails, the volvulus is untwisted at laparotomy and the bowel is decompressed via a rectal tube threaded upwards from the anus. If gangrene has occurred, the affected segment is excised and the two open ends are brought out as a double-barrelled colostomy, which is later closed (Paul–Mikulicz procedure[3]).

Recurrent sigmoid volvulus is an indication for elective resection of the redundant sigmoid loop.

Caecal volvulus

Caecal volvulus is usually associated with a congenital malrotation where, in contrast to the incomplete rotation which causes volvulus neonatorum (see p. 190), the caecum and proximal ascending colon rotate beyond the right iliac fossa (RIF) during development so that, instead of being fixed in the RIF, it has a persistent mesentery.

Clinically, there is an acute onset of pain in the RIF with rapid abdominal distension. X-ray of the abdomen shows a grossly dilated caecum, which is often ectopically placed and is frequently located in the left upper quadrant of the abdomen.

Treatment

At laparotomy, the volvulus is untwisted. Right hemicolectomy is necessary if the caecum is infarcted, and it is also the most reliable way to prevent recurrence.

Small intestine volvulus in adults

This may occur when a loop of the small intestine is fixed at its apex by adhesions or by a fibrous remnant of the vitellointestinal duct (often associated with a Meckel's diverticulum). Occasionally, the apex of the volvulus bears a tumour. In Africa, primary volvulus of the small bowel is relatively common, and may be due to the loading of a loop of gut with large quantities of vegetable foodstuffs. The clinical picture is one of acute intestinal obstruction.

Treatment

Early operation with simple untwisting and treatment of the underlying cause. If gangrene is present, resection must be carried out.

Volvulus neonatorum

This is considered on p. 190.

Mesenteric vascular occlusions

[3]Frank Thomas Paul (1851–1941), Surgeon, Liverpool Royal Infirmary, Liverpool, UK. Johann von Mikulicz-Radecki (1850–1905), Professor of Surgery, successively at Cracow, Konigsberg and Breslau, Poland.

Embolism or thrombosis of the mesenteric vessels constitutes a special variety of intestinal obstruction without occlusion of the bowel.

Aetiology

Mesenteric embolus

This may arise from the left atrium in atrial fibrillation, a mural thrombus secondary to myocardial infarction, a vegetation on a heart valve or an atheromatous plaque on the aorta. Occasionally, it may be a paradoxical embolus originating in the deep leg veins and crossing the septum of the heart through a patent foramen ovale (Figure 12.4 p. 96).

Mesenteric arterial thrombosis

This is usually thrombosis secondary to atheroma. Arterial occlusion may also be secondary to an aortic dissection (Chapter 11, p. 76).

Mesenteric venous thrombosis

This is associated with portal hypertension, or may follow splenectomy for thrombocytopenic purpura, pressure of a tumour on the superior mesenteric vessels or septic thrombophlebitis (e.g. secondary to Crohn's disease). Both mesenteric arterial and venous thrombosis are well documented in previously healthy young women on oral contraceptives, and are also associated with thrombophilias such as antithrombin III deficiency.

Non-occlusive infarction of the intestine

This may occur in patients with grossly diminished cardiac output and mesenteric blood flow consequent upon myocardial infarction or congestive cardiac failure.

Pathology

Mesenteric vascular occlusion results in infarction of the affected bowel with bleeding into the gut wall, lumen and peritoneal cavity; gangrene and subsequent perforation of the ischaemic bowel occurs. Impaired arterial blood flow to the gut without infarction may produce the symptoms of 'intestinal angina' in which severe abdominal pain follows meals; indeed, fear of eating and thus inducing pain produces rapid loss of weight. There may be an associated steatorrhoea. Minor degrees of occlusion may be overcome by development of a collateral circulation, particularly if the block develops slowly. One or even two of the three main arteries (coeliac, superior and inferior mesenteric) may be occluded without symptoms.

Clinical features

There may be some pre-existing factor such as a heart lesion or liver disease. The classical triad is acute colicky abdominal pain, rectal bleeding and shock (due to associated blood loss) in an elderly patient who has atrial fibrillation.

The abdomen is generally tender, and a vague, tender mass may be felt, which is the infarcted bowel. However, the condition is impossible to diagnose unless the clinician has a high index of suspicion.

Treatment

The shock is treated by blood transfusion. Occasionally, successes have been reported from embolectomy in very early cases before frank gangrene has occurred. Resection of the gangrenous bowel is carried out, but this is obviously impossible when the whole superior mesenteric supply (small intestine and right side of the colon) is affected, usually a fatal situation. Revascularization using a saphenous vein conduit to take blood from an iliac artery to the superior mesenteric artery may be possible. Resection of the definitely infarcted bowel is performed, and the bowel of dubious viability is left and inspected at subsequent laparotomy the following day.

Young patients who have undergone extensive resection of the small bowel can be managed by long-term total parenteral nutrition, with intestinal transplantation as an alternative in selected cases.

Neonatal intestinal obstruction

Classification

- Intestinal atresia.
- Volvulus neonatorum.
- Meconium ileus.
- Necrotizing enterocolitis.
- Hirschsprung's disease.
- Anorectal atresias.

Continuous vomiting in the newborn suggests intracranial injury, infection or obstruction. Bile vomiting in the neonate indicates, almost without exception, intestinal obstruction.

In addition to vomiting, there may be constipation, abdominal distension and visible peristalsis.

Plain X-ray of the abdomen shows distended loops of intestine with fluid levels.

Intestinal atresia

This may be a septum, complete or partial, or a complete gap, which may be associated with a corresponding defect in the mesentery. Multiple segments may be involved.

Treatment

Resection of the stricture and anastomosis. The operation is difficult and the mortality is high.

Volvulus neonatorum

This is due to a congenital malrotation of the bowel. The caecum remains high and the midgut mesentery is narrow, and drags across the duodenum, which may thus also be obstructed. Because of the narrow attachment of mesentery, it readily undergoes volvulus. Untreated, the whole of the midgut becomes gangrenous.

Treatment

Laparotomy is performed as soon as possible. The operative procedure comprises untwisting the volvulus, and widening the narrow mesenteric attachment to the retroperitoneum. Adhesions between caecum and duodenum (Ladd's bands[4]) are divided, and the caecum and ascending colon are placed on the left side or in the midline. An appendicectomy is performed if practical, as the unusual position of the appendix may cause diagnostic difficulty in the future.

Meconium ileus

Eighty per cent of infants with meconium ileus have cystic fibrosis (mucoviscidosis), which is a generalized defect of mucus secretion of the intestine, pancreas (fibrocystic pancreatic disease) and

the bronchial tree. Because of the loss of intestinal mucus and a blockage of pancreatic ducts with loss of enzymatic digestion, the lower ileum of the fetus becomes blocked with inspissated, viscous meconium. Perforation of the bowel may occur in intrauterine life (meconium peritonitis).

Clinical features

The infant presents with acute obstruction in the first days of life, with gross abdominal distension and vomiting. The loop of ileum impacted with meconium may be palpable. X-ray of the abdomen shows, in addition to distended coils of bowel, the typical mottled 'ground glass' appearance of meconium.

Treatment

It may be possible to clear the meconium by instillation of Gastrografin per rectum under X-ray control. This material is radio-opaque and hyperosmolar (drawing fluid into the bowel lumen) and contains an emulsifying agent (Tween), which facilitates evacuation of the meconium. If this fails, or if the bowel has perforated, surgery is indicated. This comprises enterotomy and removal of the inspissated meconium by lavage. Occasionally, the impacted segment of ileum may show areas of gangrene and require resection. Postoperatively, the infant is given pancreatic enzyme supplements by mouth.

The long-term prognosis is dictated by the extent to which the chest is affected since, owing to the lack of mucus secretion of the bronchi, recurrent chest infection is almost inevitable.

Necrotizing enterocolitis

This is a condition seen in premature infants and is due to mesenteric ischaemia, which permits bacterial invasion of the mucosa. Terminal ileum, caecum and distal colon are commonly affected. The condition probably represents the culmination of a number of disorders, such as hypoxia, hypotension and hyperviscosity, which reduce distal perfusion, together with sepsis and the presence of an umbilical artery cannula.

Clinical features

The infant shows signs of generalized sepsis with vomiting and listlessness. The abdomen is distended and tense. Blood and mucus are passed

[4]William Edwards Ladd (1880–1967), Professor of Paediatric Surgery, Harvard Medical School, Boston, MA, USA.

per rectum in over half the cases. The affected bowel may perforate or the condition resolve with stricture formation.

X-rays of the abdomen show distended loops of intestine, and gas bubbles may be seen in the bowel wall. Pneumoperitoneum signifies intestinal perforation.

Treatment

Initially, this is medical. The infant is resuscitated and commenced on total parenteral nutrition and broad-spectrum antibiotics. Indications for surgery are failure to respond, profuse intestinal haemorrhage and evidence of perforation or obstruction due to stricture formation. It comprises resection of the frankly gangrenous or perforated segment or segments of intestine with primary anastomosis when possible to avoid ileostomies, which are difficult to manage in neonates. Mortality remains around 20%.

Hirschsprung's disease[5]

This may present as acute obstruction in the neonate, with an incidence of 1 in 5000. Eighty per cent of the patients are male.

Pathology

This condition, also termed congenital or aganglionic megacolon, is produced by faulty development of the parasympathetic innervation of the distal bowel. There is an absence of ganglion cells in the submucosal plexus of Auerbach[6] and intermyenteric plexus of Meissner[7] affecting the rectum, which sometimes extends into the lower colon and, rarely, affects the whole of the large bowel. The involved segment is spastic, causing a functional obstruction with gross proximal distension of the colon. Recent work suggests it is associated with a mutation in the *RET* proto-oncogene, probably interacting with another mutant gene, affecting the migration of neural crest cells in the embryo to the gut, where they normally become ganglia.

Until the true nature of the disease was determined, surgical treatment was directed, quite

fruitlessly, to resection of the dilated, normally innervated portion of the colon.

Clinical features

In the most severe cases, obstructive symptoms commence in the first few days of life with failure to pass meconium; death results if untreated. Less marked examples present with extraordinarily stubborn constipation in infancy and these children survive into adult life with gross abdominal distension and stunted growth. Many untreated infants develop severe, life-threatening enterocolitis within the first 3 months of life.

Rectal examination reveals a narrow, empty rectum above which faecal impaction may be felt; this examination is usually followed by a gush of flatus and faeces.

Special investigations

- *Abdominal X-ray* shows dilated gas-filled loops of bowel throughout the abdomen except in the pelvis.
- *Barium enema* demonstrates the characteristic narrow rectal segment, above which the colon is dilated and full of faeces.
- *Rectal wall biopsy*, deep enough to include the submucosa, shows complete absence of ganglion cells. In difficult cases, a longitudinal full-thickness biopsy is required.

Differential diagnosis

The differential diagnosis is acquired megacolon, a condition of severe constipation commencing usually at the age of 1–2 years, often in a child with mental retardation. Rectal examination in these cases is typical, impacted faeces being present right up to the anal verge. Biopsy of the rectal wall shows normal ganglion cells. This condition is relieved by regular enemas and aperients.

Treatment

If the child is obstructed in the neonatal period, colostomy is performed. Elective surgery is carried out when the infant is 6–9 months old, or until at least 3 months have elapsed after a colostomy has been established. The aganglionic segment is resected and an abdominoperineal pull-through anastomosis performed between normal colon and the anal canal.

---

[5]Harald Hirschsprung (1830–1916), Professor of Paediatrics, Queen Louisa Hospital, Copenhagen, Denmark.
[6]Leopold Auerbach (1828–1897), Neuropathologist, Breslau, Poland.
[7]Georg Meissner (1829–1905), Professor of Physiology, Göttingen, Germany.

It is important at operation to ensure by frozen section histological examination that ganglion cells are present in the remaining colon.

Anorectal atresias

Anorectal atresias are a spectrum of abnormalities from imperforate anus to complete absence of anus and rectum. They result from failure of breakdown of the septum between the hindgut and the invaginating ectoderm of the proctodaeum. Fifty per cent are associated with fistula: in the female into the vagina; in the male into the bladder or urethra. Twenty-five per cent are associated with congenital anomalies elsewhere.

Clinical features

The anus may be entirely absent or represented by a dimple or a blind canal. Diagnosis may be suspected on pre-natal ultrasound. Traditionally the extent of the defect is judged by X-raying the child, held upside down, with a metal marker such as a small coin at the site of the anus: the distance between the gas bubble in the distal colon and the marker can then be measured.

Imperforate anus is associated with vertebral and other congenital defects; any child with the diagnosis should have an ultrasound or magnetic resonance imaging of the spine.

Treatment

- If the septum is thin (less than 1 cm), it is divided with suture of the edges of the defect to the skin.
- If there is an extensive gap between the blind end and the anal verge, a colostomy is fashioned with a later attempt at a pull-through operation at about 2 years of age. Some surgeons perform an immediate pull-through procedure in the neonate.
- If a vaginal fistula is present, operation is not urgent, as the bowel decompresses through the vagina. Elective surgery is performed when the girl is older.
- If a rectourethral or vesical fistula is present (meconium escaping in the urine) the fistula must be closed urgently, with either colostomy or reconstruction of the anus, in order to prevent ascending infection of the urinary tract.

Intussusception

Definition

An intussusception is the prolapse of one portion of the intestine into the lumen of the immediately adjoining bowel. The prolapsing or invaginating bowel is called the intussusceptum.

Terminology

Different portions of the intestine may form the apex of the intussusception. The common forms, in order of frequency, are the following:

- *ileocolic:* an ileoileal intussusception extends through the ileocaecal valve into the colon; this is the commonest sort (75%);
- *ileocaecal:* the ileocaecal valve is the apex of the intussusception;
- *ileoileal:* the ileum is invaginated into the adjacent ileum;
- *colocolic:* the colon invaginates into an adjacent colon (usually because of a protruding tumour of the bowel wall).

Aetiology

Ninety-five per cent occur in infants or young children, in whom there is usually no obvious cause. The mesenteric lymph nodes in these patients are invariably enlarged. It is postulated that the lymphoid tissue in Peyer's patches[8] in the bowel wall undergoes hyperplasia because of an adenovirus; the swollen lymphoid tissue protrudes into the lumen of the bowel and acts as a 'foreign body', which is then propelled by peristalsis distally along the gut, dragging the bowel behind.

In adults and in some children, a polyp, carcinoma, intestinal lymphoma or an inverted Meckel's diverticulum may form the apex of the intussusception.

The intussusceptum has its blood supply cut off by direct pressure of the outer layer and by stretching of its supplying mesentery so that, if untreated, gangrene will occur.

---

[8]Johann Peyer (1653–1712), Anatomist, Schaffhausen, Switzerland.

Clinical features in infants

Intussusception usually occurs in previously healthy children commonly aged between 3 and 12 months. Boys are affected twice as often as girls.

The history is of paroxysms of abdominal colic typified by screaming and pallor. There is vomiting and usually the passage of blood and/or slime per rectum, giving the appearance of redcurrant jelly. On examination, the child is pale and anxious, and a typical attack of screaming may be observed. Palpation of the abdomen, after sedation if necessary, reveals a sausage-shaped tumour anywhere except in the RIF. Occasionally, the tumour cannot be felt because it is hidden under the costal margin. Rectal examination nearly always reveals 'redcurrant jelly' on the examining finger and, rarely, the tip of the intussusception can be felt.

If neglected, after 24 hours the abdomen becomes distended, faeculent vomiting occurs and the child becomes intensely toxic, owing to gangrene of the intussusception and associated peritonitis.

Treatment in the infant

Non-operative

Barium is run in per rectum, and X-ray confirmation of the diagnosis is established. If the intussusception is recent, it may be completely reduced hydrostatically by the pressure of the column of barium and this is confirmed radiologically.

Operative

The intussusception is reduced at laparotomy by squeezing its apex backwards out of the containing bowel. In late cases, reduction may be impossible or the bowel may be gangrenous so that resection may be necessary.

Mortality is very low in the first 24 hours but is very high in the irreducible or gangrenous cases. An intussusception may recur in a small percentage of children.

23

The small intestine

Learning objectives

✓ To know the varying presentations of a Meckel's diverticulum.

✓ To have knowledge of Crohn's disease of the small intestine, in particular its varying presentations and treatment.

Meckel's diverticulum

Meckel's diverticulum[1] is the remnant of the vitellointestinal duct of the embryo. It lies on the antimesenteric border of the ileum and, as an approximation, occurs in 2% of the population, arises 60 cm (2 feet) from the caecum, and averages 5 cm (2 inches) in length.

Clinical features

It may present in numerous ways:

- *A symptomless finding* at operation or autopsy.
- *Acute inflammation*, clinically identical to acute appendicitis.
- *Perforation by a foreign body*, presenting as peritonitis.
- *Intussusception* (ileoileal), often gangrenous by the time the patient comes to operation.
- *Peptic ulceration* due to contained heterotopic gastric epithelium, which bears HCl-secreting parietal cells. This particularly occurs in children and characteristically is the cause of

melaena at about the age of 10 years. Rarely, the peptic ulcer perforates or gives rise to postcibal pain. The diverticulum may also contain ectopic pancreatic tissue.

- *Patent vitellointestinal duct*, presenting as an umbilical fistula that discharges intestinal contents.
- *Raspberry tumour at the umbilicus* due to a persistent umbilical extremity of the duct.
- *Vitellointestinal band* stretching from the tip of the diverticulum to the umbilicus, which may snare a loop of intestine to produce obstruction or act as the apex of a small bowel volvulus.

Special investigations

Most diverticula are incidental findings. However, the following investigations may be indicated.

- *Technetium scan.* Radiolabelled technetium (^{99m}Tc) is taken up by gastric mucosa, and scintigraphy will outline the stomach and, in addition, the Meckel's diverticulum, usually near the right iliac fossa (RIF).
- *Barium follow-through or small bowel enema* may show the diverticulum arising from the antimesenteric border.
- *Computed tomography (CT)* scan may demonstrate the diverticulum.

Treatment involves resection of the diverticulum.

---

[1]Johann Frederick Meckel (1781–1833), Professor of Anatomy and Surgery, Halle, Germany. His grandfather and father were both Professor of Anatomy.

Lecture Notes: General Surgery, 12th edition. © Harold Ellis, Sir Roy Y. Calne and Christopher J. E. Watson. Published 2011 by Blackwell Publishing Ltd.

Crohn's disease

Crohn's disease[2] is a non-specific inflammatory disease of the alimentary canal, with diseased segments sandwiched between normal segments (i.e. it is discontinuous). Crohn first described its occurrence in the ileum and termed it 'regional ileitis'. However, this description is inaccurate, as the disease may affect any part of the alimentary tract from the mouth to the anus. Crohn's disease may affect the large bowel alone (Chapter 25, p. 210).

Aetiology

The aetiology of Crohn's disease has environmental (cigarette smoking; urban living) and genetic (20% of patients have an affected relative) components. Recent work has pointed to a genetic mutation in the *NOD* gene family. These genes are involved in the innate immune response to bacterial antigens within the gut. This observation explains the success of dietary manipulation, such as the elemental diet (see p. 196). The presence of granulomas on histology has suggested infection by a mycobacterium species, possibly *Mycobacterium avium* ssp. *paratuberculosis*. However, the success of immunosuppression in the control of Crohn's disease suggests an autoimmune rather than an infectious cause.

Acute ileitis can also be caused by the bacterium *Yersinia enterocolitica*.

Pathology

Distribution

The small bowel is affected in two-thirds of cases, with the lower ileum being the commonest site, although the disease may affect any part of the alimentary canal from the buccal mucosa to the anal verge. One-third of patients with ileal disease also have rectal or colonic manifestations.

Macroscopic appearance

In the acute stage, the bowel is bright red and swollen; mucosal ulceration and intervening oedema result in a 'cobblestone' appearance of the mucous membrane. The wall of the intestine is greatly thickened, as is the adjacent mesentery, and the regional lymph nodes are enlarged. Mesenteric fat advances over the serosal surface in affected segments. There may be skip areas of normal intestine between involved segments. Fistulae may occur into adjacent viscera.

Microscopic appearance

There is fibrosis, lymphoedema and a chronic inflammatory infiltrate through the whole thickness of the bowel with non-caseating foci of epithelioid and giant cells. Ulceration is present, with characteristic fissuring ulcers extending deep through the mucosa. These may extend through the bowel wall to form abscesses, or fistulae into adjacent viscera.

Clinical features

Crohn's disease occurs at any age, but is particularly common in young adults with a peak age of onset between 20 and 40 years of age. There is no sex difference. The typical clinical picture is a young adult with abdominal pain and diarrhoea, often with a palpable mass in the RIF. However, Crohn's disease may manifest clinically in several ways.

- *Acute Crohn's disease.* Crohn's disease may present like appendicitis with acute abdominal pain, usually in the RIF, and vomiting. Rarely, there is perforation of the bowel or acute haemorrhage. Unlike appendicitis, the history is usually of several days or weeks, and investigation may reveal anaemia, or other features of Crohn's disease may be present.
- *Intestinal obstruction.* Following inflammatory exacerbations, fibrosis of the intestinal wall occurs, leaving stenotic segments which result in intestinal obstruction. Obstruction may also follow an intraperitoneal abscess.
- *Fistula formation.* Fistulae may develop, penetrating adjacent loops of gut or the bladder, or they may be perianal. External faecal fistulae may follow operative intervention.
- *Malabsorption.* Extensive involvement of the bowel produces malabsorption with steatorrhoea and multiple vitamin deficiencies. It is exacerbated when bowel resections have already occurred.

---

[2]Burrill Bernard Crohn (1884–1983), Gastroenterologist, Mount Sinai Hospital, New York, NY, USA. The disease was first described by Morgagni (1682–1771).

- *Diarrhoea.* Diarrhoea may be due to inflammation and mucosal ulceration, colonic or rectal involvement, bacterial overgrowth in obstructed segments and malabsorption secondary to either disease or short bowel following previous surgery. Mucosal ulceration causes diarrhoea, with positive occult blood and anaemia.
- *Perianal disease.* Ten per cent of patients with small bowel Crohn's disease also have perianal disease, ranging from fissures to fistulae (Chapter 26, p. 224).

Special investigations

Crohn's disease is associated with anaemia, positive occult blood and occasionally steatorrhoea. Serum albumin is low, and inflammatory markers such as C-reactive protein and the acute phase proteins are helpful indices of disease activity. Additional investigations include the following:

- *Small bowel enema*, or enteroclysis, in which contrast is instilled into the duodenum via a nasogastric tube and followed fluoroscopically as it passes through the bowel, may demonstrate fistulae or strictures (the string sign of Kantor[3]) in the affected segment, usually the terminal ileum, and ulcerated small bowel may show a 'cobblestone' appearance.
- *CT or magnetic resonance enteroclysis* may also demonstrate extraluminal disease
- *Technetium-labelled leucocyte scan* is a sensitive way to show the extent of disease activity. Leucocytes are taken up in the inflamed segments, and also localize to abscesses.

Complications outside the gastrointestinal tract

In addition to those already mentioned, the following are associated with the disease.

- *Renal calculi:* usually oxalate stones secondary to hyperoxaluria, which occurs as a consequence of steatorrhoea.
- *Biliary calculi* are more common in patients with ileal Crohn's disease, and in whom the ileum has been resected. This is due to the interruption of the enterohepatic bile-salt circulation.
- *Primary sclerosing cholangitis, sacroiliitis, pyoderma gangrenosum and uveitis* also occur, but are more common when the colon is also involved.

Treatment

Treatment is primarily medical, although surgery is appropriate in the management of complications and chronic disease. Surgery is avoided when possible because of the malabsorption that may follow extensive resections of the bowel or the production of blind loops of intestine.

Medical management

Initial management is conservative. Nutritional support may be required, and an elemental diet may be useful. Acute episodes are treated with steroids and immunosuppressants such as azathioprine; parenteral nutrition may be required. Infliximab, a monoclonal antibody to tumour necrosis factor (TNF-α), has been shown to be effective treatment for acute exacerbations and fistulating disease.

Mild symptoms are treated with 5-aminosalicylate drugs such as sulfasalazine and mesalazine, and steroids may be required. Metronidazole may also help.

Surgical management

If found at laparotomy in the acute stage, the condition should be left undisturbed since in a high proportion the acute phase may subside completely without further episodes.

In the chronic stage of the disease, surgery is indicated for severe or recurrent obstructive symptoms, and for the treatment of fistulae into the bladder or skin. Recognizing that the disease is recurrent and that further resections may be required, surgery should be as conservative as possible. Either resection of the affected segment or a strictureplasty is performed.

Prognosis

Recurrence of the disease after resection occurs in some 50% of cases within 10 years, and repeated operations may be required over the years.

---

[3]John Leonard Kantor (1890–1947), Radiologist, Presbyterian Hospital, New York, NY, USA.

Tumours of the small intestine

One of the many mysteries of tumour formation is the rarity of growths from beyond the pylorus to the ileocaecal valve.

Classification

Benign

- Adenoma.
- Gastrointestinal stromal tumour (see Chapter 21, p. 179).
- Lipoma.
- Hamartoma (e.g. Peutz–Jeghers syndrome,[4] associated with circumoral pigmentation and multiple intestinal polyps).

Malignant

1 *Primary*:
   a adenocarcinoma;
   b lymphoma;
   c carcinoid;
   d gastrointestinal stromal tumour (see Chapter 21, p. 179).
2 *Secondary invasion* (e.g. from stomach, colon or bladder, or from a lymphoma).

Clinical features

Tumours of the small intestine may present with the following:

- intestinal bleeding;
- obstruction;
- intussusception;
- volvulus.

Carcinoid syndrome

Carcinoid tumours are APUD (amine precursor uptake and decarboxylation) tumours, and share this property with cells of neural crest origin with which they were once confused. They belong to a group of neuroendocrine tumours called gastro-enteropancreatic tumours; the other tumours in this group are pancreatic endocrine tumours such as gastrinomas and insulinomas. In 10% of cases, there is an association with the multiple endocrine neoplasia type 1 (MEN-1) syndrome (Chapter 38, p. 324). Carcinoid tumours are most commonly found in the appendix, but may be found anywhere in the alimentary canal and occasionally in the lung (10%). They commonly secrete 5-hydroxytryptamine (5-HT, also called serotonin), in addition to other hormones, but are rarely symptomatic until they have metastasized to the liver and are thus able to secrete their hormone directly into the systemic circulation, since the liver normally inactivates these hormones.

Pathology

Macroscopic appearance

The tumour appears as a yellowish submucosal nodule. The overlying mucous membrane is at first intact but later ulcerates. Extension to the serosa leads to fibrosis and obstruction. Usually, the tumour encircles the bowel at the time of diagnosis, and has infiltrated the mesenteric lymph nodes.

Microscopic appearance

The tumour is made up of Kultschitzky cells,[5] which take up silver stains and arise in the crypts of the intestinal mucosa.

The tumour is very slow growing, and usually presents after the fourth decade. Up to one-quarter are multiple. Carcinoids of the appendix are relatively benign but 4% eventually metastasize. They may present early as appendicitis by obstructing the appendix lumen. Those arising in the ileum and large bowel spread to the regional lymph nodes and the liver.

Clinical features

Carcinoid tumours present with features related to the primary tumour or metastatic spread, or with the carcinoid syndrome because of its endocrine products:

---

[4]Johannes Peutz (1886–1957), Physician, The Hague, The Netherlands. Harold Jeghers (1940–1990), Professor of Medicine, Georgetown University School of Medicine, Washington, DC, and Tufts University Medical School, Boston, MA, USA.

[5]Nicolai Kultschitzky (1865–1925), Professor of Histology, Kharkov, Russia. After the Russian Revolution he became Lecturer in Anatomy at University College, London, UK.

- flushing (90%) with attacks of cyanosis and a chronic red-faced appearance, often precipitated by stress or ingestion of food or alcohol;
- diarrhoea (70%), often profuse, with noisy borborygmi;
- bronchospasm (15%);
- abdominal pain (40%) owing to mesenteric fibrosis resulting in partial obstruction.

Abnormalities in the heart (pulmonary and tricuspid stenosis) are late manifestations; lung carcinoids also cause stenosis of the left heart valves (mitral and aortic). Hepatomegaly and a palpable abdominal mass produced by the tumour and its secondaries may also be present.

Special investigations

- *5-Hydroxyindole acetic acid (5-HIAA) urinary concentration.* 5-HT is broken down to 5-HIAA, which is excreted in the urine. A 24 hour urine collection contains raised levels of 5-HIAA.
- *Chromogranin A serum concentration* is raised in patients with neuroendocrine tumours such as carcinoids.

- *CT or ultrasound of the* liver to seek metastases. The primary tumour is often elusive, but CT may show mesenteric infiltration.
- *Radiolabelled octreotide scintigraphy* is a useful test for screening for tumour and for detection of metastases; the octreotide binds to somatostatin receptors which are often expressed on the tumour.

Treatment

Resection of the tumour in early cases. Local deposits in the liver are also occasionally resectable. Palliation of more extensive deposits can be achieved by embolizing the hepatic arterial supply via a catheter passed through the femoral artery. Cytotoxic therapy may induce worthwhile remission.

Symptoms may be controlled with octreotide, a somatostatin analogue that inhibits 5-HT release. Targeted radiotherapy, using radiolabelled octreotide, may have a place in treatment. Even if widespread deposits are present, the tumour is slow growing and the patient may survive for many years.

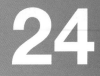

Acute appendicitis

Learning objective

✓ To know about the presentation and treatment of appendicitis, and the range of diagnoses that it can mimic.

This is the most common abdominal emergency and is estimated to affect one-sixth of the British population. It is, however, prevalent only in people on a Western diet.

Pathology

Acute appendicitis usually occurs when the appendix is obstructed by a faecolith or foreign body in the lumen, by a fibrous stricture in its wall from previous inflammation or by enlargement of lymphoid follicles in its wall secondary to inflammation of its mucosa; rarely, it is associated with an obstructing carcinoid tumour near its base. Occasionally, acute appendicitis occurs proximal to an obstructing lesion (usually carcinoma) in the caecum or ascending colon. As the appendix of the infant is wide mouthed and well drained, and as the lumen of the appendix is almost obliterated in old age, appendicitis at the two extremes of life is relatively rare. However, when it does occur in these age groups it is poorly tolerated, and often diagnosed late.

The obstructed appendix acts as a closed loop; bacteria proliferate in the lumen and invade the appendix wall, which is damaged by pressure necrosis. The vascular supply to the appendix is made up of end-arteries, which are branches of the appendicular branch of the ileocolic artery.

Lecture Notes: General Surgery, 12th edition. © Harold Ellis, Sir Roy Y. Calne and Christopher J. E. Watson. Published 2011 by Blackwell Publishing Ltd.

Once these are thrombosed, gangrene is inevitable and is followed by perforation.

There is no strict time relationship for this chain of events. An appendix may perforate in under 12 hours, but conversely it is not rare to see an acutely inflamed but not perforated appendix after 3 or 4 days.

The effects of appendicular obstruction depend on the content of the appendix lumen. If bacteria are present, acute inflammation occurs; if, as sometimes happens, the appendix is empty, then a *mucocele* of the appendix results, owing to continued secretion of mucus from the goblet cells in the mucosal wall.

Appendicitis can occur in the non-obstructed appendix. Here, there may be a direct infection of the lymphoid follicles from the appendix lumen, or in some cases the infection may be haematogenous (e.g. the rare streptococcal appendicitis). The non-obstructed acutely inflamed appendix is more likely to resolve than the obstructed form.

Pathological course

The acutely inflamed appendix may resolve, but if so a further attack is likely. It is not uncommon for a patient with acute appendicitis to confess to one or more previous milder episodes of pain, the 'grumbling appendix'. More often, the inflamed appendix undergoes gangrene and then perforates, either with general peritonitis or, more fortunately, with a localized appendix abscess. These possibilities are summarized in Figure 24.1.

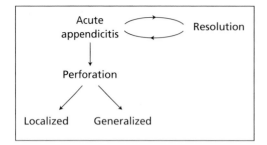

Figure 24.1 The pathological course of appendicitis.

Clinical features

History

The vast majority of patients with acute appendicitis present with marked localized pain and tenderness in the right iliac fossa (RIF).

- *Pain* – typically, the pain commences as a central periumbilical colic, which shifts after approximately 6 hours to the RIF or, more accurately, to the site of the inflamed appendix as the adjacent peritoneum becomes inflamed. The appendix is a long tube (7–10 cm long), tethered proximally to the caecum near the ileocaecal junction; distally the tip may lie anywhere from behind the caecum (retrocaecal), adjacent to the ileum or down in the pelvis lying against the rectum or bladder. Thus, if the appendix is in the pelvic position, the pain may become suprapubic, with urinary frequency as the bladder is irritated; if it is in the high retrocaecal position, the symptoms may become localized in the right loin with less tenderness on abdominal palpation. Rarely, the tip of the inflamed appendix extends over to the left iliac fossa and pain may localize there. The colicky central abdominal pain is visceral in origin; the shift of pain is due to later involvement of the sensitive parietal peritoneum by the inflammatory process. Typically, the pain is aggravated by movement and the patient prefers to lie still with the hips and knees flexed.
- *Nausea and vomiting* usually occur following the onset of pain. Murphy[1] described the

diagnostic sequence as colicky central abdominal pain, followed by vomiting, followed by movement of the pain to the RIF.
- *Anorexia* is almost invariable.
- *Constipation* is usual, but diarrhoea may occur (particularly when the ileum is irritated by the inflamed appendix).

There may be a history of previous milder attacks of similar pain.

With perforation of the appendix, there may be temporary remission or even cessation of pain as tension in the distended organ is relieved; this is followed by more severe and more generalized pain with profuse vomiting as general peritonitis develops.

Examination

- Pyrexia (around 37.5°C) and tachycardia are usual.
- The patient is flushed, may appear toxic and is obviously in pain.
- Movement exacerbates the pain.
- The tongue is usually coated, and a fetor oris is present.
- The abdomen shows localized tenderness in the region of the inflamed appendix. There is usually guarding of the abdominal muscles over this site with release tenderness. Coughing mimics the release test for rebound tenderness.
- Rectal examination reveals tenderness when the appendix is in the pelvic position or when there is pus in the rectovesical or Douglas pouch.[2]
- In late cases with generalized peritonitis, the abdomen becomes diffusely tender and rigid, bowel sounds are absent and the patient is obviously very ill. Later still, the abdomen is distended and tympanitic, and the patient exhibits the hippocratic facies of advanced peritonitis.

Special investigations

- *Leucocyte count:* a mild polymorph leucocytosis is the rule.
- *Computed tomography (CT)* is increasingly being used to evaluate atypical presentations of appendicitis and its complications.

---

[1]John Benjamin Murphy (1857–1916), Professor of Surgery, North Western University, Chicago, IL, USA.

[2]James Douglas (1675–1742), Obstetrician and Anatomist, London, UK.

- *Ultrasound of the RIF*, in experienced hands, may be diagnostic.

In general, the investigations are directed at excluding the differential diagnoses, as well as confirming appendicitis.

Differential diagnosis

The differential diagnosis of appendicitis includes most of the causes of acute abdominal pain. They should be considered systematically under the following headings.

- other intra-abdominal causes of acute pain;
- the urogenital tract;
- the chest;
- gynaecological emergencies in female patients;
- the central nervous system.

Intra-abdominal disease

The following commonly simulate appendicitis.

- *Non-specific mesenteric adenitis*, particularly in young children, following upper respiratory tract infection. This may coexist with appendicitis, so the diagnosis is best confirmed at the time of appendicectomy.
- *Meckel's diverti*culitis, often indistinguishable from appendicitis; the presence of an inflamed Meckel's diverticulum (see Chapter 23, p. 194) should always be excluded if the appendix is normal at exploration.
- *Acute Crohn's ileitis* (see Chapter 23, p. 195), affects young adults, usually with a long history of recurrent pain.
- *Acute intestinal obstruction*, with colicky pain and vomiting, but noisy bowel sounds and distended bowel on X-ray.
- *Gastroenteritis*, with diarrhoea and vomiting but more diffuse and less severe tenderness. Vomiting usually precedes any colic.
- *Perforated peptic ulcer*, normally a sudden onset; RIF pain may occur as fluid tracks down the right paracolic gutter.
- *Acute cholecystitis*, in which the initial colicky pain is foregut pain, experienced in the epigastrium. A distended, inflamed gallbladder may descend to the RIF.
- *Pancreatitis*, a central pain with central and sometimes RIF tenderness, diagnosed by a raised serum amylase concentration.
- *Acute colonic diverticulitis*, usually affecting the left colon but may give RIF pain if the

sigmoid colon is sufficiently mobile, or if there is inflammation of a solitary caecal diverticulum. The age group differs from the usually younger patient with appendicitis.

The urogenital tract

- *Ureteric colic and acute pyelonephritis.* The urine must be tested for blood and pus cells in every case of acute abdominal pain. The patient with ureteric colic is usually restless and moving about, with pain radiating from loin to groin. Remember, however, that an inflamed appendix adherent to the ureter or bladder may produce dysuria and microscopic haematuria or pyuria; if reasonable doubt exists, it is safer to perform a diagnostic laparoscopy to visually assess the appendix.
- *Testicular torsion* may occasionally present with periumbilical pain and vomiting. It is mandatory to examine the testes of all boys with abdominal pain, to exclude both torsion and maldescent (Chapter 46, p. 379).

The chest

Basal pneumonia and pleurisy may give referred abdominal pain, which may be surprisingly difficult to differentiate, especially in children. Auscultation may reveal a rub, and chest X-ray may demonstrate pneumonia.

Gynaecological emergencies

The commonest gynaecological pitfalls are acute salpingitis, ectopic pregnancy and ruptured cyst of the corpus luteum. A ruptured or torted ovarian cyst presents with sudden severe RIF pain radiating to the loin, and the patient with salpingitis has a more diffuse bilateral lower abdominal pain and a vaginal discharge. Ultrasound helps to visualize the distended fallopian tube in salpingitis and ectopic pregnancy. A pregnancy test (serum β-HCG) may help confirm the presence of an ectopic pregnancy. In women of childbearing age, laparoscopic pelvic examination may be helpful in resolving the differential diagnosis, and appendicectomy may be performed at the same time.

The central nervous system

The pain preceding the eruption of herpes zoster affecting the 11th and 12th dorsal segments, the irritation of these posterior nerve roots in spinal disease (invasive tumour or tuberculosis) and the lightning pains of tabes dorsalis all occasionally mimic appendicitis.

Nothing can be so easy, nor anything so difficult, as the diagnosis of acute appendicitis. The tyro may smile indulgently at the long list of differential diagnoses given in the textbooks but, as year follows year, he or she will experience the chagrin of making most, if not all, of these errors.

Treatment

The treatment of acute appendicitis is appendicectomy; nowadays, usually performed at laparoscopy to enable formal confirmation of the diagnosis particularly in women. Immediate appendicectomy is not indicated in the following circumstances:

- The patient is moribund with advanced peritonitis. In this case the patient should be aggressively resuscitated with intravenous fluids, antibiotics and analgesia; inotropes may also be required.
- The attack has already resolved; in such a case, appendicectomy can be advised as an elective procedure, but there is no immediate emergency.
- An appendix mass has formed without evidence of general peritonitis (see below).
- When circumstances make operation difficult or impossible, e.g. at sea. Here reliance must be placed on a conservative regimen and the hope that resolution or local abscess will form, rather than on one's surgical skill with a razor blade and a bent spoon.

Antibiotic prophylaxis is given preoperatively. When at operation peritonitis is discovered, antibiotic therapy is continued; metronidazole and gentamicin, or a cephalosporin, are effective for both the anaerobic and aerobic bowel organisms, but this regimen may need to be supplemented or changed when the bacteriological sensitivities of the cultured pus become available after 24–48 hours. After appendicectomy, a drain is inserted when there is severe inflammation of the appendix bed, when a local abscess is present or when closure of the appendix stump is not perfectly sound. Very occasionally, the inflamed and adherent appendix cannot be safely removed; in such

circumstances, the area of the appendix requires adequate drainage and subsequent 'interval appendicectomy' in about 3 months.

The appendix mass (Box 24.1)

Not uncommonly, the patient will present with a history of 4 or 5 days of abdominal pain and with a localized mass in the RIF. The rest of the abdomen is soft, bowel sounds are present and the patient obviously has no evidence of general peritonitis. In these circumstances, the inflamed appendix is walled off by adhesions to the omentum and adjacent viscera, with or without the presence of a local abscess. Immediate surgery in such circumstances is difficult and dangerous, with a risk of damage to adjacent bowel loops.

Box 24.1 A mass in the right iliac fossa

The causes of a mass in the right iliac fossa are best thought of by considering the possible anatomical structures in this region.

- Appendix abscess or appendix mass
- Carcinoma of caecum: differentiated from the above by usually an older age group, a longer history, often the presence of diarrhoea, anaemia with positive occult blood and finally the barium enema examination
- Crohn's disease: always to be thought of when there is a local mass in a young patient with diarrhoea
- A distended gallbladder, which may extend down as far as the right iliac fossa
- Pelvic kidney (or renal transplant)
- Ovarian or tubal mass
- Aneurysm of the common, internal or external iliac artery
- Retroperitoneal tumour arising in the soft tissues or lymph nodes of the posterior abdominal wall or from the pelvis
- Ileocaecal tuberculosis (rare in the UK, common in India)
- Psoas abscess – now rare

Treatment

Initial treatment is conservative. The outlines of the mass are marked on the skin, the patient is put to bed on a fluid diet and a careful watch kept on the general condition, temperature and pulse. Metronidazole is commenced, but prolonged antibiotics are not given, as these may merely produce a chronic inflammatory mass honeycombed with abscesses (the so-called 'antibioticoma').

On this regimen, 80% of appendix masses resolve. In the remaining cases, the abscess obviously enlarges over the next day or two and the temperature fails to subside. In these circumstances, drainage of the abscess is instituted. In neglected cases, an appendix abscess may burst spontaneously through the abdominal wall, into the rectum, or into the general peritoneal cavity.

If resolution occurs, appendicectomy is carried out after an interval of 3 months to allow the inflammatory condition to settle completely.

Unless interval appendicectomy is performed, there is considerable risk of a further attack of acute appendicitis.

Appendicitis in pregnancy

Appendicitis in pregnancy is no more rare or common than appendicitis in the general community, but it has a higher mortality and morbidity because it is confused with other complications of pregnancy. Differentiation must be made from pyelonephritis, vomiting of pregnancy, red degeneration of a fibroid or torsion of an ovarian cyst.

Because the appendix is displaced by the enlarging uterus, pain and tenderness are higher and more lateral than in the usual circumstances. There is considerable danger of abortion, particularly in the first trimester.

25

The colon

Constipation and diarrhoea

Constipation and diarrhoea are two symptoms frequently attributable to diseases of the large bowel. There are, of course, many causes of these common complaints, owing not only to lesions of the large intestine but also to other parts of the alimentary canal being affected or to general diseases. It is useful here to consider the commoner causes of these two symptoms.

Constipation

1 *Organic obstruction:*
   a carcinoma of the colon;
   b diverticular disease.
2 *Painful anal conditions:*
   a fissure *in ano*;
   b prolapsed piles.
3 *Adynamic bowel:*
   a Hirschsprung's disease;[1]
   b senility;
   c spinal cord injuries and disease;
   d myxoedema;
   e Parkinson's disease.

[1]Harald Hirschsprung (1830–1916), Professor of Paediatrics, Queen Louisa Hospital, Copenhagen, Denmark.

Lecture Notes: General Surgery, 12th edition. © Harold Ellis, Sir Roy Y. Calne and Christopher J. E. Watson. Published 2011 by Blackwell Publishing Ltd.

4 *Drugs:*
   a aspirin;
   b opiate analgesics;
   c anticholinergics;
   d ganglion blockers.
5 *Habit and diet:*
   a dyschezia (rectal stasis due to suppression of urge to defaecate);
   b dehydration;
   c starvation;
   d lack of bulk in diet.

Diarrhoea

1 *Specific infections:*
   a food poisoning (e.g. *Salmonella*);
   b dysentery (amoebic and bacillary);
   c cholera;
   d viral enterocolitis.
2 *Inflammation or irritation of the intestine:*
   a ulcerative colitis;
   b tumours of the large bowel;
   c diverticular disease;
   d Crohn's disease.
3 *Drugs:*
   a antibiotics and antibiotic-induced colitis;
   b erythromycin (stimulates the motilin receptor);
   c purgatives;
   d digoxin.
4 *Loss of absorptive surface:*
   a bowel resections and short circuits;
   b sprue and coeliac disease;
   c idiopathic steatorrhoea.

5 *Pancreatic dysfunction:* steatorrhoea due to lipase deficiency.
6 *Postgastrectomy and vagotomy.*
7 *General diseases:*
a anxiety states;
b hyperthyroidism;
c uraemia;
d carcinoid syndrome (Chapter 23, p. 197);
e Zollinger–Ellison syndrome (Chapter 32, p. 284).

Diverticulosis and diverticulitis

Background (Table 25.1)

Diverticula of the colon consist of outpouchings of mucous membrane through the muscle wall of the bowel. Because they lack the normal muscle coats, they are examples of 'false' diverticula, in contrast to a Meckel's diverticulum of the small bowel, which is a true diverticulum. They lie alongside the taenia coli, often overlapped by the appendices epiploicae. In the colon, diverticula are found most commonly in the sigmoid and descending colon, and become increasingly rare in passing from the left to the right side of the colon. They are unusual before the age of 40 years, but they are found in about 30% of all autopsies in the elderly. The sex distribution is roughly equal. Although colonic diverticula are common in Western communities, they are extremely rare among people of the developing countries.

Pathogenesis

Hypertrophy of the muscle of the sigmoid colon produces high intraluminal pressures, which cause herniation of the mucosa at the sites of potential weakness in the bowel wall, corresponding to the points of entry of the supplying vessels to the bowel (Figure 25.1). The aetiology of the

Table 25.1 Diverticulum terminology

True diverticulum	An outpouching covered by all the layers of the bowel wall (e.g. Meckel's diverticulum, jejunal diverticulum)
False diverticulum	Lacking the normal muscle coat of the bowel (e.g. colonic diverticula)
Diverticula	Plural of diverticulum
Diverticulosis	The presence of (usually colonic) diverticula
Diverticular disease	Complicated diverticulosis
Diverticulitis	Inflammation of a diverticulum

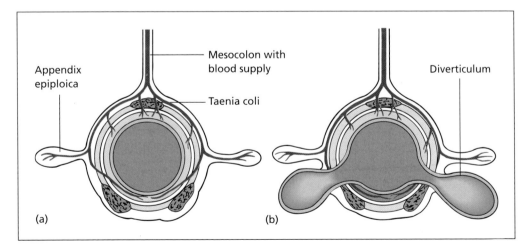

Figure 25.1 The relationship of diverticula of the colon to the taenia coli and to the penetrating blood vessels. (a) Normal colon. (b) Colon with diverticula. Both shown in transverse section.

muscular hypertrophy is unclear, but may relate to the nature of the intraluminal contents. Diets that are low in bulk tend not to distend the sigmoid colon, permitting high intramural pressures to develop, whereas high-fibre diets or bulking agents distend the colon and reduce intraluminal pressure. It may be that the modern, refined, low-roughage diet may be responsible for the Western nature of the disease.

Diverticulitis

This results from infection of one or more diverticula. An inflamed diverticulum may do one of three things.

1 *Perforate into:*
   a the general peritoneal cavity to cause peritonitis;
   b the pericolic tissues with formation of a pericolic abscess;
   c adjacent structures (e.g. bladder, small bowel, vagina), forming a fistula.
2 *Produce chronic infection* with inflammatory fibrosis, resulting in obstructive symptoms – acute, chronic or acute on chronic.
3 *Haemorrhage,* as a result of erosion of a vessel in the bowel wall. The bleeding varies from acute and profuse to a chronic occult loss.

Clinical features

Acute diverticulitis

This is well nicknamed 'left-sided appendicitis': an acute onset of low central abdominal pain, which shifts to the left iliac fossa (LIF) accompanied by fever, vomiting and local tenderness and guarding. A vague mass may be felt in the LIF and also on rectal examination. Perforation into the general peritoneal cavity produces the signs of general peritonitis. A pericolic abscess is comparable to an appendix abscess but on the left side: a tender mass accompanied by a swinging fever and leucocytosis.

Chronic diverticular disease

This exactly mimics the local clinical features of carcinoma of the colon (see p. 212); there may be:

1 *Change in bowel habit*, with diarrhoea alternating with constipation.
2 *Large bowel obstruction* with vomiting, distension, colicky abdominal pain and constipation. Small bowel obstruction from

adhesion of a loop of small intestine to the inflammatory mass is not uncommon.
3 *Blood and mucus per rectum.* There may be episodes of pain in the LIF, passage of mucus or bright red blood per rectum or of melaena, or there may be anaemia due to chronic occult bleeding.

Examination reveals tenderness in the LIF and there is often a thickened mass in the region of the sigmoid colon, which may also be felt per rectum. More unusual presentations are the following:

- *Sudden severe rectal haemorrhage:* bleeding from a diverticulum is the most likely cause of a sudden, profuse, bright red bleed in an elderly, often hypertensive, patient.
- *Colovesical fistula:* fistula into the bladder with the passage of gas bubbles (pneumaturia) and faecal debris in the urine. Diverticulitis is the commonest cause of colovesical fistula, others being carcinoma of the colon, carcinoma of the bladder, Crohn's disease and trauma.

Special investigations

- *Computed tomography (CT)* is the investigation of choice in the acute stage and can help exclude other causes of lower abdominal pain in difficult cases.
- *Sigmoidoscopy:* if the affected segment is low in the colon, there may be an oedematous block to the passage of the instrument beyond about 15 cm. Rigid sigmoidoscopes view only the rectum, and so do not visualize colonic diverticula. Fibreoptic sigmoidoscopes are longer and flexible, and do allow full visualization of the sigmoid colon.
- *Colonoscopy*, like flexile sigmoidoscopy, may allow the affected segment of sigmoid colon to be inspected, but often the rigid and narrow sigmoid in this condition makes onward passage of the instrument impossible.
- *Barium enema* demonstrates diverticula as globular outpouchings, which often show a signet-ring appearance because of the filling defect produced by contained pellets of faeces (faecoliths). Diverticular disease is characterized by stricture formation, which may closely simulate an annular carcinoma. More often, the oedema and thickening produce a 'saw-tooth' narrowed segment in the sigmoid. This examination should not be performed in the acute phase to prevent

iatrogenic perforation of friable and inflamed bowel.

Differential diagnosis

The important differential diagnosis is from neoplasm of the colon. It is impossible to be certain of this differentiation clinically or even on special investigations, unless a positive biopsy is obtained by flexible sigmoidoscopy or colonoscopy to establish definitively the diagnosis of carcinoma. Even at laparotomy, it is difficult to be sure whether one is dealing with carcinoma or diverticular disease; indeed, these two common conditions may coexist.

Treatment

Acute diverticulitis

This is managed conservatively; the patient is placed on a fluid diet and antibiotics (metronidazole with penicillin and gentamicin, or ciprofloxacin, are the combinations of choice). The great majority settle on this regimen.

- *A pericolic abscess* is diagnosed by CT, and may be drained percutaneously. This may occasionally be complicated by formation of a faecal fistula. Once the sepsis is controlled a laparotomy and resection of the diseased segment can be performed.
- *General peritonitis* from rupture of an acute diverticulitis is a dangerous condition. When peritonitis is the result of perforation of a diverticular abscess, laparoscopic lavage and drainage may suffice; otherwise, laparotomy is performed and the affected segment of colon resected. A primary anastomosis may be performed after intraoperative colonic lavage, but more commonly a colostomy is fashioned, usually as a Hartmann's procedure. Full antibiotic therapy is given.
- *Acute obstruction* due to diverticulitis requires laparotomy to establish the diagnosis. It is important to determine whether or not the obstruction is caused by an adherent loop of small intestine, which is by no means uncommon. The affected segment of colon is resected and the bowel brought out as an end colostomy (see p. 216). In experienced hands, an intraoperative antegrade colonic lavage may be performed followed by a primary anastomosis, with or without a 'covering' loop

ileostomy to divert the faecal stream until the anastomosis has healed; the ileostomy is subsequently closed.

Chronic diverticular disease

If the diagnosis is made with considerable certainty and symptoms are mild, this can be treated conservatively. The bowels are regulated by means of a lubricant laxative (e.g. Milpar). A high-roughage diet (fruit, vegetables, wholemeal bread and bran) is prescribed. If symptoms are severe or if carcinoma cannot be excluded, laparotomy and resection of the sigmoid colon is performed.

Colovesical fistula is treated by resection of the affected segment of the colon and bladder wall; a primary colonic anastomosis is fashioned and the defect in the bladder oversewn. The anastomosis may be defunctioned by a 'covering' loop ileostomy to permit healing without further fistula formation.

Angiodysplasia

This term is applied to one or multiple small (<5 mm) mucosal or submucosal vascular malformations, usually a dilated vein or sheaf of veins. Because they occur most commonly in the elderly, they are considered to be degenerative vascular anomalies. The caecum and ascending colon are the sites most usually involved, although they may be found anywhere in the small or large bowel.

Clinical features

They are usually asymptomatic, and were unknown before the advent of mesenteric angiography and colonoscopy. Their only clinical manifestation is bleeding, which may take the form of continuous chronic intestinal blood loss, presenting with anaemia, or recurrent acute dark or bright red rectal haemorrhage, which may occasionally be severe and life-threatening. Recurrent bleeding is common. They account for some 5% of such emergency cases.

Special investigations

- *Colonoscopy* is the investigation of choice, although it is often difficult to visualize the caecum in these elderly patients. The lesions appear as bright red 0.5–1 cm diameter submucosal lesions with small, dilated vessels visible on close inspection. They are invisible on barium enema.

- *Mesenteric angiogram.* Actively bleeding angiodysplasias may be detected on angiography as contrast medium leaks into the bowel lumen.

Treatment

Blood transfusion is necessary if haemorrhage is severe. Colonoscopic electrocoagulation or argon plasma coagulation may be curative. Resection, usually a right hemicolectomy, is sometimes required.

Colitis

Colitis, inflammation of the colon, presents with diarrhoea and often lower abdominal pain, and blood and mucus per rectum. The five main causes of colitis are as follows:

1 *ulcerative colitis;*
2 *Crohn's colitis;*
3 *antibiotic-associated colitis,* e.g. pseudomembranous colitis due to *Clostridium difficile* (see Chapter 4, p. 18);
4 *infective colitis,* e.g. *Campylobacter* and amoebic colitis;
5 *ischaemic colitis,* owing to mesenteric ischaemia, occurring spontaneously or following ligation of the inferior mesenteric artery in aortic surgery.

Ulcerative colitis

Ulcerative colitis is an inflammatory disease of the rectum extending for a variable distance proximally in the colon. Women are more often affected than men, and it is found in any age from infancy to the elderly, but the maximum incidence is between the ages of 20 and 40 with a second peak between 55 and 65.

Aetiology

The aetiology of ulcerative colitis is unknown, although it appears to combine environmental stimuli, autoimmune responses and genetic factors (there is an association with the human leucocyte antigen HLA-B27); it is one of the few diseases in which smoking appears to be protective.

Pathology

The rectum and sigmoid colon are principally affected, but the whole colon may be involved. (Note that the sigmoid is the site of election for all the major diseases of the colon: colitis, volvulus, carcinoma, polyposis and diverticulitis. Why it deserves this notoriety is unknown.)

Initially, there is oedema of the mucosa, with contact bleeding and petechial haemorrhage, proceeding to ulceration; the ulcers are shallow and irregular. Oedematous islands of mucosa between the ulcers form pseudopolyps. The wall of the colon is oedematous and fibrotic and is therefore rigid with loss of its normal haustrations. The changes are confluent, with no unaffected 'skip lesions' as found in Crohn's disease. Surprisingly, the inflamed colon does not become adherent to its neighbouring intra-abdominal viscera.

Microscopically, the principal locus of the disease is mucosal; small abscesses form within the mucosal crypts ('crypt abscesses'). These abscesses break down into ulcers whose base is lined with granulation tissue. The walls of the colon are infiltrated with polymorphs and round cells; there is oedema and submucosal fibrosis. In the chronic, burnt-out disease the mucosa is smooth and atrophic; the bowel wall is thinned.

Clinical features

Manifestations of ulcerative colitis may be fulminant, intermittent or chronic. The commonest scenario is of diarrhoea, with blood and mucus. There may be accompanying cramp-like abdominal pains. Examination reveals nothing except some tenderness in the LIF, and blood on the glove of the examining finger after rectal examination. The rectal mucosa may feel oedematous.

In severe attacks there is fever, toxaemia, severe bleeding and risk of perforation. Anorexia and loss of weight occur in the acute episodes.

Special investigations

Investigations aim to make the diagnosis, differentiate it from Crohn's colitis, exclude complications and assess the proximal extent.

- *Sigmoidoscopy* reveals oedema of the mucosa with contact bleeding in the early mild cases, proceeding to granularity of the mucosa and then frank ulceration with pus and blood in the bowel lumen. Biopsy will give confirming histological evidence of the diagnosis.

- *Colonoscopy* enables the whole of the large bowel to be inspected, the proximal extent to be noted and biopsy material to be obtained.
- *Barium enema* shows a ragged surface, indicating ulceration. Oedema and fibrosis produce loss of haustration and in the chronic case the typical smooth, narrow 'drainpipe' colon.
- *Examination of the stools* reveals pus and blood visible to the naked eye or under the microscope; no specific organism has ever been grown.

Differential diagnosis

Ulcerative colitis may be difficult to differentiate from other causes of diarrhoea (Chapter 25, p. 204), especially the dysenteries and carcinoma, or Crohn's disease of the large bowel (Table 25.2). Differentiation from colonic Crohn's disease may be particularly difficult, even when the resected colon is examined by an expert pathologist. Indeed, about 10% of cases have to be labelled 'non-specific colitis'.

Complications

Local

- Toxic dilatation, in which the colon dilates in a fulminant colitis, leading to perforation.
- Haemorrhage (acute, or chronic with progressive anaemia).
- Stricture.
- Malignant change (see below).
- Perianal disease: anal fissures are common; fistula *in ano*, fistula into the vagina and perianal abscesses do occur, but are less common than in Crohn's disease.

General

- Toxaemia.
- Weight loss and anaemia.
- Arthritis (including ankylosing spondylitis) and uveitis.
- Dermatological manifestations: pyoderma gangrenosum, erythema nodosum, other skin rashes and ulceration of the legs.
- Primary sclerosing cholangitis is also associated with ulcerative colitis, as it is with Crohn's disease.

Malignant change

Patients with ulcerative colitis who have had chronic total colitis (affecting the whole large

Table 25.2 Crohn's and ulcerative colitis*

	Crohn's colitis	Ulcerative colitis
Clinical features	Perianal disease, e.g. fissure *in ano* and fistula *in ano* common	Perianal disease rare
	Gross bleeding uncommon	Often profuse haemorrhage
	Small bowel may also be affected	Small bowel not affected
Pathology		
Macroscopic differences	Any part of colon may be involved (skip lesions)	Disease extends proximally from rectum
	Transmural involvement	Mucosal involvement only
	Fistulae in adjacent viscera	No fistulae
	No polyps	Pseudo-polyps of regenerating mucosa
	Thickened bowel wall	No thickening of bowel wall
	Malignant change rare	Malignant change common in long-standing cases
Microscopic differences	Granulomas present	No granulomas

*10% of cases cannot be assigned clearly to one or other disease and are labelled as 'non-specific colitis'.

bowel), particularly if the first attack was in childhood, have a high risk of developing carcinoma of the colon. Statistics indicate that 5–12% of patients with colitis of 20 years' duration will develop malignant change. Patients should therefore be offered annual or biannual colonoscopy with multiple biopsies to seek the dysplasia that heralds malignant change.

Even in the absence of a total or pan-colitis, patients with ulcerative colitis are at far greater risk of developing carcinoma of the large bowel than a normal individual. Moreover, the tumours occurring in colitics are more likely to affect a younger age group, be anaplastic and be multiple compared with those arising in previously healthy bowels. Often, the condition is only diagnosed late, as both the patient and doctor attribute the symptoms (bleeding, diarrhoea and pus) to the colitis.

Treatment

Initially this is medical in the uncomplicated case, but surgery is required when medical treatment fails or when complications supervene.

Medical treatment

A high-protein diet is prescribed with vitamin supplements, iron and potassium (the last to replace electrolyte loss in the stools). Blood transfusion is given if the patient is severely anaemic. Diarrhoea may be controlled with codeine phosphate or loperamide. Corticosteroids given systemically, by rectal infusion or in combination, will often produce remission in an acute attack. Salicylates such as mesalazine or sulfasalazine (sulphonamide/salicylate combination) are used to maintain a remission. In more severe cases the anti-tumour necrosis factor antibodies infliximab or adalimumab, or immunosuppressants such as azathioprine or ciclosporin, may be required.

Patients with ulcerative colitis are often highly intelligent, tense and anxious, and treatment should be supplemented with sympathy and reassurance.

Surgery

The indications for surgery are the following:

- *Fulminating disease* not responding to medical treatment (defined as the passage of more than six bloody motions per day, with fever, tachycardia and hypoalbuminaemia).
- *Chronic disease* not responding to medical treatment.
- *Prophylaxis against malignant change* with long-standing disease.
- *Complications of colitis* already listed.

The procedure usually comprises total removal of the colon and rectum with either a permanent ileostomy or an ileoanal anastomosis with an interposed pouch of ileum (Parks' pouch[2]).

Most patients requiring surgery for ulcerative colitis are either on corticosteroids or have recently received them. Surgical procedures must therefore be covered by an increased dosage of corticosteroids to compensate for presumed suppression of endogenous glucocorticoids, which can then be tailed off gradually in the postoperative period.

Crohn's colitis

Crohn's disease,[3] although most commonly found in the terminal ileum (Chapter 23, p. 195), may occur anywhere in the alimentary tract from the mouth to the anus. It may be confined to the large bowel, or there may be involvement of both the small and large intestine.

Clinical features

Colonic Crohn's disease closely mimics ulcerative colitis in its clinical manifestations. Unlike ulcerative colitis, the affected segment of colon commonly becomes adherent to adjacent structures with abscess formation and fistulation. Perianal inflammation with abscesses and multiple fistulae *in ano* is also common and indeed may be the first manifestation of the disease.

Treatment

This is similar to that of Crohn's disease of the small intestine (Chapter 23, p. 195). Resection of involved large bowel may require segmental colectomy if small areas are involved or total excision with a permanent ileostomy for extensive disease. Restorative proctocolectomy and Parks' pouch formation is not performed for Crohn's disease because of the immediate risks of sepsis and fistulation, and the chance of recurrence.

---

[2]Sir Alan Parks (1920–1982), Surgeon, St Mark's Hospital, London, UK.
[3]Burrill Bernard Crohn (1884–1983), Gastroenterologist, Mount Sinai Hospital, New York, NY, USA.

Tumours

Classification

Benign

- Adenomatous polyp.
- Papilloma.
- Lipoma.
- Neurofibroma.
- Haemangioma.

Malignant

1 *Primary:*
   a carcinoma;
   b lymphoma;
   c carcinoid tumour (Chapter 23, p. 197).
2 *Secondary*: invasion from adjacent tumours, e.g. stomach, bladder, uterus and ovary.

Carcinoma

Carcinomas affecting the large bowel are common. They are the second most common cause of death from malignant disease in this country, next in frequency to cancers of the lung in men and cancer of the breast in women.

Tumours may occur at any age. Women are affected more often than men (although, interestingly, the incidence of rectal cancer is roughly equal in the two sexes). The sigmoid is the most common site in the colon, although the rectum accounts for one-third of all the large bowel cancers. Five per cent of tumours of the large bowel are multiple (synchronous).

Predisposing factors

Pre-existing polyps, ulcerative colitis and a number of inherited colorectal cancer syndromes are risk factors for the development of carcinoma of the large bowel. Inherited syndromes such as familial adenomatous polyposis and hereditary non-polyposis colon cancer account for a significant proportion of colorectal cancers, and potential carriers should be offered screening (see below). Family history alone is sufficient to increase the risk, and it has been estimated that one first-degree relative contracting colon cancer aged over 45 years increases one's lifetime risk from 1 in 50 to 1 in 17; if the relative was diagnosed before 45, the lifetime risk increases to 1 in 10.

Familial adenomatous polyposis

This is a rare disease, but it is important because it invariably proceeds to carcinoma of the colon unless treated and accounts for 0.5% of all colon cancers. It has an autosomal dominant inheritance, and is associated with mutation in the familial adenomatous polyposis (FAP) gene. The polyps first appear in adolescence; symptoms of bleeding and diarrhoea commence about the age of 21 years and malignant change occurs between 20 and 40 years of age. Affected individuals usually have hypertrophy of the retinal pigment layer which is a useful, non-invasive screening test. Variants such as *Gardner's syndrome*[4] exist in which colonic polyps are associated with desmoid tumours and osteomas of the mandible and skull.

Treatment comprises a total colectomy with excision of the rectum, and formation of an ileo-anal pouch. If the polyps are not profuse in the lower rectum, it is possible to resect the colon while leaving a stump of rectum to which an ile-orectal anastomosis is performed, and then carry out regular diathermy of the polyps in the rectal stump through a sigmoidoscope.

Hereditary non-polyposis colon cancer

This accounts for around 5% of colorectal cancers, and is also dominantly inherited. It results from a gene mutation affecting DNA mismatch repair, which leads to genomic instability. Tumours tend to occur in the right colon, and arise before the age of 50. Occurrence of colon cancer in at least three family members spanning two generations, with one before the age of 50, strongly suggests this syndrome. It is also associated with tumours of the ovary, uterus and stomach.

Pathology

Macroscopically, the tumours can be classified into the following groups:

- papilliferous;
- malignant ulcer;
- annular;

[4]Eldon John Gardner (1909–1989), Geneticist, later Professor of Zoology, Utah State University, Logan, UT, USA.

- diffuse infiltrating growth;
- mucinous tumour.

Microscopically, these are all adenocarcinomas.

Spread

- *Local:* encircling the wall of the bowel and invading the coats of the colon, eventually involving adjacent viscera (small intestine, stomach, duodenum, ureter, bladder, uterus, abdominal wall, etc.).
- *Lymphatic:* to the regional lymph nodes, eventually spreading via the thoracic duct, and may involve supraclavicular nodes in late cases.
- *Bloodstream:* to the liver via the portal vein, and thence to the lung.
- *Transcoelomic:* producing deposits of malignant nodules throughout the peritoneal cavity.

Staging

Traditionally carcinoma of the colon has been staged according to the classification of Dukes,[5] and depends upon the extent of transmural extension and lymph node spread (Chapter 26, p. 227), although TNM staging (Chapter 7, p. 39) is more commonly used nowadays.

Clinical features

The manifestations of carcinoma of the colon can be divided, as with any tumour, into those produced by the tumour itself, those arising from the presence of secondaries and the general effects of the tumour.

Local effects

1 *Change in bowel habit* is the most common symptom, either constipation or diarrhoea or the two alternating with each other. The diarrhoea may be accompanied by mucus (produced by the excessive secretion of mucus from the tumour) or bleeding, which may be bright, melaena or occult.
2 *Intestinal obstruction* due to a constricting neoplasm, commonly found in the left (descending) colon (see Chapter 22, p. 183).

3 *Perforation* of the tumour, either into the general peritoneal cavity or locally with the formation of a pericolic abscess, or by fistulae into adjacent viscera, e.g. a gastrocolic fistula or colovesical fistula, is an occasional presentation.

The effects of secondary deposits

The patient may present with jaundice, abdominal distension due to ascites or hepatomegaly.

The general effects of malignant disease

Presenting features may be anaemia, anorexia or loss of weight.

Tumours of the left side of the colon, where the contained stool is solid, are typically constricting growths, so obstructive features predominate. In contrast, tumours of the right side tend to be proliferative and here the stools are semiliquid, and therefore obstructive symptoms are relatively uncommon and the patient with a carcinoma of the caecum or ascending colon often presents with anaemia and loss of weight.

Examination

This should seek evidence of the following:

1 The presence of a mass palpable either per abdomen or per rectum (a sigmoid tumour may prolapse into the pouch of Douglas[6]).
2 Clinical evidence of intestinal obstruction.
3 Evidence of spread (hepatomegaly, ascites, jaundice or supraclavicular lymphadenopathy).
4 Clinical evidence of anaemia or loss of weight suggesting malignant disease.

Special investigations

- *Occult blood in the stool* is frequently present.
- *Sigmoidoscopy* will reveal tumours in the rectosigmoid region and allow positive evidence by biopsy to be obtained. Even if the tumour is not reached directly, the presence of blood or slime coming down from above is strongly suspicious of malignant disease.

[5]Cuthbert Esquire Dukes (1890–1977), Pathologist, St Mark's Hospital, London, UK.

[6]James Douglas (1675–1742), Obstetrician and Anatomist, London, UK.

- *Colonoscopy*, using the fibreoptic colonoscope, enables the higher reaches of the colon to be inspected and a biopsy to be obtained.
- *Barium enema* will usually reveal the growth, as either a stricture or filling defect ('apple-core' deformity). It is important to remember that a negative barium enema does not definitely exclude the presence of a small tumour, particularly in the presence of extensive diverticulosis. False-positive X-rays may result from the presence of faecal material in the bowel lumen. It is by no means easy to differentiate radiologically between a carcinomatous stricture and one produced by diverticular disease; indeed, these two common conditions may coexist.
- *CT.* In elderly patients who tolerate bowel preparation poorly, CT may give sufficient information for the diagnosis of colonic cancer, and identify any liver involvement.

Rarely, if there is reasonable doubt as to the diagnosis, laparotomy is indicated.

Differential diagnosis

Diseases producing local symptoms

- Diverticular disease.
- Ulcerative colitis.
- The dysenteries and other causes of diarrhoea and constipation (Chapter 25, p. 204).

Treatment

- *Preoperative.* The bowel is cleared by enemas and oral stimulant laxatives (e.g. Picolax). Metronidazole and gentamicin (or a cephalosporin) are given at the time of surgery. The haemoglobin level is checked and blood transfusion given if necessary.
- *Operative.* The principle of operative treatment is wide resection of the growth together with its regional lymphatics. In the unobstructed case, the bowel can be prepared beforehand and primary resection with restoration of continuity can be achieved. In the obstructed case, in which bowel preparation is contraindicated, the primary goal is to relieve obstruction. It may be possible to achieve primary resection with restoration of continuity at the same time, but the poor vascularity and high incidence of colonic anastomotic breakdown means that

this is undertaken only after serious consideration. The options would be to use an extended right colonic resection round to the splenic flexure, or bring out a defunctioning colostomy or ileostomy.
- *Postoperative.* Adjuvant chemotherapy with 5-fluorouracil (5-FU), in combination with folinic acid, may reduce the risk of recurrent disease; for metastatic disease, the combination of 5-FU together with folinic acid and irinotecan may prolong survival.
- *Follow-up cross-sectional imaging* is performed to detect local recurrence and the appearance of liver metastases; metastatic spread to one lobe of the liver in the absence of other disease may be treated by resection of the affected liver lobe.
- *Follow-up surveillance colonoscopy* is undertaken at intervals to detect new tumours and local recurrence.

The incurable case

Even if secondary spread is present, the best palliation is achieved by resection of the primary tumour. If this is impossible, the tumour may be stented to relieve obstruction. Where stenting is not possible a palliative short-circuit or colostomy is performed. Irradiation and cytotoxic therapy may give temporary alleviation of symptoms.

Prognosis

Dukes' A tumours are usually curable with over 90% 5 year survival. Survival with Dukes' B tumours, in which the disease is still confined to the bowel wall, is around 65%, and the presence of lymph node metastases gives a 30% survival. If the apical lymph node, i.e. the node at the highest point of lymphatic drainage, is free from disease (C1), the prognosis is better than in C2 disease, in which the apical node is involved.

Colonic surgery (Figure 25.2)

The different colonic resections are based on the blood supply to the colon coming from the superior mesenteric artery (midgut components, i.e. caecum, ascending colon and two-thirds of the transverse colon) and the inferior mesenteric artery (hindgut components, i.e. distal transverse colon, descending colon, sigmoid and rectum) together with a free anastomosis between the principal arteries via the marginal artery (of

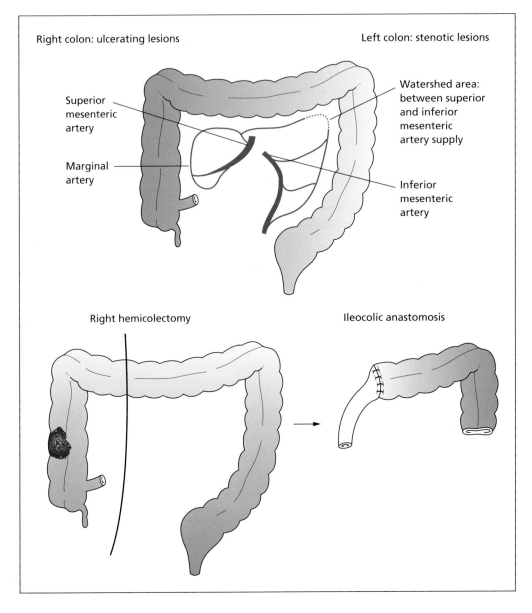

Right colon: ulcerating lesions

Left colon: stenotic lesions

Superior mesenteric artery

Watershed area: between superior and inferior mesenteric artery supply

Marginal artery

Inferior mesenteric artery

Right hemicolectomy

Ileocolic anastomosis

Figure 25.2 Typical colonic operations. For a lesion in the right colon a right hemicolectomy is performed, with an ileocolic anastomosis. For a lesion in the left colon a left hemicolectomy or sigmoid colectomy is performed, with anastomosis of the colon to the rectum; in an emergency situation, with unprepared bowel, a Hartmann's operation can be performed with the bowel end exteriorized as a colostomy and the rectum oversewn. At a second stage the continuity of the bowel can be restored by colorectal anastomosis.

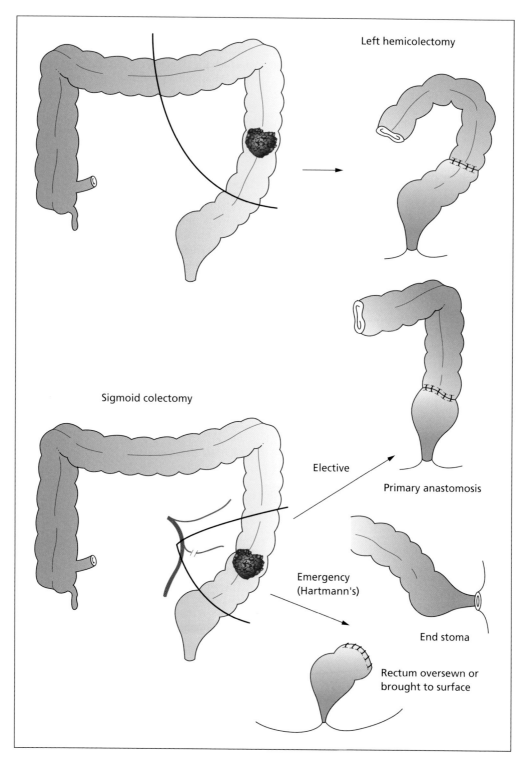

Figure 25.2 *Continued*

Drummond[7]). Since survival of colonic cancer is, in the case of Dukes' C disease, dependent upon the adequacy of resection (clearing all affected lymph nodes), surgery for cancer involves taking as much of the lymphatic drainage as possible. In practice, this means resecting as far down the principal artery as possible, as the lymphatic drainage runs alongside the arterial inflow. In non-cancer operations, more conservative surgical techniques may be employed.

Colostomy

When the bowel is brought to the surface and opened, it is termed a stoma (meaning mouth); in the case of the colon, such an opening is termed a colostomy. Stomas may be permanent, e.g. when the distal bowel has been removed, or temporary, when there is a possibility of restoring continuity at a future date.

Indications for colostomy formation

The common indications for colostomy formation are the following:

- to divert faeces to allow healing of a more distal anastomosis or fistula;
- to decompress a dilated colon, as a prelude to resection of the obstructing lesion;
- removal of the distal colon and rectum.

Types of colostomy

Loop colostomy

The colon is brought to the surface and the antimesenteric border opened. A rod or similar device is often used to stop the opened bowel loop from falling back inside. A loop colostomy is used temporarily to divert faeces and is simple to reverse; more commonly nowadays, a loop ileostomy is preferred because of the better blood supply to the bowel facilitating subsequent closure.

End colostomy

An end (or terminal) colostomy is fashioned by dividing the colon and bringing the proximal end

to the surface. It may be used as a definitive procedure in a patient undergoing total rectal excision, or following perforated diverticular disease in which the diseased bowel is removed and gross faecal contamination makes performing a primary anastomosis to restore continuity undesirable. In the latter, the distal bowel may be closed off and left within the abdomen (a Hartmann's procedure[8]) or brought to the surface at a separate place as a mucous fistula.

Double-barrelled colostomy

A double-barrelled (Paul–Mikulicz[9]) colostomy comprises proximal and distal ends of colon brought out adjacent to each other, rather like a loop colostomy but with the intervening colon removed. This type of colostomy is not commonly used because the distal bowel is usually too short, but it is useful in the treatment of sigmoid volvulus, in which there is usually sufficient distal colon.

Complications of colostomy formation

- *Retraction*, in which the colon disappears down the hole out of which it was brought. Retraction is either real and due to tension or apparent and due to necrosis of the terminal bowel.
- *Stenosis*, in which the opening becomes smaller. This may be due to ischaemia or poor apposition of colonic mucosa with the skin edge.
- *Paracolostomy hernia*, in which peritoneal contents herniate through the abdominal wall defect made to accommodate the stoma.
- *Prolapse*, in which the colon intussuscepts out of the stoma.
- *Lateral space small bowel obstruction*, which is caused by failure to obliterate the space between the terminal colon and the lateral abdominal wall.

In addition, there are psychological problems, excess gas production with certain foods, and leakage and skin excoriation due to ill-fitting stoma appliances or poorly constructed stomas.

[7]Sir David Drummond (1852–1932), Professor of Medicine, University of Durham, Durham, UK.

[8]Henri Hartmann (1860–1952), Professor of Surgery, Hôtel-Dieu, Paris, France.
[9]Frank Thomas Paul (1851–1941), Surgeon, Liverpool Royal Infirmary, Liverpool, UK. Johann von Mikulicz-Radecki (1850–1905), Professor of Surgery, successively at Cracow, Konigsberg and Breslau, Poland.

Stoma appliances: principles

Modern-day stoma appliances have made the management of stomas straightforward. The principal components are the collecting pouch, or bag, into which the faeces are collected, and the adhesive flange, which adheres to the skin and keeps the pouch in position. The flange is cut to fit the stoma closely, and any exposed skin is covered with a barrier paste. Colostomies contrast with ileostomies by the nature of the effluent. Ileostomy effluent is very irritant and causes severe skin excoriation. For this reason, an ileostomy is constructed with a spout to keep the effluent off the skin, in contrast to a colostomy, which is flush.

Management of a colostomy

In the first few weeks after performing a colostomy, the faecal discharge is semiliquid, but this gradually reverts to normal, solid stools. The colostomy appliances, which are both waterproof and windproof, allow the patient to lead a normal life with little risk of leakage or unpleasant odour.

Although there is obviously no sphincteric control of the colostomy opening, most patients find that they pass a single stool a day, usually after breakfast. This can be helped by preparations such as Fybogel or Celevac, which produce a bulky, formed stool. Patients are best advised to avoid large amounts of vegetables or fruit, which may produce diarrhoea and excessive flatus.

26

The rectum and anal canal

Learning objectives
✓ To know the causes and treatment of rectal bleeding.
✓ To know the presentations and management of rectal cancer.

The distribution around the anal canal of various conditions is shown in Figure 26.1.

Bright red rectal bleeding (Table 26.1)

The passage of bright red blood per rectum is a common symptom, which the patient usually attributes to 'piles'; indeed, haemorrhoids are by far the commonest cause of rectal bleeding. It is important, however, to bear in mind a list of possible causes of this symptom.

General causes

- Bleeding diatheses (rare).

Local causes

- Haemorrhoids.
- Fissure *in ano*.
- Tumours of the colon and rectum:
  - benign;
  - malignant.

Lecture Notes: General Surgery, 12th edition. © Harold Ellis,
Sir Roy Y. Calne and Christopher J. E. Watson. Published 2011 by
Blackwell Publishing Ltd.

- Diverticular disease.
- Ulcerative colitis.
- Trauma.
- Angiodysplasia of the colon.
- Rarely, massive haemorrhage from higher up the alimentary canal – even a bleeding duodenal ulcer may produce bright red blood per rectum instead of the usual melaena, although such cases are commonly accompanied by haematemesis.

Haemorrhoids

Functional anatomy

Continence is partly a function of the anal sphincters, and partly a consequence of the anal cushions. The anal cushions comprise highly vascular tissue lining the anal canal, with a rich blood supply from the rectal arteries, which anastomose with the draining veins both through capillaries and through direct arteriovenous shunts. The draining veins form saccules, commonly just below the dentate line, which then drain via the superior rectal vein. The venous saccules are supported by smooth muscle to form the cushions. Apposition of these subepithelial vascular cushions is important for continence of flatus and fluid.

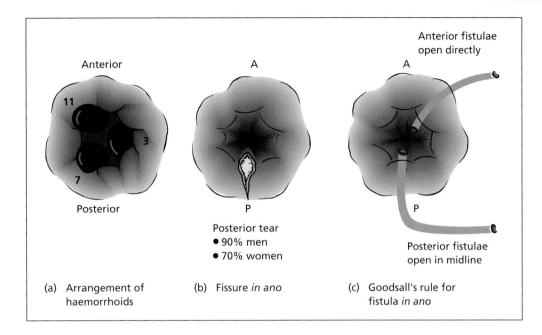

(a) Arrangement of haemorrhoids

(b) Fissure *in ano*

(c) Goodsall's rule for fistula *in ano*

Figure 26.1 Distribution of different conditions around the anal canal.

Table 26.1 Rectal bleeding

	Blood	Pain
Piles	Bright red blood on paper and in pan. May prolapse	Painless, unless prolapsed and thrombosed
Fissure	Bright red blood on paper and outside of stool	Painful, pain lasting long after passing stool
Colon and rectal cancer	Blood often mixed in with stool, especially if proximal tumour	Usually painless, unless distally placed in rectum or in anal canal, when causes tenesmus
Diverticular disease	Large volume of blood in the pan	Painless
Ulcerative colitis	Blood and mucus mixed with loose stool	Painless, unless coexistent fissure

Classification

Haemorrhoids (or piles; the words are synonymous) may be classified according to their relationship to the anal orifice into internal, external and interoexternal. Internal haemorrhoids are congested vascular cushions with dilated venous components draining into the superior rectal veins. External haemorrhoids is a term that should be abandoned, as it is applied to a conglomeration of quite different entities including perianal haematoma ('thrombosed external pile'), the 'sentinel pile' of fissure *in ano* and perianal skin tags.

Strictly speaking, internal piles that prolapse should be termed interoexternal haemorrhoids, but this term is seldom used except by literary perfectionists. In this chapter, which aims at being neither archaic nor pedantic, the terms 'external' and 'interoexternal' haemorrhoids will not be used further.

Pathology

Internal haemorrhoids, or piles, are abnormal anal cushions, usually congested as a result of straining at stool, and traumatized by the passage of hard stool. The anal cushions are particularly prominent in pregnancy owing to the venous congestion caused by the large gravid uterus and the laxity of the supporting tissues caused by the influence of progesterone. With the patient in the lithotomy position, the usual arrangement is that three major piles occur at 3, 7 and 11 o'clock.

Grading haemorrhoids

- *First-degree haemorrhoids* are confined to the anal canal – they bleed but do not prolapse.
- *Second-degree haemorrhoids* prolapse on defaecation, then reduce spontaneously.
- *Third-degree haemorrhoids* prolapse outside the anal margin on defaecation; they may be manually replaced by the patient.
- *Fourth-degree haemorrhoids* remain prolapsed outside the anal margin at all times.

Predisposing factors

Most haemorrhoids are idiopathic, but they may be precipitated or aggravated by factors that produce congestion of the superior rectal veins. These include compression by any pelvic tumour (of which the commonest is the pregnant uterus), cardiac failure, excessive use of purgatives, chronic constipation and a rectal carcinoma.

Occasionally, anorectal varices, similar in appearance to oesophageal varices, coexist with haemorrhoids in patients with portal hypertension since the anorectal area is the site of portosystemic anastomoses between the superior and inferior rectal veins (Chapter 30, p. 259).

Clinical features

Rectal bleeding is almost invariable; this is bright red and usually occurs at defaecation. In the case of first-degree piles, this is the only symptom. More extensive piles prolapse and may produce a mucus discharge and pruritus ani. The prolapsed piles may result in soiling.

Note that pain is not a feature of internal haemorrhoids except when these undergo thrombosis (see below). When a patient complains of 'an attack of piles', it often means that some acute painful condition has developed at the anal margin. The most common and dramatic is strangulation of prolapsing piles leading to thrombosis; apart from this, acute pain may be due to the following:

- fissure *in ano*;
- perianal haematoma;
- perianal or ischiorectal abscess;
- tumour of the anal margin;
- proctalgia fugax: benign episodic pain relieved by digital dilatation of the anal sphincter.

Every patient presenting with the story suggestive of internal haemorrhoids is submitted to the following procedure:

1 *Examination of the abdomen* to exclude palpable lesions of the colon or aggravating factors for haemorrhoids, e.g. an enlarged liver or a pelvic mass, including the pregnant uterus.
2 *Rectal examination*. Internal haemorrhoids are not palpable but prolapsing piles are immediately obvious. The presence of prolapsing piles does not exclude a lesion higher in the bowel.
3 *Proctoscopy*, which will visualize the internal haemorrhoids.
4 *Sigmoidoscopy* is performed routinely, again to eliminate a lesion higher in the rectum – proctitis, polyp or carcinoma.
5 *Colonoscopy or flexible sigmoidoscopy* is carried out when symptoms such as alteration in bowel habit point to a more sinister condition than internal haemorrhoids. A barium enema is carried out when colonoscopy is not readily available.

Complications

- *Anaemia*: following severe or continued bleeding.
- *Thrombosis*: this occurs when prolapsing piles are gripped by the anal sphincter ('strangulated piles'). The venous return is occluded and thrombosis of the pile occurs. The prolapsed haemorrhoids are swollen often to the size of large plums, purplish-black and tense, and are accompanied by considerable pain and distress. Suppuration or ulceration may occur. After 2–3 weeks, the thrombosed piles become fibrosed, often with spontaneous cure.

Treatment

Before commencing treatment, it is essential to exclude either any predisposing cause or an associated and more important lesion, e.g. carcinoma of the rectum.

Conservative management

Ideally, the patient should avoid straining at stool, and aim to pass a firm, soft motion daily. A bulk laxative, together with advice on an adequate fluid intake, are often required.

Sclerotherapy

This is suitable for first- and second-degree piles; 2–3 mL of 5% phenol in almond oil (or arachis oil) is injected above each pile as a sclerosing submucous perivenous injection. (The phenol sterilizes the oil, which is the main sclerosant.) Because the injection is placed high in the anal canal above the dentate line, it is painless. One or more repeat injections may be required at monthly intervals.

Banding

Application of a small O-ring rubber band to areas of protruding mucosa results in strangulation of the mucosa, which falls away after a few days. It can be successfully applied to first-, second- and third-degree piles, but care must be taken to position the bands above the dentate line, lest the patient should feel the application.

Surgery

Haemorrhoidectomy is performed for third- and fourth-degree piles.

Thrombosed strangulated piles

Conservative management is instituted for these. The patient is placed in bed with the foot of the bed elevated. Opiate analgesia is given for the severe pain, which is also eased by local cold compresses. Often the thrombosed piles fibrose completely with spontaneous cure. Many surgeons carry out haemorrhoidectomy at once in these patients.

Specific complications of haemorrhoidectomy

Acute retention of urine

This is the result of acute anal discomfort postoperatively.

Stricture

This only occurs when excessive amounts of mucosa and skin are excised. It is important to leave a bridge of epithelium between each excised haemorrhoid.

Postoperative haemorrhage

This may be reactionary, usually on the night of the operation, or secondary, on about the seventh or eighth day. The bleeding may not be apparent externally, as the source of haemorrhage may be above the anal sphincter, with the blood filling the large bowel with only a little escaping to the exterior.

General treatment comprises blood transfusion if haemorrhage is severe as evidenced by the general appearance of the patient, a pulse raised above 100 and a systolic blood pressure below 100 mmHg.

Local treatment is carried out under general anaesthetic in the operating theatre. The blood is washed out of the rectum with warm saline. Occasionally in reactionary haemorrhage, a bleeding point is seen and can be diathermied or suture-ligated. More often, there is a general oozing from the operation field and the anal canal requires packing with gauze around a wide-bored rubber tube, which allows evacuation of flatus and escape of any blood from the bowel. The tube and gauze are removed after 48 hours.

Perianal haematoma

This lesion, which is also termed a thrombosed external pile, is produced by thrombosis within the inferior rectal venous plexus. Unlike internal haemorrhoids, it is covered by squamous epithelium supplied by somatic nerves and is therefore painful. The onset is acute, often after straining at stool, with sudden pain and the appearance of a lump at the anal verge. Local examination shows a tense, smooth, dark-blue, cherry-sized lump at the anal margin.

Untreated, this perianal haematoma either subsides over a few days, eventually leaving a fibrous tag, or ruptures, discharging some clotted blood.

Treatment

In the acute phase, immediate relief is produced by evacuating the haematoma through a small incision, conveniently performed under local anaesthetic. If the patient is seen when the haematoma is already discharging or becoming absorbed, hot baths are prescribed and reassurance given that all will soon be well.

Fissure *in ano*

A fissure is a tear at the anal margin, which usually follows the passage of a constipated stool. The site is usually posterior in the midline (90% of men, 70% of women), occasionally anteriorly in the midline and rarely multiple. The posterior position of the majority of fissures has traditionally been explained by the anatomical arrangement of the external anal sphincter; its superficial fibres pass forward to the anal canal from the coccyx, leaving a relatively unsupported V posteriorly. However, mucosal tears are probably quite common and, while most heal spontaneously, those occurring posteriorly (or anteriorly) are slow to heal because of the relatively poor blood supply to the anal mucosa posteriorly. The anterior fissures of women may be associated with weakening of the perineal floor following tears at childbirth. Multiple fissures may complicate Crohn's disease[1] of the colon.

Clinical features

Acute anal pain is characteristic. It is stinging in nature and lasts for a while after the passage of stool, sometimes 2 or more hours later. Fissure is the commonest cause of pain at the anal verge (see p. 220). There is often slight bleeding and, because of the pain, the patient is usually constipated. On examination, the anal sphincter is in spasm, and there may be a 'sentinel pile' protruding from the anus, which represents the torn tag of anal epithelium. The fissure can usually be seen by gently pulling open the anal verge. It may be impossible to do a rectal examination without anaesthetic; the fissure may then be palpable as a crack in the anal canal.

Treatment

Early small fissures may heal spontaneously. A local anaesthetic ointment together with a lubri-

[1]Burrill Bernard Crohn (1884–1983), Gastroenterologist, Mount Sinai Hospital, New York, NY, USA. The disease was first described by Morgagni (1682–1771).

cant laxative may give relief. Application of glyceryl trinitrate (GTN) or diltiazem cream relaxes the anal sphincter, allowing the torn epithelium to heal.

More intractable cases usually respond to dividing the internal sphincter submucosally under general anaesthetic. It is important to take a detailed history of continence and to assess the anal tone prior to performing a sphincterotomy, as incontinence may result, particularly in patients who have suffered previous obstetric injury. It is for the same reason that an anal stretch is now seldom performed. A newer alternative is a chemical sphincterotomy using an injection of botulinum toxin (Botox) into the internal sphincter. This has the advantage that the sphincter paralysis is short lived, but gives a more sustained effect than GTN or diltiazem cream.

A chronic recurring fissure *in ano* requires excision.

Anorectal abscesses

Classification (Figure 26.2)

- *Perianal*: resulting from infection of a hair follicle, a sebaceous gland or perianal haematoma.
- *Submucous*: infected fissure or laceration of the anal canal.
- *Ischiorectal*: from infection of an anal gland leading from the anal canal into the submucosa, spread of infection from a perianal abscess, or penetration of the ischiorectal fossa by a foreign body. The abscess may form a track like a horse shoe behind the rectum to the opposite ischiorectal fossa.
- *Pelvirectal*: spread from pelvic abscess (rare).

Treatment

Early surgical drainage to prevent rupture and the possible formation of a fistula *in ano*.

Fistula *in ano*

Definitions

- A *fistula* is an abnormal communication between two epithelial surfaces, e.g. between a

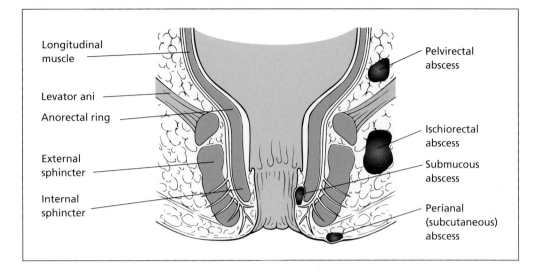

Longitudinal muscle

Levator ani

Anorectal ring

External sphincter

Internal sphincter

Pelvirectal abscess

Ischiorectal abscess

Submucous abscess

Perianal (subcutaneous) abscess

Figure 26.2 The anatomy of perianal abscesses.

hollow viscus and the surface of the body or between two hollow viscera.
- A *sinus* is a granulating track leading from a source of infection to a surface.

Aetiology

The term fistula *in ano* is loosely applied to both fistulae and sinuses in relation to the anal canal. The great majority result from an initial abscess forming in one of the anal glands that pass from the submucosa of the anal canal to open within its lumen. Growth of bowel organisms, as opposed to skin flora, from an anorectal abscess is suggestive of the presence of a fistula. Rarely, fistulae are associated with Crohn's disease, ulcerative colitis and carcinoma of the rectum (occasionally, also, tuberculosis).

Anatomical classification (Figure 26.3)

Anal fistulae are classified according to their position and relation to the internal and external anal sphincters.

- Submucous ⎫ Superficial
- Subcutaneous ⎭
- Intersphincteric ⎫ Low anal
- Trans-sphincteric ⎭
  - Suprasphincteric—high anal
  - Anorectal (extrasphincteric).

Superficial fistulae may be either subcutaneous or submucous, and are superficial tracks resulting from rupture, respectively, of subcutaneous and submucous abscesses. Intersphincteric and trans-sphincteric fistulae are examples of *low anal fistulae,* in which the track is below the anorectal ring; they constitute 95% of all fistulas. They differ in their penetration through the external sphincter, and most are at a low level with the track passing through the subcutaneous part of the sphincter. Suprasphincteric fistulae pass via the intersphincteric space to open into the anus above the puborectalis and are *high anal fistulae.* Anorectal fistulae, fortunately rare, extend through levator ani to open above the anorectal junction.

Fistulae with external openings posterior to the meridian in the lithotomy position usually open in the midline of the anus, whereas those with anterior external openings usually open directly into the anus – Goodsall's law[2] (Figure 26.1).

Clinical features

There is usually a story of an initial anorectal abscess, which discharges. Following this, there are recurrent episodes of perianal infection with persistent discharge of pus. Examination reveals the external opening of a fistula. The internal

[2]David Goodsall (1843–1906), Surgeon, St Mark's Hospital, London, UK.

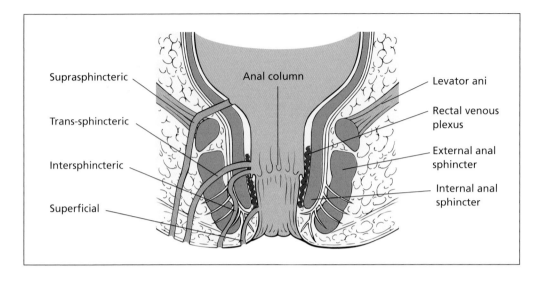

Figure 26.3 The anatomy of perianal fistulae.

opening may be felt per rectum, but probing of the track is painful and should be deferred until the patient is anaesthetized. Accurate assessment of the extent of the fistula track, in particular its relation to the anal sphincter, is crucial. Where doubt exists, endoanal ultrasound or magnetic resonance (MR) can demonstrate the anatomy of a fistula very clearly.

Treatment

Superficial and low-level anal fistulae are laid open and allowed to heal by granulation. Because no sphincter, or only the subcutaneous part of the external and internal sphincters, is divided in this procedure, there is no loss of anal continence. Fistulae can only be treated in this manner when they quite definitely lie below the level of the anorectal ring; careful assessment is therefore important.

In high fistulae (suprasphincteric, and trans-sphincteric close to the anorectal ring) the fistula track is either injected with fibrin glue or a bio-prosthetic 'fistula plug' is passed along the track. If either of these sphincter-preserving treatments fails, the lower part of the track is laid open and a non-absorbable strong ligature (e.g. nylon), termed a seton, is passed through the upper part of the track and left in place for 2–3 weeks so that the sphincter is fixed by scar tissue; the track is then divided by repeated tightening of the liga-

ture. Laying open of the whole track of a suprasphincteric fistula in error will completely divide the sphincters and result in incontinence.

Recurrent fistulae that are associated with Crohn's disease may respond to long-term antibiotics and treatment with an anti-tumour necrosis factor (TNF) antibody such as infliximab.

Stricture of the anal canal

Classification

- *Congenital.*
- *Traumatic*, particularly postoperative, after too radical excision of the skin and mucosa in haemorrhoidectomy.
- *Inflammatory*: lymphogranuloma inguinale (mostly female), Crohn's disease, ulcerative colitis.
- *Post irradiation.*
- *Infiltrating neoplasm.*

Treatment

Depends on the underlying pathology and may call for repeated dilatation, plastic reconstruction, defunctioning colostomy or, in the case of malignant disease, excision of the rectum.

Prolapse of the rectum

This may be partial or complete.

- *Partial prolapse* is confined to the mucosa, which prolapses 2–5 cm from the anal verge. Palpation of the prolapse between the finger and thumb reveals that there is no muscular wall within it. It may occur in infants who, unlike the usual textbook description, are not wasted but often perfectly healthy. Treatment of these babies requires nothing more than reassurance of the parents that the condition is self-curing. In adults, it usually accompanies prolapsing piles or sphincter incompetence, and may present with pruritus ani.
- *Complete prolapse* involves all layers of the rectal wall. It usually occurs in elderly women. Apart from the discomfort of the prolapse, there is associated incontinence owing to the stretching of the sphincter and mucus discharge from the prolapsed mucosal surface.

Treatment

Treatment of partial prolapse in adults comprises excision of the redundant mucosa, or a submucosal phenol-in-oil injection in order to produce sclerosis. In children, as already mentioned, self-cure without active treatment is the fortunate rule.

Repair of a rectal prolapse may be performed either transabdominally or perineally; the former being preferred in younger patients, the latter in the more elderly. Transabdominal mesh rectopexy, in which prosthetic mesh is partly wrapped around the mobilized rectum and sutured to the presacral fascia, relies on the resultant brisk fibrous reaction to fix the rectum to the pelvic tissues. The classic perineal approach was anal encirclement with a Thiersch wire,[3] in which a wire or nylon suture is passed around the anal orifice to narrow it and keep the prolapse reduced. This was complicated by obstruction and erosion of the wire and fell from favour. Today, a less traumatic approach is performed (Delorme's procedure[4]), with excision of a sleeve of mucosa and pleating of the underlying muscle to form a doughnut-like ring, which holds the rectum in the pelvis rather as a ring pessary may control vaginal prolapse. An alternative is the Altemeier[5] perineal rectosigmoidectomy, in which a full thickness resection of prolapsing rectum is performed.

Pruritus ani

There are four principal causes of pruritus ani:

1 *Local causes within the anus or rectum.* Any factor that causes moisture and sogginess of the anal skin, e.g. lack of cleanliness, excessive sweating, leakage of mucus from haemorrhoids, proctitis, colitis, fistula *in ano*, rectal neoplasm or threadworms.
2 *Skin diseases*: scabies, pediculosis, fungal infections, e.g. *Candida albicans*.
3 *General diseases* associated with pruritus: diabetes mellitus, Hodgkin's disease, obstructive jaundice.
4 *Idiopathic*: here very often the original cause has disappeared but the pruritus persists because of continued scratching of the anal region by the patient.

Treatment

Directed to the underlying cause. The idiopathic group often responds dramatically to hydrocortisone ointment and attention to local hygiene.

Tumours

Pathology

Benign

- Adenoma.
- Papilloma.
- Lipoma.
- Endometrioma.

Malignant

1 *Primary:*
   a adenocarcinoma;
   b squamous carcinoma of the lower anal canal;

---

[3]Karl Thiersch (1822–1895), Professor of Surgery, Erlangen then Leipzig, Germany. Devised the split skin graft.
[4]Edmond Delorme (1843–1929), Chief of Surgery, French Army.

[5]William Arthur Altemeier (1910–1983), Professor of Surgery, Cincinnati, OH, USA.

c melanoma;
d carcinoid tumour;
e lymphoma.
2 *Secondary*: invasion from prostate, uterus or pelvic peritoneal deposits.

Rectal polyps

Rectal polyps may be divided into four categories:

1 *Hyperplastic*: formerly termed metaplastic polyps, these are small, 2–3 mm, sessile, wart-like lesions. Often multiple and virtually always benign; it is an incidental finding on sigmoidoscopy.
2 *Neoplastic (adenomatous) polyp.* There are three histological types of benign neoplastic polyp, all of which may undergo malignant change. Multiple polyps are present in familial adenomatous polyposis (Chapter 25, p. 211):
   a tubular adenoma – usually small and rounded, the most common type of adenomatous polyp; the epithelium is arranged in tubular fashion;
   b tubulovillous adenoma;
   c villous adenoma: appears like an anemone with many fronds growing from its base on the rectal wall. Often grows very large, and produces large amounts of mucus. Greatest potential for malignant change, so best completely removed.
3 *Hamartomatous*, e.g. the juvenile polyp; a developmental malformation which presents in children and adolescents and which looks like a cherry on a stalk. It is always benign, presents with bleeding and may prolapse during defaecation.
4 *Inflammatory (pseudopolyp)*: associated with colitis; is not a true polyp but is oedematous mucosa against a background of ulcerated, mucosa-denuded, bowel wall.

Diagnosis is by biopsy. Because of the propensity for malignant change of neoplastic polyps, particularly villous adenomas, these should always be excised in full to ensure that no area of malignant change is missed. Small polyps may be excised in the clinic; larger polyps will require an operating sigmoidoscope with diathermy coagulation.

Carcinoma of the rectum

Pathology

The sexes are equally affected. It occurs in any age group from the twenties onwards, but is particularly common in the age range 50–70 years. Carcinoma of the rectum accounts for approximately one-third of all tumours of the large intestine. Predisposing factors (as with carcinoma of the colon) are pre-existing adenomas, familial adenomatous polyposis and ulcerative colitis.

Macroscopic appearance

The tumours may be as follows:

- papilliferous;
- ulcerating (commonest);
- stenosing (usually at rectosigmoid);
- mucinous (colloid).

Microscopic appearance

Rectal carcinomas are adenocarcinomas; about 9% are associated with profuse mucus secretion ('colloid tumours') and 1% are highly anaplastic adenocarcinomas. At the anal verge, squamous carcinoma may occur, but a malignant tumour protruding through the anal canal is more likely to be an adenocarcinoma of the rectum invading the anal skin.

Spread

1 *Local*:
   a circumferentially around the lumen of the bowel;
   b invasion through the muscular coat;
   c penetration into adjacent organs, e.g. prostate, bladder, vagina, uterus, sacrum, sacral plexus, ureters and lateral pelvic wall.
2 *Lymphatic*: to regional lymph nodes along the inferior mesenteric vessels. At a late stage, there is invasion of the iliac lymph nodes and of the groin lymph nodes (by retrograde spread) and involvement of the supraclavicular nodes via the thoracic duct.
3 *Blood*: via the superior rectal venous plexus, thence the portal vein to the liver and then lungs.
4 *Transcoelomic*: seeding of the peritoneal cavity.

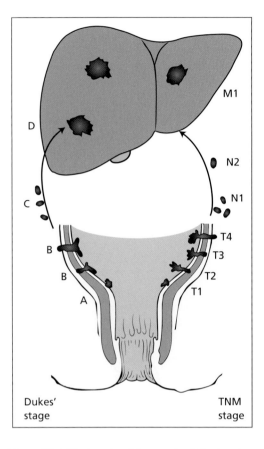

Tis The tumour involves the mucosa only.
T1 The tumour is confined to submucosa.
T2 The tumour invades the muscle wall.
T3 The tumour invades through the muscle wall into the serosa or pericolic/perirectal tissue.
T4 The tumour invades other organs or has perforated into the peritoneal cavity.

N0 No regional lymph nodes.
N1 Tumour involves one to three lymph nodes in pericolic or perirectal tissue.
N2 Tumour involves more than three lymph nodes in pericolic or perirectal tissue or any nodes more than 3 cm away from the primary tumour.

M0 No distant metastasis.
M1 Distant metastasis.

Prognosis

Depends largely on the stage of progression of the tumour and its histological degree of differentiation. The more advanced its spread and the more anaplastic its cells, the worse the prognosis.

Clinical features

The patient may present with the following:

- local disturbances owing to the presence of the tumour in the rectum;
- manifestations of secondary deposits;
- the general effects of malignant disease.

Effects of secondary deposits and malignant disease are similar to those of carcinoma of the colon (Chapter 25, p. 212) with the addition that, rarely, carcinoma of the rectum may spread to the groin nodes as a late phenomenon. With carcinoma at the anal verge, this commonly occurs.

Local symptoms

Bowel disturbance (constipation and/or diarrhoea occur in 80% of cases) and bleeding, which is almost invariable and is the presenting complaint in about 60% of patients. There may also be mucus discharge, rectal pain and tenesmus.

Examination

Abdominal palpation is negative in early cases, but careful attention must be paid to the detection of hepatomegaly, ascites or abdominal distension. Other general features that may be detected in late

Figure 26.4 Staging of rectal cancer by Dukes' and TNM classifications. Dukes' A, confined to the bowel wall; B, penetrating the wall; C, involving regional lymph nodes; D, distant spread.

Staging

The extent of spread of rectal tumours is traditionally classified by Dukes' method[6] (Figure 26.4).

A The tumour is confined to the mucosa and submucosa.
B There is invasion of the muscle wall.
C The regional lymph nodes are involved.
D Distant spread has occurred, e.g. to the liver or invasion into the bladder.

More recently, colonic and rectal cancers have been staged using the TNM system (see Chapter 7, p. 39).

[6]Cuthbert Esquire Dukes (1890–1977), Pathologist, St Mark's Hospital, London, UK.

cases are enlarged supraclavicular nodes, nodes in the groin or jaundice. Rectal examination reveals the tumour in 90% of cases.

Special investigations

- *Sigmoidoscopy* enables the great majority of tumours to be inspected and a biopsy to be taken.
- *Colonoscopy* is indicated to rule out synchronous tumours if a second tumour is suspected (5% of tumours in the large bowel are multiple) or if there is ulcerative colitis or familial polyposis. Barium enema is indicated when colonoscopy is not readily available.
- *Computed tomography (CT)* of the chest, abdomen and pelvis is performed to detect metastatic spread.
- *Magnetic resonance (MR) imaging* of the pelvis is useful for preoperative staging of the tumour and for planning preoperative radio- and chemotherapy.

Differential diagnosis of a rectal tumour

Differential diagnosis of a palpable tumour in the rectum must be made from the following:

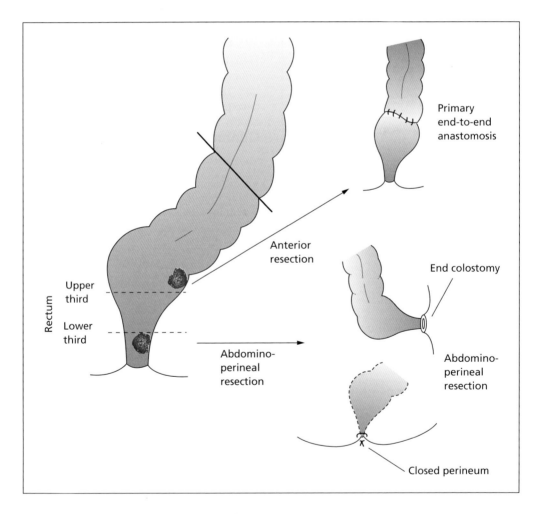

Figure 26.5 Surgical procedures for carcinoma of rectum.

- benign tumours;
- carcinoma of the sigmoid colon prolapsing into the pouch of Douglas and felt through the mucosal wall;
- secondary deposits in the pelvis;
- ovarian or uterine tumours;
- extension from carcinoma of the prostate or cervix;
- diverticular disease;
- endometriosis;
- lymphogranuloma inguinale;
- amoebic granuloma;
- the rare malignant tumours of the rectum (see p. 226);
- faeces (these give the classical physical sign of indentation).

The beginner may mistake the normal cervix for a palpable tumour, and should not be caught out by the presence of a ring pessary or tampon in the vagina, which are readily felt per rectum.

Treatment

Curative

Surgery depends upon the distance of the tumour from the anal verge (Figure 26.5).

- *Upper third tumours* can be resected with restorative anastomosis between the sigmoid colon and the lower rectum (anterior resection).
- *Lower third tumours*, less than 5 cm from the anal verge, are usually treated by abdominoperineal excision of the rectum, with a terminal colostomy. Adjunctive radiotherapy may reduce the incidence of local recurrence after abdominoperineal resection.
- *Mid-third rectal tumours* can usually be treated by anterior resection, provided satisfactory distal clearance can be obtained. The operation is easier in women, in whom the wider pelvis facilitates dissection.

Palliative procedures

Even if secondaries are present, palliation is best achieved when possible by excision of the primary tumour. A colostomy may be necessary for intestinal obstruction, but this does not relieve the bleeding, mucus discharge and sacral pain.

In completely inoperable cases, radiotherapy, diathermy or laser of the tumour may give temporary relief, as may cytotoxic drugs.

27

Peritonitis

Learning objective
✓ To know the causes and manifestations of peritonitis and of localized collections of pus.

General characteristics of peritonitis

Aetiology

Bacteria may enter the peritoneal cavity via four portals:

1 *From the exterior*: penetrating wound, infection at laparotomy, peritoneal dialysis.
2 *From intra-abdominal viscera*:
   a gangrene of a viscus, e.g. acute appendicitis, acute cholecystitis, diverticulitis or infarction of the intestine;
   b perforation of a viscus, e.g. perforated duodenal ulcer, perforated appendicitis, rupture of the intestine from trauma;
   c postoperative leakage of an intestinal suture line.
3 *Via the bloodstream*: as part of a septicaemia (pneumococcal, streptococcal or staphylococcal). This has been wrongly termed primary peritonitis; in fact, it is secondary to some initial source of infection.
4 *Via the female genital tract*: acute salpingitis or puerperal infection.

Approximately 30% of all cases of peritonitis in adults result from postoperative complications: 20% from acute appendicitis and 10% from a perforated peptic ulcer.

Lecture Notes: General Surgery, 12th edition. © Harold Ellis, Sir Roy Y. Calne and Christopher J. E. Watson. Published 2011 by Blackwell Publishing Ltd.

Pathology

Peritonitis of bowel origin usually shows a mixed faecal flora (*Escherichia coli*, *Streptococcus faecalis*, *Pseudomonas*, *Klebsiella* and *Proteus*, together with the anaerobic *Clostridium* and *Bacteroides*). Gynaecological infections may be chlamydial, gonococcal or streptococcal. Blood-borne peritonitis may be streptococcal, pneumococcal, staphylococcal or tuberculous. In young girls, a rare gynaecological infection is due to pneumococcus.

The pathological effects of peritonitis are as follows:

1 Widespread absorption of toxins from the large, inflamed surface.
2 The associated paralytic ileus (Chapter 28, p. 236) with the following:
   a loss of fluid;
   b loss of electrolytes;
   c loss of protein.
3 Gross abdominal distension with elevation of the diaphragm, which produces a liability to lung collapse and pneumonia.

Clinical features

Peritonitis is inevitably secondary to some precipitating lesion, which may itself have definite clinical features, e.g. the onset may be an attack of acute appendicitis or a perforated duodenal ulcer, with appropriate symptoms and signs.

Early peritonitis is characterized by severe pain; the patient wishes to lie still because any movement aggravates the agony. Irritation of the diaphragm may be accompanied by pain referred to the shoulder tip. Vomiting is frequent. The temperature is usually elevated and the pulse rises progressively. Examination at this time shows localized or generalized tenderness, depending on the extent of the peritonitis. The abdominal wall is held rigidly and rebound tenderness is present. The abdomen is silent, or the transmitted sounds of the heart beat and respiration may be detected. Rectal examination may show tenderness in the pouch of Douglas.

In advanced peritonitis, the abdomen becomes distended and tympanitic, signs of free fluid are present, the patient becomes increasingly toxic with a rapid, feeble pulse, vomiting is faeculent and the skin is moist, cold and cyanosed (the hippocratic facies).

Special investigations

These are of only limited value; diagnosis depends on the clinical features.

- *Full blood count* usually reveals a marked leucocytosis.
- *Serum amylase* will identify acute pancreatitis and prevent unnecessary surgery.
- *Chest X-ray* (performed with the patient erect) may reveal free gas under the diaphragm in cases of a perforated abdominal viscus (seen in 70% of perforated peptic ulcers). It may also exclude pulmonary infection as a differential diagnosis.
- *Abdominal X-ray* may also demonstrate free gas, or may demonstrate another cause of peritonitis.
- *Computed tomography (CT)* is excellent at detecting free gas, and is most likely to pinpoint the cause of peritonitis.

Differential diagnosis

This is from intestinal obstruction and from ureteric or biliary colic, in all of which the patient tends to be restless. Basal pneumonia, myocardial infarction, intraperitoneal haemorrhage and leakage of an aortic aneurysm are other fairly common misdiagnoses.

Principles of treatment

In this section, only an outline of treatment is given, as specific causes of peritonitis may require specific therapy; these are dealt with in their appropriate chapters. The standard principles of resuscitation are followed, after an initial assessment of the patient's general condition.

1 *Oxygen therapy* if the patient is hypoxic, or haemoglobin oxygen saturations are less than 95%.
2 *Intravenous fluid and electrolyte replacement*; plasma expanders or blood may be required in the presence of shock.
3 *Antibiotic therapy*, with specificity to treat the broad spectrum of bowel organisms, e.g. penicillin and gentamicin or a cephalosporin together with metronidazole; therapy is guided, where possible, by checking the sensitivity of the responsible organisms isolated on a peritoneal swab or from blood cultures.
4 *Relief of pain* with opiates, e.g. intravenous morphine.
5 *Gastric aspiration* by means of a nasogastric tube reduces the risk of inhalation of vomit under anaesthesia and prevents further abdominal distension by removing swallowed air.
6 *Surgery* is indicated if the source of infection can be removed or closed, e.g. the repair of a perforated ulcer or removal of the gangrenous, perforated appendix.

Any localized collection of pus requires drainage, and later surgery may be required for the evacuation of residual abscesses, e.g. subphrenic or pelvic collections.

Conservative treatment is indicated, at least initially, when the infection has been localized, e.g. an appendix mass, or when the primary focus is irremovable, as in pancreatitis or postpartum infection. When the patient is moribund or when there is a lack of surgical facilities, as on board a ship, reliance is placed on intravenous therapy, gastric aspiration and antibiotics.

Specific causes of peritonitis are detailed below.

Peritoneal dialysis peritonitis

Patients with chronic renal failure on peritoneal dialysis are prone to peritonitis either from organisms entering via the indwelling dialysis catheter (usually skin flora such as *Staphylococcus* spp.) or from perforation of a viscus, in which case the flora are generally a mixture of colonic organisms. Diagnosis is made by the presence of abdominal pain and turbid dialysate. Single organisms are treated by intravenous and intra-peritoneal antibiotics. Multiple organisms, particularly if gut flora, suggest perforation and require laparotomy as well as antibiotics. Once infected, the peritoneal dialysis catheter may form a focus for sepsis, in which case it should be removed.

Non-specific bacterial peritonitis

Patients with hepatic cirrhosis and ascites are at risk of developing spontaneous bacterial peritonitis. Such patients are immunosuppressed by their disease, and the protein-rich ascitic fluid forms an efficient culture medium for organisms. Infection occurs when enteric organisms translocate across the bowel wall. It is confirmed by a peritoneal tap rich in leucocytes and is treated with intravenous antibiotics. Such infections often precipitate encephalopathy, renal failure and hepatic decompensation.

Pneumococcal peritonitis

This may be secondary to the septicaemia accompanying a pneumococcal lung infection or, uncommonly these days, may result from an ascending infection from the vagina in girls between the ages of 4 and 10.

Clinically, there is peritonitis of sudden onset accompanied by severe toxaemia and fever. The white cell count is elevated above 20×10^9/L.

Treatment

Usually, laparotomy is performed because perforated appendicitis is suspected. Clear or turbid fluid containing fibrin flakes is discovered without an obvious primary cause. A slide made of the pus shows the characteristic Gram-positive pneumococci lying in pairs. The condition responds to penicillin therapy.

Haemolytic streptococcal peritonitis

This may occur in children, secondary to streptococcal infection of the tonsil, otitis media, scarlet fever or erysipelas.

Staphylococcal peritonitis

This very rarely complicates staphylococcal septicaemia, which more often produces intra-abdominal or perinephric abscesses.

Tuberculous peritonitis

Always secondary to tuberculosis elsewhere, the primary focus may no longer be active. It usually occurs as a result of local spread from the mesenteric lymph nodes or via the female genital tract, although it may complicate generalized miliary tuberculosis.

With the diminution of tuberculosis elsewhere, tuberculous peritonitis is becoming increasingly rare in this country. It is seen most often in immigrants from developing countries and in patients who are immunosuppressed, either therapeutically or by disease (e.g. human immunodeficiency virus (HIV)).

Pathology

The peritoneum is studded with tubercles in the initial phase, with an accompanying serous effusion. Later, the tubercles coalesce, local abscesses may develop and the intra-abdominal viscera become matted together with dense fibrous adhesions.

Clinical features

It may present as acute peritonitis, ascites or intestinal obstruction secondary to gross adhesions. Diagnosis is usually made only at operation.

Treatment

Treatment comprises antituberculous chemotherapy. Operation may be required for the relief of intestinal obstruction from adhesions.

Bile peritonitis

This may occur as a result of the following:

- traumatic rupture of the gallbladder or its ducts, e.g. open or closed injury, iatrogenic damage from liver biopsy or percutaneous cholangiography;
- leakage from the liver, the gallbladder or its ducts after a biliary tract operation;
- perforation of an acutely inflamed gallbladder;
- transudation of the bile through a gangrenous but non-perforated gallbladder;
- spontaneous perforation of the gallbladder; or it may be
- idiopathic – a rare but well-recognized condition in which bile peritonitis occurs without obvious cause, possibly a small perforation due to a calculus, which then becomes sealed.

Bile peritonitis is only a rare accompaniment of acute cholecystitis, because unlike the appendix, which when inflamed rapidly undergoes gangrene, the inflamed gallbladder is usually thickened and walled off by adhesions. In addition, again unlike the appendix, which only receives an end-artery supply from the ileocolic artery, the gallbladder has an additional blood supply from the liver bed, and therefore frank gangrene of the gallbladder is unusual.

The patient presents with all the features of general peritonitis. Laparotomy is required to deal with the underlying cause, but the mortality associated with bile peritonitis is up to 50%. As with all other causes of peritonitis, it is the elderly patient with late disease who does badly.

Localized intraperitoneal collections of pus

Following peritonitis, pus may collect in the subphrenic spaces or in the pelvis. These are the most dependent parts of the peritoneal cavity when the patient lies supine.

Subphrenic abscess

Anatomy (Figure 27.1)

The subphrenic region lies between the diaphragm above and the transverse colon with

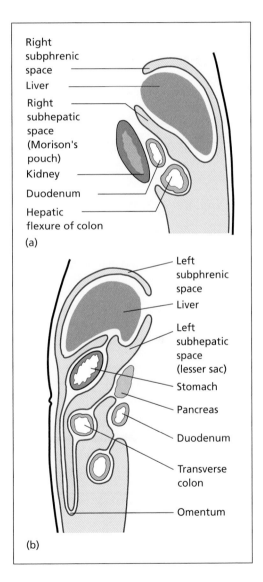

Right subphrenic space
Liver
Right subhepatic space (Morison's pouch)
Kidney
Duodenum
Hepatic flexure of colon
(a)

Left subphrenic space
Liver
Left subhepatic space (lesser sac)
Stomach
Pancreas
Duodenum
Transverse colon
Omentum
(b)

Figure 27.1 The anatomy of the subphrenic spaces: (a) right; (b) left.

mesocolon below and is divided further by the liver and its ligaments. The right and left *subphrenic spaces* lie between the diaphragm and the liver and are separated from each other by the falciform ligament. The right and left *subhepatic spaces* are below the liver, the right forming Morison's pouch[1] and the left being the lesser sac, which communicates with the former through the foramen of Winslow.[2] The right *extraperitoneal space* lies between the bare area of the liver and the diaphragm. About two-thirds of subphrenic abscesses occur on the right side. Rarely, they are bilateral.

Aetiology

A localized collection of pus may occur in the subphrenic region following general peritonitis. Usually, the underlying cause is a peritonitis involving the upper abdomen – leakage following biliary or gastric surgery or a perforated peptic ulcer. Rarely, infection occurs from haematogenous spread or from direct spread from a primary chest lesion, e.g. empyema.

Clinical features

Subphrenic infection usually follows general peritonitis after 10–21 days, although, if antibiotics have been given, an abscess may be disguised and may only become manifest weeks or even months after the original episode. There may be no localizing symptoms, the patient presenting with malaise, nausea, loss of weight, anaemia and pyrexia; hence, the aphorism 'pus somewhere, pus nowhere else, pus under the diaphragm'. At least half the patients have a fever, which continues from the original peritonitis, although the standard description is of a swinging temperature, which commences some 10 days after the initial illness.

Localizing features are pain in the upper abdomen or lower chest or referred to the shoulder tip with localized upper abdominal or chest wall tenderness. There may be signs of fluid or collapse at the lung base. In late cases, a swelling may be detected over the lower chest wall or upper abdomen.

Special investigations

- *Full blood count*: the white count is raised in the region of $15–20 \times 10^9$/L, with a polymorph leucocytosis.
- *Chest X-ray* may show the following (Figure 27.2):
  - elevation of the diaphragm on the affected side;
  - pleural effusion and/or collapse of the lung base;
  - gas and a fluid level below the diaphragm.
- *Ultrasound* may show diminished or absent mobility of the diaphragm, and may demonstrate the subphrenic abscess.
- *CT* will demonstrate an abscess, and also locate any other intraperitoneal collections of pus.

Treatment

In early cases, where there is absence of gas and free fluid on X-ray, the patient is placed on broad-spectrum antibiotic therapy. If there is a rapid response, the diagnosis is one of a spreading cellulitis of the subphrenic space.

If there is clinical or radiological evidence of a localized abscess, or if resolution fails to occur on chemotherapy, percutaneous drainage may be carried out under ultrasound or CT guidance. If this fails, or the abscess is loculated, surgical drainage is performed. Depending on the location of the abscess, this is carried out either by a posterior extraperitoneal approach through the bed of, or just below, the twelfth rib or by an anterior approach via a subcostal incision.

Pelvic abscess

A pelvic abscess may follow any general peritonitis, but it is particularly common after acute appendicitis (75%) or after gynaecological infections. In men, the abscess lies between the bladder and the rectum; in women, it lies between the uterus and posterior fornix of the vagina anteriorly and the rectum posteriorly (pouch of Douglas[3]).

Left untreated, the abscess may burst into the rectum or vagina, or may discharge onto the

---

[1]James Rutherford Morison (1853–1939), Professor of Surgery, University of Durham, Durham, UK.
[2]Jacob Winslow (1669–1760), Danish; became Professor of Anatomy and Surgery in Paris, France.

[3]James Douglas (1675–1742), Obstetrician and Anatomist, London, UK.

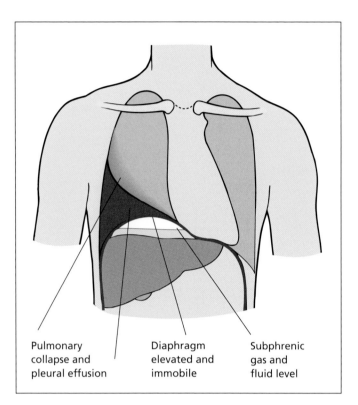

Pulmonary collapse and pleural effusion

Diaphragm elevated and immobile

Subphrenic gas and fluid level

Figure 27.2 Diagram of the radiological appearance of a right subphrenic abscess. The diaphragm is raised (and fixed on screening), a fluid level is present beneath it and there is a sympathetic pleural effusion with compression and/or collapse of the lung base.

abdominal wall, particularly if there has been a previous abdominal laparotomy incision at the time of the original episode of peritonitis. Occasionally, the abscess may rupture into the peritoneal cavity.

Clinical features

- *General*: swinging pyrexia, toxaemia, weight loss with leucocytosis.
- *Local*: diarrhoea, mucus discharge per rectum and the presence of a mass felt on rectal or vaginal examination, which is occasionally large enough to be palpated abdominally.

Treatment

An early pelvic cellulitis may respond rapidly to a short course of antimicrobial chemotherapy, but there is the risk that the prolonged antibiotic treatment of an unresolved infection may produce a chronic inflammatory mass studded with small abscess cavities in the pelvis. It is safer therefore, when there is an established pelvic abscess, to withhold chemotherapy and await pointing into the vagina or rectum through which surgical drainage can be carried out. Very often, even this is not required, as firm pressure by the finger in the rectum may be followed by rupture of the abscess through the rectal wall.

28

Paralytic ileus

Learning objective
✓ To know the causes and management of paralytic ileus.

The word ileus comes from the Greek verb 'to roll', from which it became applied to colic and hence to obstruction. Obstructions are subdivided into mechanical and paralytic, the latter produced by lack of intestinal motility. It is therefore a bad habit to say that a patient has 'an ileus' when one really means a 'paralytic ileus', as the word ileus alone implies merely intestinal obstruction.

Paralytic (or adynamic or neurogenic) ileus can be defined as a state of atony of the intestine. Its principal clinical features are the following:

- abdominal distension.
- absolute constipation.
- vomiting.
- absence of intestinal movements and, hence, absence of colicky pain.

Aetiology

The state of paralytic ileus may be produced by a large number of factors, sometimes coexisting.

Peritonitis

Perhaps as a result of toxic paralysis of intrinsic nerve plexuses, the bowel in peritonitis becomes atonic. There may be an associated mechanical obstruction produced by kinking of loops of bowel by fibrinous adhesions, so that frequently the

Lecture Notes: General Surgery, 12th edition. © Harold Ellis, Sir Roy Y. Calne and Christopher J. E. Watson. Published 2011 by Blackwell Publishing Ltd.

paralytic ileus is complicated by mechanical obstruction.

Metabolic factors

Severe potassium depletion, uraemia and diabetic coma may result in paralytic ileus.

Drugs

Paralytic ileus is produced by heavy dosages of anticholinergic agents and antiparkinsonian drugs.

Postoperative

Some degree of paralytic ileus occurs after every laparotomy. Its aetiology is complex, including sympathetic overaction, the effects of manipulation of the bowel, potassium depletion (when there has been excessive preoperative vomiting), peritoneal irritation from blood or associated peritonitis and the atony of stomach and the large bowel, which occurs after every abdominal operation for a period of some 24–48 hours.

The distension that occurs on the first and second postoperative day is probably produced by swallowed air. This air passes through the small intestine (where peristalsis usually returns quickly) to the colon, which is atonic and produces a functional hold-up.

Paralytic ileus that persists for more than 48 hours postoperatively probably has some other aetiological factor present.

Pathology

The deleterious effects of paralytic ileus are similar to those of a simple mechanical obstruction.

- There is severe loss of fluid, electrolytes and protein into the gut lumen and in the vomitus or gastric aspirate.
- Gross gaseous distension of the gut, produced mainly from swallowed air that cannot pass through the bowel, impairs the blood supply of the bowel wall and allows toxin absorption to occur.

Clinical features

Paralytic ileus is most commonly seen in the post-operative stage of peritonitis or of major abdominal surgery. There is abdominal distension, absolute constipation and effortless vomiting. Pain is not present, apart from the discomfort of the laparotomy wound and the abdominal distension. On examination, the patient is anxious and uncomfortable. The abdomen is distended, silent and tender. A plain X-ray of the abdomen will show gas distributed throughout the small and large bowel and some fluid levels may be present on an erect abdominal X-ray.

The paralytic ileus may merge insidiously into a mechanical obstruction produced by adhesions or bands following abdominal surgery, and an important, often extremely difficult, differential diagnosis lies between these two conditions. The diagnosis is important, since paralytic ileus is treated conservatively whereas mechanical obstruction usually calls for urgent operation.

Differential diagnosis

Differentiation of paralytic ileus from mechanical obstruction is based on the following criteria:

- *Duration.* Paralytic ileus rarely lasts more than 3 or 4 days; persistence of symptoms after this time is suspicious of mechanical obstruction.
- *Bowel sounds.* The presence of bowel sounds is important. An absolutely silent abdomen is diagnostic of paralytic ileus, whereas noisy bowel sounds indicate mechanical obstruction.
- *Pain.* Paralytic ileus is relatively painless, whereas colicky abdominal pain is present in mechanical obstruction.
- *Timing.* If symptoms commence after the patient has already passed flatus or had a bowel action, it is very likely that a mechanical obstruction has supervened. The other possibility to consider is that there has been a leakage from an anastomosis and that peritonitis is now present.

- *X-ray appearances.* A plain X-ray of the abdomen showing a localized loop of distended small intestine without gas shadows in the colon or rectum is strongly suggestive of mechanical obstruction, in contrast to the diffuse appearance of gas throughout the small and large bowel in paralytic ileus.

Treatment

Prophylaxis

Biochemical imbalance is corrected preoperatively. The bowel is handled gently at operation. Postoperatively, gastric distension due to air swallowing may require nasogastric suction.

In the established case

Nasogastric suction is employed to remove swallowed air and prevent gaseous distension. The aspiration of fluid also helps to relieve the associated gastric dilatation. Intravenous fluid and electrolyte therapy is instituted with careful biochemical control. Pethidine, which has relatively little effect on intestinal motility compared with the other opioids, may be used to allay discomfort, and is combined with a phenothiazine such as prochlorperazine for nausea. Eventually, patience is rewarded and recovery from the ileus will occur unless it is secondary to some underlying cause, such as infection.

In the absence of any evidence of mechanical obstruction or infection, prolonged stubborn ileus is occasionally treated pharmacologically. Motility stimulants such as metoclopramide, together with erythromycin (which stimulates the motilin receptor), may be tried. Metoclopramide is a dopamine antagonist that stimulates gastric emptying and small intestinal transit.

Pseudo-obstruction

Pseudo-obstruction, also known as adynamic ileus or Ogilvie's syndrome,[1] is a particular form of paralytic ileus which mainly affects the large bowel. It results from interference with the autonomic supply to the gut in which there is

---

[1] Sir William Heneage Ogilvie (1887–1971), Surgeon, Guy's Hospital, London, UK.

predominant sympathetic activity. It typically complicates fractures of the spine or pelvis, retroperitoneal haemorrhage and retroperitoneal surgery, intestinal ischaemia, ureteric colic and occasionally parturition; Ogilvie described it first in patients with malignant infiltration of the coeliac plexus. Usually, the small bowel is unaffected and peristalsis continues and passes intestinal contents into the colon. The large bowel is atonic, so the colon, in particular the caecum, distends enormously, becomes ischaemic and, if unrelieved, will perforate.

Symptoms are typical of large bowel obstruction, with colicky abdominal pain, distension and absolute constipation. Examination confirms abdominal distension, and digital examination reveals a capacious empty rectum.

Treatment

The patient is made nil by mouth and identifiable causes, such as electrolyte imbalances, are addressed. The colon is decompressed either at colonoscopy or pharmacologically with the administration of the cholinesterase inhibitor neostigmine. Laxatives, particularly stimulant laxatives, should be avoided since they are likely to precipitate perforation.

29

Hernia

Learning objective

✓ To know the common sites of abdominal wall hernias, their anatomy, how they present and their treatment.

Definition

A hernia is the protrusion of an organ or part of an organ through a defect in the wall of the cavity containing it, into an abnormal position. The term is usually used with reference to the abdomen.

Abdominal wall hernias

Most hernias occur as a diverticulum of the peritoneal cavity and therefore have a sac of parietal peritoneum. The common varieties of hernias through the abdominal wall, in order of frequency, are as follows:

- inguinal (indirect or direct);
- femoral;
- umbilical and paraumbilical;
- incisional;
- ventral and epigastric.

Aetiology

Hernias occur at sites of weakness in the abdominal wall. This weakness may be congenital, e.g. persistence of the processus vaginalis of testicular descent giving rise to a congenital inguinal hernia, or failure of complete closure of the umbilical scar. It may occur at the site of penetration of structures through the abdominal wall, e.g. the femoral

Lecture Notes: General Surgery, 12th edition. © Harold Ellis, Sir Roy Y. Calne and Christopher J. E. Watson. Published 2011 by Blackwell Publishing Ltd.

canal, or the layers of the abdominal wall may be weakened following a surgical incision (incisional hernia), either by poor healing as a result of infection, haematoma formation or poor technique or by damage to nerves that results in paralysis of the abdominal muscles.

Hernias should also be thought of as portents of other diseases or conditions, as they are often associated with pathological increases in intra-abdominal pressure by conditions such as the following:

- *chronic cough*, secondary to chronic bronchitis;
- *constipation*, perhaps due to colonic carcinoma;
- *urinary obstruction*, due to prostatic disease;
- *pregnancy*;
- *abdominal distension* with ascites;
- *weak abdominal muscles*, e.g. in gross obesity or muscle wasting in cachexia.

Varieties

A hernia at any site may be (Figure 29.1)

- reducible;
- irreducible;
- strangulated.

Reducible hernia

The contents of a reducible hernia can be replaced completely into the peritoneal cavity.

Irreducible hernia

A hernia becomes irreducible usually because of adhesions of its contents to the inner wall of the

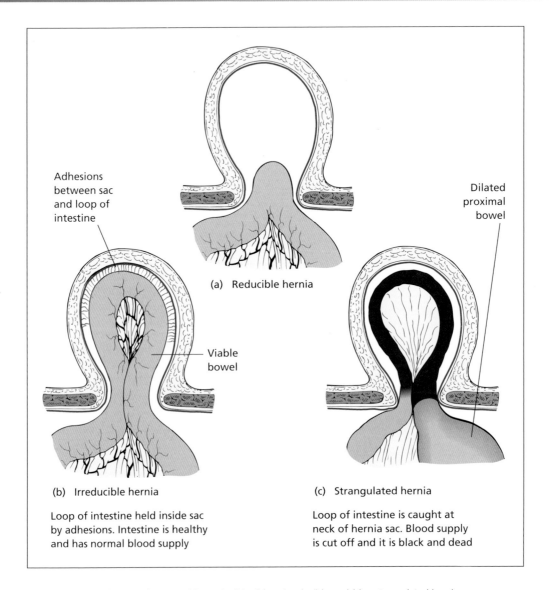

Adhesions
between sac
and loop of
intestine

Dilated
proximal
bowel

(a) Reducible hernia

Viable
bowel

(b) Irreducible hernia

Loop of intestine held inside sac
by adhesions. Intestine is healthy
and has normal blood supply

(c) Strangulated hernia

Loop of intestine is caught at
neck of hernia sac. Blood supply
is cut off and it is black and dead

Figure 29.1 The differences between (a) a reducible, (b) an irreducible and (c) a strangulated hernia.

sac, or sometimes as a result of adhesions of its contents to each other to form a mass greater in size than the neck of the sac. Occasionally, inspissated faeces within the loops of bowel in the hernia prevent reduction.

Strangulated hernia

When strangulation occurs, the contents of the hernia are constricted by the neck of the sac to such a degree that their circulation is cut off. Unless relieved, gangrene is inevitable and, if gut is involved, perforation of the gangrenous loop will eventually occur.

Clinical features

Reducible hernia (Box 29.1)

A reducible hernia simply presents as a lump that may disappear on lying down and that is usually not painful, although it may be accompanied by some discomfort. Examination reveals a reducible lump with a cough impulse.

Irreducible hernia

If the hernia will not reduce but is painless and there are no other symptoms, irreducibility is diagnosed. The absence of a cough impulse alone does not indicate strangulation, because in an irreducible femoral hernia, for example, the neck is often plugged by omentum, which prevents the cough impulse from being felt.

Strangulated hernia

If strangulation supervenes, the patient complains of severe pain in the hernia and also of central abdominal colicky pain. The other symptoms of intestinal obstruction – vomiting, distension and absolute constipation – soon appear. Examination reveals a tender, tense hernia that cannot be reduced and has no cough impulse. The overlying skin becomes inflamed and oedematous and there are are other features of intestinal obstruction with abdominal tenderness and noisy bowel sounds. These features are much less marked when omentum rather than intestine is contained within the sac.

The three common types of hernia to strangulate are, in order of frequency, femoral, indirect inguinal and umbilical.

> **Box 29.1 A lump in the groin**
>
> A patient presenting with a lump in the groin is a common clinical problem. Whenever one considers the differential diagnosis of a mass situated in a particular area, a two-stage mental process is required: first, what are the anatomical structures in that particular region, and, second, what pathological entities may arise therefrom?
>
> In considering the groin, let these possibilities pass through your mind:
>
> 1 The hernial orifices:
>
>   a inguinal hernia
>
>   b femoral hernia
>
> 2 The testicular apparatus:
>
>   a hydrocele of the cord
>
>   b ectopic testis
>
> 3 The vein: saphena varix
>
> 4 The artery: femoral aneurysm
>
> 5 The lymph nodes: lymphadenopathy due to infection, neoplasm or lymphoma
>
> 6 The psoas sheath: psoas abscess
>
> 7 The skin and subcutaneous tissues: lipoma

Inguinal hernia

May be classified into the following:

- *indirect*: entering the internal inguinal ring and traversing the inguinal canal;
- *direct*: pushing through the posterior wall of the inguinal canal medial to the internal ring.

See Table 29.1 for a summary of the differences between indirect and direct inguinal hernias.

The anatomy of the inguinal canal is the key to the understanding of these hernias.

Table 29.1 Characteristic differences that help differentiate indirect and direct inguinal hernias

	Indirect	Direct
Origin	Pass through internal ring, lateral to inferior epigastric vessels	Pass through posterior wall of inguinal canal, medial to inferior epigastric vessels
Congenital or acquired	May be congenital	Always acquired, rare in childhood and adolescence
Control by pressure over internal ring	Yes	No
Strangulates	Commonly, because of narrow neck (internal ring)	Rarely, because usually wide necked
Extends down into scrotum	Often	Rarely
Reduces on lying	Not readily	Spontaneously
Recurrence after surgery	Uncommon	More common

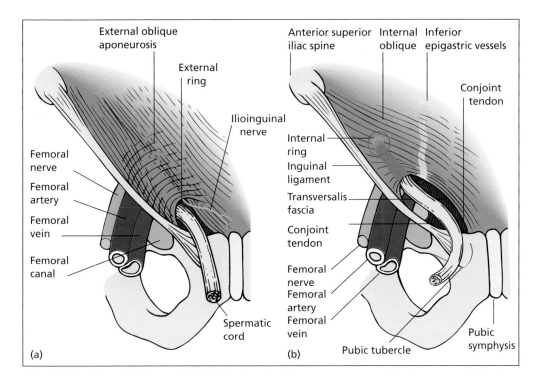

Figure 29.2 The anatomy of the inguinal canal: (a) with the external oblique aponeurosis intact; (b) with the external oblique removed.

Anatomy (Figure 29.2)

The inguinal canal represents the oblique passage taken through the lower abdominal wall by the testis and cord (the round ligament in the female). It is 4 cm long and passes downwards and medially, and from deep to superficial, from the internal to the external inguinal rings, lying parallel to, and immediately above, the inguinal ligament.

- *Anteriorly*: skin, superficial fascia and external oblique aponeurosis cover the full length of the canal; the internal oblique covers its lateral third.
- *Posteriorly*: the conjoint tendon (representing the fused common aponeurotic insertion of the internal oblique and transversus abdominis muscles into the pubic crest) forms the posterior wall of the canal medially; the transversalis fascia lies laterally.
- *Above*: the lowest fibres of the internal oblique and transversus abdominis.
- *Below*: lies the inguinal ligament.

The internal ring represents the point at which the spermatic cord pushes through the transversalis fascia; it is demarcated medially by the inferior epigastric vessels as they pass upwards from the external iliac artery and vein.

The external ring is an inverted V-shaped defect in the external oblique aponeurosis and lies immediately above and medial to the pubic tubercle.

The inguinal canal transmits the spermatic cord (round ligament in the female) and the ilioinguinal nerve.

Indirect inguinal hernia

This passes through the internal ring, along the canal in front of the spermatic cord and, if large enough, emerges through the external ring and descends into the scrotum. If reducible, such a hernia can be completely controlled by pressure with one fingertip over the internal inguinal ring, which lies 1–2 cm above the point where the femoral artery passes under the inguinal ligament, i.e. 1–2 cm above the femoral pulse. This can be felt at the mid-inguinal point, halfway between the anterior superior iliac spine and the symphysis pubis.

If the hernia protrudes through the external ring, it can be felt to lie above and medial to the pubic tubercle and is thus differentiated from a femoral hernia, which emerges through the femoral canal below and lateral to this landmark (Figure 29.3).

Indirect hernias may be congenital, due to persistence of the processus vaginalis; these present at or soon after birth or may arise in adolescence. The acquired variety may occur at any age in adult life and here the sac is formed as an outpushing of the abdominal peritoneum.

The narrow internal opening through the internal inguinal ring accounts for two important features of the indirect hernia. First, the hernia often does not reach its full size until the patient has been up and around for a little time, and then does not reduce immediately when the subject lies down, because it takes a little time for the hernial contents to pass in or out of the sac through its narrow neck. Second, the indirect hernia has a distinct tendency to strangulate at the site of this narrow orifice.

Direct inguinal hernia

This pushes its way directly forwards through the posterior wall of the inguinal canal. Because it lies medial to the internal ring, it is not controlled by digital pressure applied over the ring immediately above the femoral pulse. On inspection, the hernia is seen to protrude directly forwards (hence its name), compared with the oblique route downwards towards the scrotum of an indirect inguinal hernia.

Other points that differentiate a direct from an indirect hernia are that the direct is always acquired and is therefore extremely rare in infancy or adolescence; it usually has a large orifice and therefore appears immediately on standing, disappearing again at once when the patient lies down. Moreover, because of this large opening, strangulation is extremely rare. It is uncommon in women.

Although clinically it is usually quite easy to tell the difference between the two types of inguinal hernia, the ultimate differentiation can only be made at operation: the inferior epigastric vessels demarcate the medial edge of the internal ring; therefore, an indirect sac will pass lateral, and a direct hernia medial, to these vessels. Quite often,

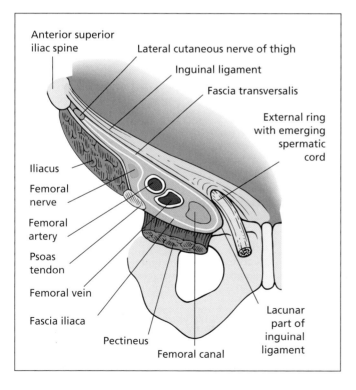

Anterior superior iliac spine

Lateral cutaneous nerve of thigh

Inguinal ligament

Fascia transversalis

External ring with emerging spermatic cord

Iliacus

Femoral nerve

Femoral artery

Psoas tendon

Femoral vein

Fascia iliaca

Pectineus

Femoral canal

Lacunar part of inguinal ligament

Figure 29.3 The anatomy of the femoral canal and its surrounds to show the relationships of a femoral hernia.

a direct and an indirect hernia coexist; they bulge on either side of the inferior epigastric vessels like the legs of a pair of pantaloons.

Sixty per cent of inguinal hernias occur on the right side, 20% on the left and 20% are bilateral.

Treatment

Congenital inguinal hernias in infants do not obliterate spontaneously; the patent processus vaginalis is ligated and the hernial sac excised at the age of about 1 year (herniotomy). In adults, operation is usually advised. This comprises excision of the sac and repair of the weakened inguinal canal, commonly performed either by plicating the transversalis fascia in the posterior wall with a nylon suture (Shouldice repair[1]) or by reinforcing the posterior wall with a nylon or poly-propylene mesh (Lichtenstein repair[2]). An alternative technique is to place a mesh from within the abdomen laparoscopically, covering the hernial orifice. The laparoscopic technique has particular advantages in the treatment of recurrent or bilateral hernias.

A truss is only prescribed in patients who are of very poor general condition and are unable to withstand an operation, although they often have difficulty keeping a truss correctly in place. But, even in such cases, a painful hernia that threatens strangulation is much better repaired as an elective procedure, if necessary under local anaesthesia, rather than as an emergency, should strangulation supervene.

Recurrent inguinal hernias may be caused by, for example, infection, haematoma or poor technique, and also by a failure to appreciate the underlying cause of the increased intra-abdominal pressure that initiated the hernia in the first place (e.g. continuing constipation or bladder neck obstruction by a large prostate).

Femoral hernia

Anatomy

A femoral hernia passes through the femoral canal. This is a gap normally about 1.5 cm in length, which just admits the tip of the little finger and which lies at the medial extremity of the femoral sheath containing the femoral artery and vein. The boundaries of the femoral canal (Figure 29.3) are as follows:

- *Anteriorly*: the inguinal ligament.
- *Medially*: the sharp edge of the lacunar part of the inguinal ligament (Gimbernat's ligament[3]).
- *Laterally*: the femoral vein.
- *Posteriorly*: the pectineal ligament (of Astley Cooper[4]), which is the thickened periosteum along the superior pubic ramus.

The canal contains a plug of fat and a lymph node (the node of Cloquet[5]).

Clinical features

Femoral hernias occur more commonly in women than in men because of the wider female pelvis (but note that indirect inguinal hernias are more common than femoral in women). They are never due to a congenital sac but are invariably acquired; although cases do rarely occur in children they are usually seen in the middle-aged and elderly.

A non-strangulated hernia presents as a globular swelling below and lateral to the pubic tubercle. It enlarges on standing and on coughing and may disappear when the patient lies down. However, in most cases, even when the hernia is completely reduced, a swelling can still be palpated and this is due to extraperitoneal fat around the femoral sac.

As the hernia enlarges, it passes through the saphenous opening in the deep fascia (the site of penetration of the great saphenous vein to join the femoral vein), and then turns upwards so that it may project above the inguinal ligament. There should not, however, be any difficulty in differentiating between an irreducible femoral and inguinal hernia – the neck of a femoral hernia always lies below and lateral to the pubic tubercle, whereas the sac of an indirect inguinal hernia extends above and medial to this landmark (Figure 29.4).

The neck of the femoral canal is narrow and has a particularly sharp medial border. For this reason,

---

[1]Edward Earle Shouldice (1890–1965), Surgeon, Toronto, Canada.
[2]Irving L. Lichtenstein, (1920-2000), Surgeon, Cedars-Sinai Medical Center, Los Angeles, CA, USA.

[3]Manuel Gimbernat (1734–1816), Anatomist and Surgeon to King Carlos III of Spain.
[4]Sir Astley Paston Cooper (1768–1841), Surgeon, Guy's Hospital, London, UK.
[5]Jules Germain Cloquet (1790–1883), Professor of Surgery, Paris, France.

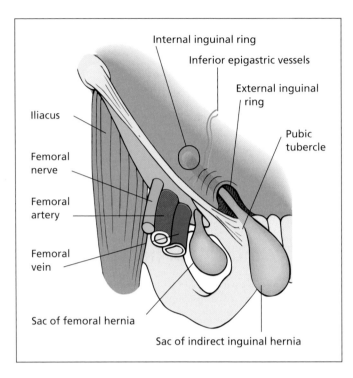

Internal inguinal ring

Inferior epigastric vessels

External inguinal ring

Iliacus

Pubic tubercle

Femoral nerve

Femoral artery

Femoral vein

Sac of femoral hernia

Sac of indirect inguinal hernia

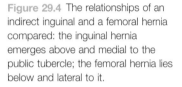

Figure 29.4 The relationships of an indirect inguinal and a femoral hernia compared: the inguinal hernia emerges above and medial to the public tubercle; the femoral hernia lies below and lateral to it.

irreducibility and strangulation are extremely common in this type of hernia.

Richter's hernia

A Richter's hernia[6] is particularly likely to occur in the femoral sac. In this type of hernia, only part of the wall of the small intestine herniates through the defect, where it is then strangulated. Because the lumen of the bowel is not completely encroached upon, symptoms of intestinal obstruction do not occur, although the knuckle of bowel may become completely necrotic and indeed perforate into the hernial sac and thence into the peritoneal cavity causing acute peritonitis.

Treatment

All femoral hernias should be repaired by excision of the sac and closure of the femoral canal because

[6]August Gottlieb Richter (1742–1842), Surgeon, Göttingen, Germany.

of their great danger of strangulation. This is usually accomplished by suturing a plug of rolled up polypropylene mesh in the canal.

Umbilical hernia

Exomphalos

This is a rare condition in which there is failure of all or part of the midgut to return to the abdominal cavity in fetal life. The bowel is contained within a translucent sac protruding through a defective anterior abdominal wall. Untreated, this ruptures with fatal peritonitis, or rupture may occur during delivery.

Treatment

Immediate surgical repair if possible. When the sac is massive, it is protected with a dressing soaked in mild antiseptic. Gradual epithelialization takes place and later repair may then be undertaken.

Congenital umbilical hernia

This results from failure of complete closure of the umbilical cicatrix. It is especially common in black children. The vast majority close spontaneously during the first year of life.

Treatment

Surgical repair should not be carried out unless the hernia persists after the child is 2 years old. The parents of an infant with a congenital umbilical hernia should be reassured that the majority disappear spontaneously. Strapping the hernia or providing a rubber truss are only required to allay parental anxiety.

Paraumbilical hernia

This is an acquired hernia that occurs just above or below the umbilicus. It especially occurs in obese, multiparous, middle-aged women. The neck is narrow and, like a femoral hernia, it is particularly prone to become irreducible or strangulated. The contents are nearly always the omentum, and often in addition transverse colon and small intestine.

Treatment

The sac is excised and the edges of the rectus sheath are overlapped above and below the hernia (Mayo's operation[7]), or, for large defects, a polypropylene mesh is sewn across the defect.

Ventral hernia

An upper midline ventral hernia may exist as an elongated gap between the recti (divarication of the recti). In the majority of cases, no treatment is required.

[7]William Mayo (1861–1939), Surgeon, Rochester, MN, USA.

Epigastric hernia

A particular variety of ventral hernia is the epigastric hernia, which consists of one or more small protrusions through defects in the linea alba above the umbilicus. These usually contain only extraperitoneal fat, but are often surprisingly painful.

Treatment

Simply suturing the defect is all that is required.

Incisional hernia

An incisional hernia occurs through a defect in the scar of a previous abdominal operation. The causes, which are the same as those of a burst abdomen, are given in Chapter 4, p. 23.

There is usually a wide neck, and strangulation is, in consequence, rare.

Treatment

If the general condition of the patient is good, the hernia is repaired by dissecting out and suturing the individual layers of the abdominal wall. Large hernias are repaired with a sheet of nylon or polypropylene mesh. If operation is considered inadvisable, an abdominal belt is prescribed.

Unusual hernias

Obturator hernia

These are found particularly in thin, elderly women. The hernia develops through the obturator canal where the obturator nerve and vessels traverse the membrane covering the obturator foramen. Pressure of a strangulated obturator hernia upon the nerve may cause referred pain in its area of cutaneous distribution, so that intestinal obstruction associated with pain along the medial side of the thigh in a thin, elderly woman should suggest this diagnosis. The hernia is often of the Richter type. Contrast-enhanced computed tomography (CT) will confirm the diagnosis.

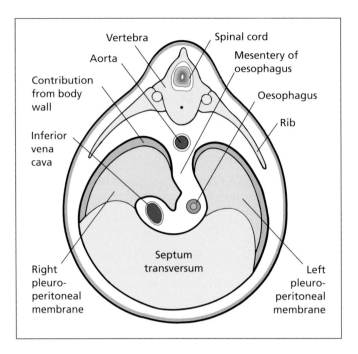

Figure 29.5 The development of the diaphragm. The drawing shows the four contributory elements: septum transversum, dorsal mesentery of the oesophagus, body wall and pleuroperitoneal membrane.

Spigelian hernia

A Spigelian hernia[8] passes upwards through the arcuate (semilunar) line into the lateral border of the lower part of the posterior rectus sheath. It presents as a tender mass to one side of the lower abdominal wall. CT will confirm the diagnosis if doubt exists.

Gluteal hernia

Traverses the greater sciatic foramen.

Sciatic hernia

Passes through the lesser sciatic foramen.

Lumbar hernia

A lumbar hernia is most commonly an incisional hernia following an operation on the kidney, but may rarely occur through the inferior lumbar triangle bounded by the crest of the ilium below, the latissimus dorsi medially and the external oblique on the lateral side.

[8]Adriaan van den Spiegel (Spigelius) (1578–1625), Professor of Anatomy and Surgery, Padua, Italy.

Diaphragmatic hernias

The diaphragmatic hernias can be classified as:

1 *Congenital.*
2 *Acquired:*
    a traumatic;
    b hiatal.

Congenital diaphragmatic hernia

Embryology

These hernias can best be understood by reference to the embryology of the diaphragm (Figure 29.5). The diaphragm is developed by fusion of the following:

- *The septum transversum*, which forms the central tendon, and which develops from mesoderm lying in front of the head of the embryo. With the folding of the head, this mesodermal mass is carried ventrally and caudally to lie in its definitive position at the anterior part of the diaphragm. During this migration, the cervical myotomes and cervical nerves contribute muscle and nerve supply, respectively; thus accounting for the long course of the phrenic nerve (C3, 4, 5) from the neck to the diaphragm.

- *The dorsal oesophageal mesentery.*
- *The pleuroperitoneal membranes*, which close the primitive communication between the pleural and peritoneal cavities.
- *A peripheral rim* derived from the body wall.

In spite of this complex story, congenital abnormalities of the diaphragm are unusual. They may manifest as hernias through the following defects:

- the foramen of Morgagni,[9] between the xiphoid and costal origins;
- the foramen of Bochdalek,[10] a defect in the pleuroperitoneal canal;
- a deficiency of the whole central tendon;
- a congenitally large oesophageal hiatus.

Clinical features

Hernias through the foramen of Morgagni are usually small and unimportant. Those through the foramen of Bochdalek or through the central tendon are large and present as respiratory distress shortly after birth. Urgent surgical repair is required.

The congenital hiatal hernias present with regurgitation, vomiting, dysphagia and progressive loss of weight in small children; they usually respond to conservative treatment and nursing the child in a sitting position. If this fails, surgical repair is necessary.

Traumatic diaphragmatic hernias

These are comparatively rare and follow blunt (crush) injuries to the chest or abdomen, or penetrating injuries such as stab wounds, which implicate the diaphragm. The left diaphragm is far more often affected than the right (which is protected by the liver) and is accompanied by herniation of the stomach and spleen into the thoracic cavity. The gas-filled stomach lying in the left chest after a crush injury may be mistaken for a tension pneumothorax on chest X-ray. Passage of a nasogastric tube or ingestion of a small amount of contrast material confirm the diagnosis.

[9]Giovanni Battista Morgagni (1682–1771), Professor of Anatomy, Padua, Italy.
[10]Vincent Bochdalek (1801–83), Professor of Anatomy, Prague, Czech Republic.

Treatment comprises urgent surgical repair, through either the chest or abdomen.

Acquired hiatal hernias

Classification

These are divided into the following:

- sliding (90%);
- rolling (10%).

In the *sliding* variety, the stomach slides through the hiatus and is covered in its anterior aspect with a peritoneal sac while the posterior part is extraperitoneal. It thus resembles an inguinal hernia *en glissade* (Figure 29.6a). This type of hernia produces both the effects of a space-occupying lesion in the chest and disturbances of the cardio-oesophageal sphincter mechanism.

In the *rolling* (or paraoesophageal) hernia, the cardia remains in position but the stomach rolls up anteriorly through the hiatus, producing a partial volvulus. Because the cardio-oesophageal mechanism is intact, there are no symptoms of regurgitation (Figure 29.6b).

These hernias probably represent a progressive weakening of the muscles of the hiatus. They occur in the obese, middle-aged and elderly, and are four times more common in women than in men.

Clinical features

Most are symptomless, but, when they occur, symptoms fall into three groups:

1 *Mechanical*, produced by the presence of the hernia within the thoracic cavity: cough, dyspnoea, palpitations, hiccough.
2 *Reflux*, resulting from incompetence of the cardiac sphincter: burning retrosternal or epigastric pain aggravated by lying down or stooping, and which may be referred to the jaw, or arms, thus simulating myocardial ischaemia. Alkalis provide relief. In severe cases, spillover into the trachea may cause pneumonitis.
3 *The effects of oesophagitis*: stricture formation with dysphagia and bleeding, which may be acute or occult.

Treatment

Sliding hiatus hernias are treated symptomati-

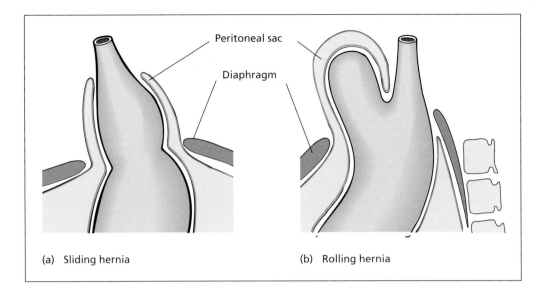

Peritoneal sac

Diaphragm

(a) Sliding hernia

(b) Rolling hernia

Figure 29.6 (a) Sliding hiatus hernia: the stomach and lower oesophagus slide into the chest through a patulous oesophageal hiatus. (b) Rolling hiatus hernia: the stomach rolls up through the hiatus alongside the lower oesophagus (paraoesophageal hernia).

cally; if symptoms persist, laparoscopic repair is performed. Paraoesophageal (rolling) hernias are usually asymptomatic, but potentially more serious with the risk of complete gastric volvulus into the chest. Should this occur, urgent surgical repair is indicated.

Reflux oesophagitis

This is discussed in Chapter 20, p. 163.

The liver

Liver enlargement

Physical signs

The normal liver in the adult is impalpable. In contrast, an infant's liver is normally palpable two finger breadths below the right costal margin.

The enlarged liver extends downwards below the right costal margin and may fill the subcostal angle or even extend beneath the left costal margin in gross hepatomegaly. The liver moves with respiration, is dull to percussion and the liver dullness may extend above the normal upper level of the fifth right interspace.

Causes of hepatomegaly

1 *Congenital*:
  a Riedel's lobe;[1]
  b polycystic liver disease (which develops in adult life).
2 *Infective*:
  a viral hepatitis;
  b liver abscess;
  c malaria;
  d amoebic hepatitis and abscess;
  e hydatid;
  f leptospirosis (Weil's disease[2]);
  g actinomycosis.
3 *Vascular*:
  a right heart failure;
  b venous outflow obstruction, e.g. Budd–Chiari syndrome;
4 *Neoplastic*:
  a primary tumour;
  b secondary deposits.
5 *Haematological*:
  a Hodgkin's disease;[3]
  b non-Hodgkin's lymphoma;
  c leukaemia;
  d myeloproliferative disorders.
6 *Autoimmune*:
  a autoimmune hepatitis;
7 *Biliary tract disease*:
  a primary biliary cirrhosis;
  b primary sclerosing cholangitis.
8 *Metabolic diseases*:
  a fatty infiltration (non-alcoholic and alcoholic fatty liver disease);
  b haemochromatosis;
  c amyloid;
  d glycogen storage diseases (e.g. Gaucher's disease[4]).

---

[1]Bernhard Riedel (1846–1916), Professor of Surgery, Jena, Germany. Also described Riedel's thyroiditis.

Lecture Notes: General Surgery, 12th edition. © Harold Ellis, Sir Roy Y. Calne and Christopher J. E. Watson. Published 2011 by Blackwell Publishing Ltd.

[2]Adolf Weil (1848–1916), Professor of Medicine, Berlin, Germany.
[3]Thomas Hodgkin (1798–1866), Curator of Pathology, Guy's Hospital, London, UK.
[4]Phillipe Gaucher (1854–1918), Physician, Hôpital St Louis, Paris, France.

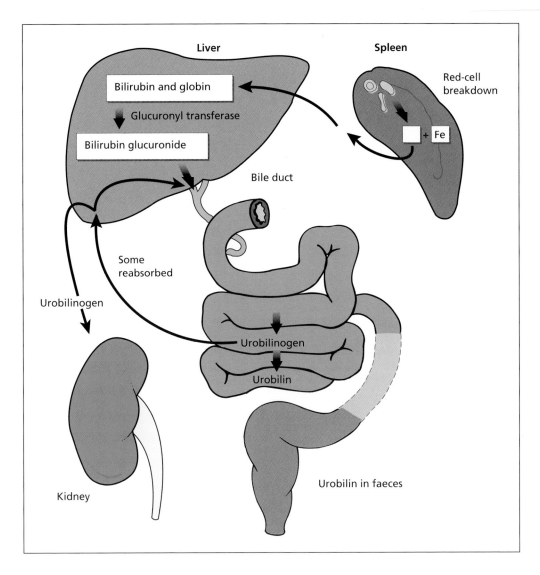

Figure 30.1 The metabolism of bilirubin.

Whenever the liver is palpable, the patient must be examined to detect any accompanying splenomegaly or lymphadenopathy. If the spleen is palpable in addition to the liver, consider cirrhosis, haematological malignancy or amyloid as possible diagnoses. If, in addition, the lymph nodes are enlarged, the diagnosis is often lymphoma, but may be due to viral infection such as Epstein–Barr virus.[5]

[5]Michael Anthony Epstein (b. 1921), Professor of Pathology, University of Bristol, Bristol, UK. Yvonne Barr (b. 1932), Epstein's assistant, Middlesex Hospital, London, UK.

Jaundice

The normal serum bilirubin is below $17\,\mu mol/L$ (1 mg/dL). Excess bilirubin becomes clinically detectable when the serum level rises to over $35\,\mu mol/L$ (2 mg/dL), and gives a yellow tinge to the sclera and skin, termed jaundice (or icterus).

Bilirubin metabolism (Figure 30.1)

Knowledge of bile pigment metabolism and excretion is essential if the pathogenesis, presentation, investigation and treatment of jaundice are to be understood.

When red cells reach the end of their life in the circulation (approximately 120 days), they are destroyed in the reticuloendothelial system. The porphyrin ring of the haemoglobin molecule is disrupted and a bilirubin–iron–globin complex produced. The iron is released and used for further haemoglobin synthesis. The bilirubin–globin fraction reaches the liver as a lipid-soluble, water-insoluble substance. In the liver, the bilirubin is conjugated with glucuronic acid in the hepatocytes and excreted in the bile as the now water-soluble bilirubin glucuronide.

In the bowel lumen, bilirubin is reduced by bacterial action to the colourless urobilinogen. Most of the urobilinogen is excreted in the faeces, where it is broken down into urobilin, which is pigmented and which, with the other breakdown products of bilirubin, gives the stool its normal colour.

A small amount of urobilinogen is reabsorbed from the intestine into the portal venous tributaries and passes to the liver, where most of it is excreted once more in the bile back into the gut. Some, however, reaches the systemic circulation and this is excreted by the kidney into the urine. When urine is exposed to air, the urobilinogen it contains is oxidized to urobilin, which is darker.

Classification and pathogenesis

The causes of jaundice are classified according to which was the abnormal stage in the metabolism of bilirubin that resulted in its accumulation.

Prehepatic jaundice

Increased production of (unconjugated) bilirubin by the reticuloendothelial system, as may result from excessive destruction of red cells in haemolysis, exceeds the ability of the liver to conjugate; therefore, the unconjugated bilirubin accumulates in the blood. There is no increase in conjugated bilirubin in the blood, so none is found in the urine. However, there is an increase in the amount of urobilinogen produced in the gut, so more is resorbed and 'overflows' into the systemic circulation, where it is excreted by the kidney.

Hepatic jaundice

In the presence of hepatocellular damage, the liver is unable to conjugate bilirubin efficiently, and less is excreted into the canaliculi. Thus, both unconjugated and conjugated bilirubin accumulate in the blood.

Posthepatic (obstructive) jaundice

Obstruction of the intrahepatic or extrahepatic bile ducts prevents excretion of conjugated bilirubin. Without pigment, the stools become pale, and the conjugated bilirubin builds up in the blood and is excreted in the urine, turning it dark brown.

Sometimes the hepatic and posthepatic forms coexist. For example, a stone in the common bile duct may produce jaundice partly by obstructing the outflow of bile and partly by secondary damage to the liver (biliary cirrhosis). Similarly, tumour deposits in the liver and cirrhosis may both result in jaundice partly by actual destruction of liver tissue and partly by intrahepatic duct compression.

Causes

Prehepatic jaundice

This is caused by increased production of bilirubin owing to increased red blood cell destruction. The most common cause is haemolysis (e.g. spherocytosis or incompatible blood transfusion), but it may occur during reabsorption of a large haematoma.

Hepatic jaundice

This is a result of impaired bilirubin conjugation owing to the following:

- hepatitis: viral (hepatitis viruses A, B, C), leptospirosis, glandular fever;
- cirrhosis;
- cholestasis from drugs, e.g. chlorpromazine;
- liver poisons, e.g. paracetamol overdosage, chlorinated hydrocarbons such as carbon tetrachloride, chloroform and halothane; phosphorus;
- liver tumours.

Posthepatic jaundice

This is caused by obstruction to biliary drainage owing to the following:

1 *Obstruction within the lumen*: gallstones.
2 *Pathology in the wall*:

a congenital atresia of the common bile duct;
b traumatic stricture;
c primary or secondary sclerosing cholangitis;
d tumour of the bile duct
   (cholangiocarcinoma).
3 *External compression*:
   a pancreatitis;
   b tumour of the head of the pancreas;
   c tumour of the ampulla of Vater;
   d hilar lymphadenopathy.

Diagnosis

This is based on history, examination and special investigations.

History

A family history of anaemia, splenectomy or gallstones suggests a congenital red cell defect. Clay-coloured stools and dark urine accompanying the episodes of jaundice indicate hepatic or posthepatic causes. Enquire after recent blood transfusions, drugs (chlorpromazine, paracetamol, methyldopa, repeated exposure to halothane), injections and alcohol consumption. Has there been contact with cases of viral hepatitis? What is the patient's occupation? (Farmers and sewer workers are at risk of leptospirosis – Weil's disease.)

Usually painless jaundice of sudden onset with liver tenderness in a young person is viral in origin. Attacks of severe colic, rigors and intermittent jaundice suggest a stone. Remorselessly progressive jaundice, often accompanied by continuous pain radiating to the back, is suspicious of malignant disease. Recent onset of diabetes suggests carcinoma of the pancreas.

Examination

The colour of the jaundice is important; a lemon-yellow tinge suggests haemolytic jaundice (owing to combined anaemia and mild icterus). Deep jaundice suggests the hepatic or posthepatic types.

Other signs of cirrhosis should be sought: spider naevi, gynaecomastia, testicular atrophy, encephalopathy, splenomegaly, liver palms, flapping tremor, leuconychia (white nails) and, occasionally, finger clubbing. There may also be ascites and leg oedema, but these may be associated with intra-abdominal malignant disease as well as cirrhosis.

Examination of the liver itself is helpful. In viral hepatitis, the liver is slightly enlarged and tender; in cirrhosis, the liver edge is firm and may be irregular, although the liver may be shrunken and impalpable. A grossly enlarged, knobbly liver may also be present in malignant disease.

If the gallbladder is palpable and distended, it is probable that the cause of the jaundice is not a stone (Courvoisier's law,[6] Chapter 31, p. 271). The liver may be smoothly enlarged in posthepatic obstructive jaundice.

A pancreatic tumour may be palpable or a separate primary focus of malignant disease may be obvious, e.g. a melanoma.

Splenomegaly suggests cirrhosis of the liver, blood disease or a lymphoma. In the last, there may also be obvious lymphadenopathy.

Special investigations (Table 30.1)

The prehepatic causes of jaundice are relatively easy to distinguish from hepatic and posthepatic, but the last two are often very difficult to differentiate one from the other and, as already stated, may be associated with each other. Laboratory tests are of some help but are by no means diagnostic. Imaging techniques are valuable in visualizing the liver, gallbladder and pancreas, whereas endoscopic cannulation of the bile ducts or transhepatic duct puncture enable the bile duct system to be outlined. Percutaneous biopsy will usually confirm the hepatic cause of jaundice.

Bilirubin is not excreted by the kidney except in its water-soluble (conjugated) form. It is therefore absent from the urine in prehepatic jaundice (hence the old term 'acholuric jaundice'), although present when there is posthepatic obstruction.

In *prehepatic jaundice*, large amounts of bilirubin are excreted into the gut; therefore, the urobilinogen in the faeces is raised, the amount absorbed from the bowel increases and there is therefore greater spill over into the urine.

In *hepatic damage*, the urinary urobilinogen may also be raised because of the inability of the liver to re-excrete the urobilinogen reabsorbed from the bowel.

In *posthepatic obstruction*, very little bile can enter the gut; therefore, the urobilinogen must be low in both the faeces and the urine.

The important laboratory findings in the various types of jaundice can now be summarized:

---

[6]Ludwig Courvoisier (1843–1918), Professor of Surgery, Basle, Switzerland.

Table 30.1 Diagnosis of jaundice

Test	Prehepatic	Hepatic	Obstructive
Urine	Urobilinogen	Urobilinogen	No urobilinogen Bilirubin present
Serum bilirubin	Unconjugated bilirubin	Conjugated and unconjugated	Conjugated bilirubin
ALT (SGPT) and AST (SGOT)	Normal	Raised	Normal or moderately raised
ALP	Normal	Normal or moderately raised	Raised
Blood glucose	Normal	Low if liver failure	Sometimes raised if pancreatic tumour
Reticulocyte count	Raised in haemolysis	Normal	Normal
Haptoglobins	Low due to haemolysis	Normal or low if liver failure	Normal
Prothrombin time	Normal	Prolonged due to poor synthetic function	Prolonged due to vitamin K malabsorption; corrects with vitamin K
Ultrasound	Normal	May be abnormal liver texture, e.g. cirrhosis	Dilated bile ducts

- *Urine*: the presence of bilirubin indicates obstructive jaundice, either intra- or posthepatic. Excess of urobilinogen indicates prehepatic jaundice or sometimes liver damage, whereas an absence of urobilinogen suggests obstructive causes.
- *Faeces*: absence of bile pigment indicates intra- or posthepatic causes.
- *Haematological investigations*: red blood cell fragility, Coombs' test[7] and reticulocyte count confirm haemolytic causes.
- *Serum bilirubin* is rarely higher than 100 μmol/L (5 mg/dL) in prehepatic jaundice, but may be considerably higher in obstructive cases. In late malignant disease, it may exceed 1000 μmol/L.
- *Conjugated bilirubin*: in prehepatic jaundice, bilirubin is present in the unconjugated form. In pure posthepatic obstructive jaundice, the bilirubin is mainly in the conjugated form, whereas in hepatic jaundice it is present in the mixed conjugated and unconjugated forms owing to a combination of liver destruction and intrahepatic duct blockage.

- *Alkaline phosphatase (ALP)* is produced by cells lining the bile canaliculi. It is normal in prehepatic jaundice, raised in hepatic jaundice and considerably raised in posthepatic jaundice and in primary biliary cirrhosis. A raised ALP level and normal bilirubin are features of obstruction of some, but not necessarily all, of the intrahepatic bile ducts (note that a different isoenzyme of ALP is produced by bone and placenta, and isolated elevated levels should be isotyped to determine origin).
- *Serum proteins* are normal in prehepatic jaundice, have a reversed albumin/globulin ratio with depressed albumin synthesis in hepatic jaundice and are usually normal in posthepatic jaundice, unless associated with liver damage.
- *Haptoglobin* concentrations are low in haemolysis. Haptoglobin binds free haemoglobin released after haemolysis, and, once bound, the complex is catabolized faster than haptoglobin alone. It is also low in severe liver disease owing to impaired synthesis.
- *Serum transaminases* such as alanine transaminase (ALT) and aspartate transaminase (AST) are raised with hepatocyte inflammation such as occurs in viral hepatitis and in the active phase of cirrhosis. Gamma

[7]Robin Royston Amos Coombs (1921–2006), Professor of Immunology, Cambridge, UK. Described the test for detecting the presence of antibodies to red blood cells.

glutamyl transferase (GGT) is a more sensitive indicator of liver disease, and is often raised before the transaminases.

- *Prothrombin time* is normal in prehepatic jaundice, prolonged but correctable with vitamin K in posthepatic jaundice (in which functioning liver tissue is still present) and prolonged but not correctable in advanced hepatic jaundice, in which not only is absorption of fat-soluble vitamin K impaired but the damaged liver is also unable to synthesize prothrombin.
- *Ultrasound scanning* is extremely useful as well as non-invasive. Gallstones within the gallbladder can be demonstrated with a high degree of accuracy. Unfortunately, stones within the distal bile ducts are often missed because of overlying duodenal gas. Dilatation of the duct system within the liver is a good indication of duct obstruction; thus, if the ducts are not dilated, an obstructive cause for the jaundice is unlikely.
- *Computed tomography (CT)* and *magnetic resonance (MR)* scans are useful in addition to ultrasound in the demonstration of intrahepatic lesions (e.g. tumour deposits, abscess, cyst), which may then be accurately needle biopsied under imaging control. A mass in the pancreas may also be demonstrated, but differentiation between carcinoma and chronic pancreatitis is difficult.
- *Abdominal X-ray* may show gallstones (10% are radio-opaque).
- *Magnetic resonance cholangiopancreatography (MRCP)* affords non-invasive high-resolution imaging of the biliary tree. However, it does not permit therapeutic intervention.
- *Endoscopic retrograde cholangiopancreatography (ERCP)*, in which the ampulla of Vater[8] is cannulated using an endoscope passed via the mouth, may demonstrate the location and indicate the nature of an obstructing lesion within the bile ducts. A periampullary tumour is also directly visualized at this examination, and can be biopsied.
- *Percutaneous transhepatic cholangiography (PTC)*, in which a needle is passed percutaneously into the liver substance and a dilated bile duct is cannulated, may be necessary where ERCP is not possible.

Both ERCP and PTC may be used to introduce stents across obstructing bile duct lesions to decompress the bile ducts and resolve jaundice.

- *Needle biopsy*. If the ultrasound scan reveals no dilatation of the duct system, an obstructive lesion is unlikely and needle biopsy of the liver may give valuable information regarding hepatic pathology (e.g. hepatitis or cirrhosis). If the ultrasound demonstrates focal lesions in the liver, an ultrasound-guided biopsy of one of the lesions can be obtained. Needle biopsy is potentially dangerous in the presence of jaundice, particularly where there is biliary dilatation or ascites. The prothrombin time, if prolonged, should first be corrected by administration of vitamin K, and fresh frozen plasma and platelet transfusions may also be indicated; a transjugular liver biopsy may be appropriate in the presence of severe coagulopathy. Should bleeding occur following biopsy, angiographic embolization or immediate laparotomy may be necessary.

Summary of investigations of jaundice

The investigations of jaundice may be grouped as follows:

- *Exclusion of prehepatic causes*: haptoglobin level, reticulocyte count, Coombs' test; split bilirubin (conjugated/unconjugated).
- *Liver synthetic function* (hepatocellular dysfunction): prothrombin time, albumin.
- *Liver cell damage*: transaminases, γ-glutamyl transferase.
- *Bile duct obstruction*: alkaline phosphatase, ultrasound of bile ducts, PTC, ERCP, MRCP and CT for pancreatic lesion.
- *Intrahepatic mass*: cross-sectional imaging, such as ultrasound and CT, with needle biopsy.

Congenital abnormalities

Riedel's lobe

This anatomical variant is a projection downwards from the right lobe of the liver of normally functioning liver tissue. It may present as a puzzling and symptomless abdominal mass.

---

[8]Abraham Vater (1648–1751), Professor of Anatomy, Wittenberg, Germany.

Polycystic liver

This is often associated with polycystic disease of the kidneys (and occasionally pancreas), and comprises multiple cysts within the liver parenchyma. The liver may reach a very large size, but functions normally. The commonest symptoms are discomfort and awareness of the grossly enlarged liver in the abdomen. Haemorrhage into the cysts and cholangitis are occasional complications.

Liver trauma

This may be due to penetrating wounds (gunshot or stab) or closed crush injuries, often associated with fractures of the ribs and injuries to other intra-abdominal viscera, especially the spleen. Severe abdominal trauma is becoming increasingly common, and accurate preoperative diagnosis of the source of the haemorrhage may be impossible.

Clinical features

Following injury, the patient complains of abdominal pain. Examination reveals shock (pallor, tachycardia, hypotension), generalized abdominal tenderness together with the signs of progressive bleeding.

CT is essential to assess the severity of the injury and to identify any additional injuries, such as a ruptured spleen. Occasionally, there is delayed rupture of a subcapsular haematoma, so that abdominal pain and shock may not be in evidence until some hours or days after the initial injury.

Treatment

If the patient's vital observations are stable, and a definite diagnosis made by CT, the patient can initially be managed conservatively with blood transfusion and careful observation. Repeat CT is undertaken to monitor progress.

If bleeding continues, as denoted by falling blood pressure, rising pulse and falling haemoglobin, and/or there is the risk of overlooking damage to other viscera, a laparotomy is performed. Minor liver tears can be sutured. Packing of the injury with gauze packs, removed after 48 hours, may be life-saving in severe trauma when the patient's condition is deteriorating. If bleeding continues, the relevant main hepatic arterial branch should be tied, and, if the bleeding continues in spite of this, major hepatic lobar resection may be necessary.

Antibiotic cover must be given because of the danger of infection of areas of devitalized liver, and is particularly important when packing is used.

Acute infections of the liver

Possible sources of infection are the following:

- *portal*, from an area of suppuration drained by the portal vein, usually diverticular sepsis or appendicitis;
- *biliary*, resulting from an ascending cholangitis;
- *arterial*, as part of a general septicaemia – this is unusual;
- *adjacent infections* spreading into the liver parenchyma, e.g. subphrenic abscess or acute cholecystitis.

Pyogenic liver abscess

Pyogenic liver abscess is a consequence of infection either in the portal territory, leading to a portal pyaemia (pyelophlebitis), or in the biliary tree. Multiple abscesses are common. Common infecting organisms include *Escherichia coli*, *Streptococcus faecalis* and *Streptococcus milleri*.

Clinical features

The condition should be suspected in patients who develop rigors, high swinging fever, a tender palpable liver and jaundice. A previous history of abdominal sepsis, such as Crohn's disease,[9] appendicitis or diverticulitis may be obtained. The clinical course is often insidious, with a non-specific malaise for over a month before presentation and diagnosis.

Special investigations

- *Blood culture*, carried out before treatment is commenced, is often positive.

[9]Burrill Bernard Crohn (1884–1983), Gastroenterologist, Mount Sinai Hospital, New York, NY, USA. The disease was first described by Morgagni (1682–1771).

- *Ultrasound or CT* of the liver may identify and localize hepatic abscesses, as well as identifying the source of the pyaemia.

Treatment

The originating site of sepsis should be dealt with appropriately. A large liver abscess can be drained percutaneously under ultrasound guidance; smaller abscesses are treated by parenteral antibiotic therapy alone.

Portal pyaemia (pyelophlebitis)

Infection may reach the liver via the portal tributaries from a focus of intra-abdominal sepsis, particularly acute appendicitis or diverticulitis. Multiple abscesses may permeate the liver; in addition, there may be septic thrombi in the intrahepatic radicles of the portal vein, and infected clot in the portal vein itself. The condition has become rare since the advent of antibiotics.

Biliary infection

Multiple abscesses in the liver may occur in association with severe suppurative cholangitis secondary to impaction of gallstones in the common bile duct. Clinically, the features are those of *Charcot's intermittent hepatic fever*[10] – pyrexia, rigors and jaundice. (Rigors represent a bacteraemia and are commonly due to infection in either the renal or biliary tract.)

Urgent drainage of the bile ducts is performed, by either endoscopic sphincterotomy or percutaneous transhepatic drainage.

Amoebic liver abscess

This particular type of portal infection is secondary to an *Entamoeba histolytica* infection of the large intestine. From there, amoebae travel via the portal circulation to the liver, where they proliferate. The amoeba produces a cytolytic enzyme that destroys the liver tissue, producing an amoebic abscess, which is sterile, although amoebae may be found in the abscess wall.

CT and ultrasound of the liver are the most valuable special investigations.

[10]Jean-Martin Charcot (1825–1893), First Professor of Neurology, Salpêtrière Hospital, Paris, France.

Treatment

The majority respond to medical treatment with metronidazole. Ultrasound-guided percutaneous drainage is required infrequently in non-responding cases.

Hydatid disease of the liver

The liver is the site of 75% of hydatid cysts in humans.

Pathology

Dogs are infected with the ova of *Echinococcus granulosus* (*Taenia echinococcus*) as a result of eating sheep offal. The tapeworms develop in the dog's small intestine from whence ova are discharged in the faeces. Humans (as well as sheep) ingest the ova from contaminated vegetables and the ova penetrate the stomach wall to invade the portal tributaries and thence pass to the liver. Occasionally, the hydatids may pass on to the lungs, brain, bones and other organs. Hydatid disease is therefore common in sheep-rearing communities, e.g. in Australia, Iceland, Cyprus, southern Europe, Africa and Wales.

Clinical features

A cyst may present as a symptomless mass. The contents may die and the walls become calcified so that this inactive structure may be a harmless postmortem finding.

The active cyst may, however,

- *rupture* into the peritoneal cavity, pleural cavity, alimentary canal or biliary tree;
- *become infected*;
- *produce obstructive jaundice* by pressure on intrahepatic bile ducts, although jaundice is much more often due to intrabiliary rupture and release of cysts into the bile ducts.

Special investigations

- *Plain X-ray* of the liver may show a clear zone produced by the cyst, or may show flecks of calcification in the cyst wall.
- *Ultrasound and CT scan* localize the cyst.

- *Serological tests* depend on the sensitization of the patient to hydatid fluid, which contains a specific antigen, leakage of which induces the production of antibodies.
- *Eosinophil count*: there may be *eosinophilia*, which, while not specific, should arouse clinical suspicion.

Treatment

A calcified cyst should be left alone. Other cysts should be treated to prevent complications. Treatment with albendazole may result in shrinkage or even disappearance of the cysts. Failure to respond or the presence of complications are indications for surgery. The cyst is exposed and aspirated. It is then possible to excise the cyst, taking care not to liberate daughter cysts that are present within the cyst.

Cirrhosis

Definition

Cirrhosis of the liver is a consequence of chronic hepatic injury, with healing by regeneration and fibrosis. Fibrosis leads to further cell damage and destruction of hepatic architecture, progressing to liver failure and portal hypertension.

Aetiology

A convenient classification of the cirrhoses is as follows:

1 *Parenchymal*:
   a alcohol;
   b viral, commonly following hepatitis B and C infections;
   c non-alcoholic fatty liver disease.
2 *Metabolic*:
   a iron overload – haemochromatosis;
   b copper overload – hepatolenticular degeneration (Kinnier Wilson's disease[11]).
3 *Biliary*:
   a primary biliary cirrhosis (Hanot's cirrhosis[12]) – an autoimmune disease characterized by raised serum antimitochondrial (M2) antibodies;

   b primary sclerosing cholangitis;
   c secondary to prolonged biliary obstruction (secondary biliary cirrhosis).
4 *Hepatic venous outflow obstruction*:
   a Budd–Chiari syndrome[13] (hepatic venous occlusion);
   b severe chronic congestive cardiac failure.
5 *Other causes*:
   a chronic active hepatitis, which is an autoimmune disease;
   b schistosomiasis;
   c nutritional (protein-deficient diet);
   d idiopathic (cryptogenic);
   e parenteral nutrition related – probably linked to the fat content.

In countries with a high consumption of alcohol (e.g. France), alcohol is the most common aetiological factor. In the tropics, schistosomiasis heads the list (Egyptian splenomegaly). In the UK, alcohol accounts for half of the cases of cirrhosis.

Consequences of cirrhosis

1 Hepatocellular failure:
   a impaired protein synthesis: prolonged prothrombin time and low albumin;
   b impaired metabolism of toxins: encephalopathy;
   c impaired bilirubin metabolism: jaundice.
2 Portal hypertension (see below).
3 Ascites due to portal hypertension.
4 Malignant change: hepatoma.

Clinical features of cirrhosis

A number of clinical signs, separate from those of portal hypertension, are seen in cirrhosis. These include gynaecomastia, testicular atrophy, amenorrhoea, spider naevi, finger clubbing and palmar erythema ('liver palms').

Hepatic encephalopathy

A neuropsychiatric condition characterized by mental changes, flapping tremor and hepatic coma. It occurs because the liver is unable to detoxify the nitrogenous breakdown products of protein metabolism combined with portosystemic shunts that divert these products directly into the systemic circulation.

[11]Samuel A. Kinnier Wilson (1877–1937), Neurologist, Hospital for Nervous Diseases, Queen Square, London, UK.
[12]Victor Charles Hanot (1844–96), Physician, Paris, France.

[13]George Budd (1808–1882), Professor of Medicine, King's College, London, UK. Hans Chiari (1851–1916), Professor of Pathology, Prague, Czech Republic.

Portal hypertension

The normal portal pressure is less than 5 mmHg. In portal hypertension, this pressure is raised.

Aetiology

Portal hypertension results from an obstruction to portal venous drainage. The causes are classified according to the site of the block.

1 *Prehepatic* (obstruction of the portal venous inflow into the liver):
   a congenital malformation;
   b portal vein thrombosis: often secondary to portal pyaemia, prothrombotic disorders, or, in the neonatal period, spreading infection from the umbilicus;
   c occlusion by tumour or pancreatitis. In adults, there is a special case in which splenic vein thrombosis caused by pancreatic pathology can result in 'segmental portal hypertension' with diversion of the splenic drainage via the short gastric veins, which results in the development of gastric and oesophageal varices.
2 *Hepatic* (obstruction of the portal flow within the liver): e.g. cirrhosis.
3 *Posthepatic* (obstruction of the hepatic veins): Budd–Chiari syndrome.
   a Idiopathic hepatic venous thrombosis in young adults of both sexes. A possible complication of oral contraceptives in women. In many cases, there is an underlying haematological cause, e.g. polycythaemia or monoclonal gammopathy.
   b Congenital obliteration.
   c Blockage of hepatic veins by tumour invasion.

By far, the commonest cause of portal hypertension is cirrhosis, yet there is no strict relationship between the severity of the liver disease and the extent of portal hypertension, which is not therefore entirely explained on the basis of mechanical obstruction.

Pathological effects

The four important effects of portal hypertension are the following:

1 collateral portosystemic venous drainage develops;
2 splenomegaly;

3 ascites (in hepatic and posthepatic portal hypertension only);
4 the manifestations of hepatic failure (in severe cirrhosis).

Collateral channels

Portal obstruction results in the development of collateral channels between the portal and systemic venous circulations (Figure 30.2). The sites of these channels are as follows:

- between the left gastric vein and the oesophageal veins, forming gastric and oesophageal varices; these are the largest and clinically the most important connections;
- along the obliterated umbilical vein to the superior and inferior epigastric veins, forming a *caput medusae* around the umbilicus;
- retroperitoneal and diaphragmatic anastomoses, which present technical hazards to the surgeon at the time of liver transplantation;
- between the superior and inferior rectal veins with development of anal canal varices;
- along any adhesions between the visceral and parietal peritoneum due to previous surgery or inflammation;
- at the site of a colostomy or ileostomy.

The oesophageal varices, and to a much lesser extent anal varices, may result in gastrointestinal haemorrhage, which is the most serious complication of portal hypertension.

Splenomegaly

Progressive splenic enlargement occurs as a result of portal congestion together with some degree of hypertrophy of the splenic substance itself. This is often associated with the haematological changes of hypersplenism: leucopenia and thrombocytopenia. Anaemia accompanying splenomegaly can be accounted for by gastrointestinal bleeding and is not necessarily a result of splenic enlargement.

Ascites

This is due to a combination of factors:

1 Splanchnic vasodilatation occurs owing to accumulation of vasoactive mediators in the splanchnic circulation secondary to the liver failure, resulting in pooling of blood. Systemic hypotension is a consequence, with renal hypoperfusion and activation of the renin–angiotensin–aldosterone system, resulting in raised serum aldosterone which leads to avid salt (sodium) and water retention.

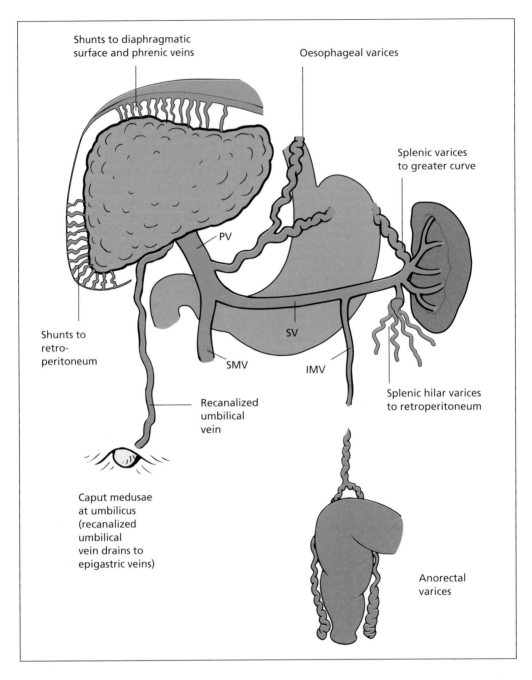

Figure 30.2 The sites of occurrence of portal–systemic communications in patients with portal hypertension. PV, portal vein; SMV, superior mesenteric vein; IMV, inferior mesenteric vein; SV, splenic vein.

2 The portal venous pressure is raised owing to compression of the portal venous radicles in the liver by the scarred surrounding hepatic tissue.

3 The serum albumin, which is synthesized by the liver, is reduced, resulting in lowering of the serum osmotic pressure.

The effects of liver failure

- Jaundice.
- Encephalopathy.

Clinical features

To the surgeon, portal hypertension presents as three problems:

1 as a differential diagnosis of jaundice or hepatomegaly;
2 as a cause of gastrointestinal haemorrhage;
3 as one of the causes of ascites (Box 30.1).

Special investigations

In addition to history and examination (which includes a careful search for the stigmata of liver disease), the following investigations are indicated:

- *Liver function tests*, particularly transaminases and alkaline phosphatase.
- *Liver synthetic function tests*, such as prothrombin time and albumin.
- *Liver biopsy* if necessary.
- *Fibreoptic endoscopy*, which may demonstrate varices and differentiate between bleeding from this source and from a peptic ulcer or multiple gastric erosions, all of which are common in patients with cirrhosis.

Box 30.1 The causes of ascites

- Liver failure and portal hypertension
- Carcinomatosis
- Heart failure
- Renal failure
- Chronic peritonitis, e.g. tuberculous
- Pancreatitis

- *Ultrasound* will demonstrate portal venous flow, splenomegaly, and the presence of intra-abdominal varices; it may also detect hepatic venous outflow occlusion.
- *Inferior vena cavagram*, which will demonstrate hepatic venous occlusion.
- *Portal pressure measurement.* This is achieved by means of a catheter passed via the transjugular route into the hepatic vein. The difference between the pressure in the vein with and without an occluding balloon inflated (the hepatic and hepatic wedge pressure) is the portal pressure, a technique akin to pulmonary pressure measurement with a Swan–Ganz catheter[14] (page 34).
- *Magnetic resonance angiography and CT angiography* for the accurate demonstration of the site of portal obstruction.

Treatment

The treatment of uncomplicated portal hypertension involves treatment of the underlying condition, e.g. cirrhosis is managed by a high-calorie, well-balanced diet with added protein in malnourished patients (provided liver damage is not severe), and with avoidance of precipitating factors such as alcohol. If oesophageal varices are visible on endoscopy, they are banded or injected with sclerosant, since the first episode of variceal haemorrhage is associated with a 15–20% mortality.

The management of haemorrhage from gastro-oesophageal varices

Haemorrhage from gastro-oesophageal varices is particularly dangerous, especially in patients with liver damage. In these subjects, the liver is further injured by the hypotension of blood loss, and encephalopathy may be precipitated owing to the absorption of large amounts of nitrogenous breakdown products from the 'meal of blood' within the intestine. Prognosis is better in the small group of patients with normal liver function and portal hypertension due to a prehepatic block, e.g. portal vein thrombosis.

---

[14]Harold James Charles ('Jeremy') Swan (1922–2005), Cardiologist, Cedars of Lebanon Hospital, Los Angles, CA, USA. William Ganz (1919–2009), Professor of Medicine, UCLA, and Senior Research Scientist, Cedars of Lebanon Hospital, Los Angeles, CA, USA.

Prophylaxis against haemorrhage

If varices are detected on screening endoscopy, pharmacological therapy with beta-blockers is instituted to reduce splanchnic blood flow and lower portal venous pressure. Large varices in patients at increased risk of haemorrhage (e.g. severe liver disease) may be treated by endoscopic band ligation (small rubber bands applied to ligate the varices) or injection with sclerosant.

Establishing the diagnosis

An attempt must be made to confirm the diagnosis. The presence of established liver disease, an enlarged spleen and proven varices does not necessarily mean that bleeding is from the varices. Such patients are prone to bleeding from gastric erosions and are commonly affected by peptic ulceration. Fibreoptic endoscopy should always be performed in order to visualize the bleeding point and to exclude non-variceal haemorrhage. Active bleeding may, however, prevent a satisfactory view at endoscopy.

Immediate treatment

The first priority is airway protection, emergency resuscitation and stabilizing the patient prior to emergency endoscopy:

- *Preventing aspiration.* Patients with liver disease have impaired consciousness and may be at risk of aspirating. They should be managed in conjunction with the critical care team.
- *Resuscitation with fluid and blood.* Coagulation abnormalities should be corrected with fresh frozen plasma and/or platelet transfusions.
- *Antimicrobial therapy.* Patients are at risk of bacterial infection and benefit from treatment with broad-spectrum antibiotics (e.g. third-generation cephalosporins) to reduce the risk of rebleeding and improve survival.

Stopping the haemorrhage

The bleeding may be arrested by a number of manoeuvres:

- *Endoscopic variceal band ligation or sclerotherapy.* These procedures can stop bleeding with minimal trauma to the patient, although there is a risk of perforation of the oesophagus, and repeated injections may produce ulceration or fibrosis and stenosis.
- *Intravenous terlipressin,* a vasopressin analogue, is given to reduce portal venous pressure and cause temporary cessation of bleeding by mesenteric arteriolar constriction. Therapeutic doses cause intestinal colic and myocardial ischaemia, which responds to glyceryl trinitrate infusion.
- *Balloon tamponade,* achieved by passing a Sengstaken–Blakemore tube[15] via the mouth into the oesophagus and cardia. The gastric balloon on the end is inflated, following which gentle traction is applied to the tube such that the balloon impacts on the oesophagogastric junction, which stops flow in the varices. Rebleeding after balloon decompression is common, so it is used to buy time pending definitive treatment.
- *Transjugular intrahepatic portosystemic shunt (TIPS):* a metal stent is inserted via the jugular vein and, under radiological control, passed through the liver substance to open up a passage between the hepatic vein and the portal vein. The resultant portosystemic shunt decompresses the portal system. TIPS has reduced the necessity for oesophageal transection or operative portosystemic shunt formation. Unfortunately, shunt procedures (surgical or radiological), in which an anastomosis is made between the portal and systemic circulations, are likely to precipitate encephalopathy.
- *Oesophageal transection,* in which the oesophagus together with the varices are divided at the cardio-oesophageal junction using a circular stapling gun in order to interrupt the communications between the two systems of veins within the wall of the lower oesophagus.
- *Surgical portocaval shunt,* by surgical anastomosis of the portal vein to the inferior vena cava or by splenic vein to the left renal vein used to be commonplace. Such procedures have now been superseded by TIPS and endoscopic control of oesophageal varices. Laparotomy should be avoided when possible if a subsequent transplant is planned, as the resulting vascular adhesions will add greatly to the dangers of the transplant operation.

---

[15]Robert Sengstaken (b. 1923), Neurosurgeon, New York, NY, USA. Arthur H. Blakemore (1897–1970), Surgeon, Columbia Presbyterian Medical Center, New York, NY, USA.

Treatment of ascites

- *Paracentesis* gives immediate relief if discomfort is intense, but it has the disadvantage that the patient loses protein, which should therefore be replaced at the time (10 g albumin per litre of ascites removed).
- *Diet*: low-sodium, high-protein diet; intravenous albumin.
- *Diuretics*: spironolactone often combined with a thiazide or loop diuretic.
- *TIPS*: see above.

Intractable ascites due to hepatic cirrhosis is an indication for liver transplantation, which is performed after failure of medical therapy.

Hepatorenal syndrome

Renal failure is often associated with ascites and liver failure, particularly alcoholic cirrhosis. It is in part a consequence of depletion of the intravascular volume, as may be caused by diuretic therapy or surgery. There is a reduction in intrarenal blood flow brought about by increased glomerular afferent arteriolar tone, but the cause of this is unknown. The glomerular filtration rate falls as the blood flow is diverted away from the renal cortex. Established renal failure in the presence of liver disease is difficult to treat, and is best avoided by maintaining hydration during surgery.

Renal failure may occur in any patient with jaundice, particularly following surgery. It is best prevented by avoiding fluid depletion and maintaining a good diuresis intraoperatively.

Liver neoplasms

Classification

Benign

- Haemangioma.
- Adenoma.
- Focal nodular hyperplasia

Malignant

1 *Primary*:
   a hepatocellular carcinoma (hepatoma);
   b fibrolamellar carcinoma, uncommon variant of hepatoma affecting young adults and children;
   c cholangiocarcinoma.
2 *Secondary* (most common):
   a portal spread (from alimentary tract);
   b systemic blood spread (from lung, breast, testis, melanoma, etc.);
   c direct spread (from gallbladder, stomach and hepatic flexure of colon).

Hepatocellular carcinoma

Hepatocellular carcinoma (HCC) exhibits marked geographical variation in incidence, being uncommon in the West but common in central Africa and south-east Asia. This distribution largely reflects the prevalence of hepatitis B and C virus infection. In the UK, the incidence of HCC is increasing, a reflection of the increasing prevalence of viral hepatitis in particular, and cirrhosis in general.

Eighty per cent of cases of HCC arise in patients with cirrhosis of the liver, and it is most common when cirrhosis is caused by one of the following:

- hepatitis B infection, the commonest cause of HCC worldwide;
- hepatitis C infection, in which the lead-time from infection to HCC may be 25 years or more;
- alcoholic liver disease;
- haemochromatosis, in which the degree of iron overload is related to HCC;
- non-alcoholic fatty liver disease (NAFLD).

Pathology

The pathogenesis of HCC, when associated with cirrhosis, is related to the chronic inflammatory process within the liver. Macroscopically, the tumour either forms a large, solitary mass or there may be multiple foci throughout the liver.

Spread occurs through the liver substance and into the vessels, so that portal vein thrombosis is a common finding. Metastasis outside the liver is late.

Clinical features

The clinical presentation varies depending on the extent of liver disease. In the absence of cirrhosis, the presentation is with massive liver swelling and possibly ascites. In the presence of advanced liver disease, malignant change in the liver may be marked by rapid deterioration and decompensation with encephalopathy, ascites and impaired synthetic function.

Special investigations

- *Serum α-fetoprotein (AFP)* may be significantly raised, but it is neither sensitive nor specific for hepatocellular carcinoma and may rise in other diseases such as hepatitis C.
- *Cross-sectional imaging* with ultrasound, CT or MR will confirm the presence of a large tumour. Small tumours, 1 cm or less in diameter, are difficult to distinguish from regenerative nodules in the presence of cirrhosis.
- *Selective hepatic angiography* may distinguish regenerative nodules from small HCCs, or may reveal multifocal cancer.

Treatment

In the absence of cirrhosis, a primary hepatocellular carcinoma confined to one lobe can be treated by hemihepatectomy. In the presence of cirrhosis, removal of any liver substance is likely to precipitate hepatic decompensation and death. Localized treatments such as radiofrequency ablation or transarterial chemoembolization (TACE) may be used, but in this situation the whole liver is 'at risk' and, even after successful destruction of one lesion, further lesions are likely to develop. The only alternative is replacement of the diseased liver by liver transplantation. Results from this procedure are good providing the tumour load is limited.

Cholangiocarcinoma

This is much less common (20% of primary tumours). It is an adenocarcinoma arising from the bile duct system that usually presents with jaundice and may complicate primary sclerosing cholangitis. Spread occurs directly through the liver substance and regional nodes with a fatal outcome.

Some tumours present early and are amenable to resection, which usually involves an extended liver resection (see below). For the more usual inoperable cases it may be possible to relieve the jaundice at ERCP by passing a plastic or an expanding metal stent upwards along the common bile duct through the growth into the dilated radicles above the obstruction or downwards by percutaneous intubation. This relieves the jaundice, often for many months.

Secondaries

The liver is an extremely common site for secondary deposits, which are often found at autopsy on patients who have died of advanced malignant disease. Necrosis at the centre of metastases leads to the typical umbilication of these tumours.

The clinical effects of secondary deposits in the liver are as follows:

- hepatomegaly: the liver is large, hard and irregular;
- jaundice: a late sign due to liver destruction and intrahepatic duct compression;
- hepatic failure, also a late sign;
- portal vein obstruction: producing oesophageal varices and ascites;
- inferior vena cava obstruction: producing leg oedema.

Treatment of secondary tumours

Resection of secondary tumours is not appropriate in the case of disseminated malignancy. However, it may be considered when deposits can be surgically excised leaving an adequate residual liver volume in the absence of any demonstrable extrahepatic disease. Following resection, the liver will hypertrophy and regain normal functional capacity. This is mostly applicable to secondary deposits from a previous colonic carcinoma. For this reason, such patients should have regular ultrasound scans postoperatively to detect potentially curable metastatic disease early. Following such a policy, 10–20% of patients who develop colorectal liver metastases can undergo resection with a 30–40% 5 year disease-free survival.

Liver surgery

Anatomical considerations

The liver has remarkable regenerative powers and, as such, will tolerate resection of up to two-thirds of its mass. However, anatomically it is not suited to resection, since the inflow structures (portal vein, hepatic artery and bile duct tributaries) cross the hepatic venous outflow. Nevertheless, there are recognized planes of resection that follow from an understanding of the segmental anatomy of the liver (Figure 30.3).

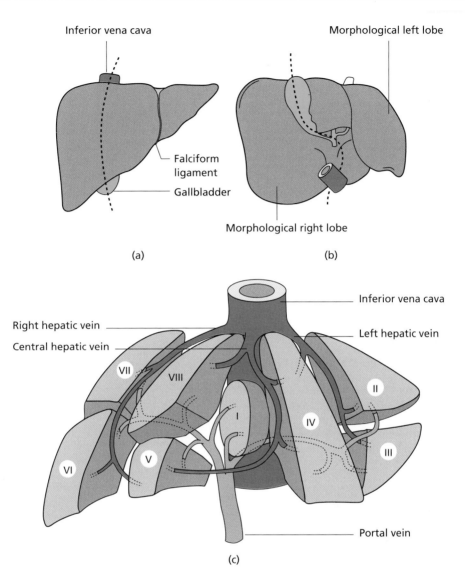

Inferior vena cava

Morphological left lobe

Falciform
ligament

Gallbladder

Morphological right lobe

(a)

(b)

Inferior vena cava

Right hepatic vein

Left hepatic vein

Central hepatic vein

VII

VIII

II

I

IV

V

III

VI

Portal vein

(c)

Figure 30.3 (a–c) Segmental anatomy of the liver showing inflow vessels (hepatic artery, portal vein and bile ducts) to the eight liver segments and the hepatic venous drainage via the three main hepatic veins. (Reproduced from Ellis H, Mahadevan V. (2010) *Clinical Anatomy*, 12th edn. Oxford: Wiley-Blackwell.)

Surgical resections

The following are the common liver resections performed for primary and secondary (usually colonic) tumours of the liver:

- right lobectomy involves removal of segments V to VIII by dividing the liver along a line between the gallbladder fossa and vena cava, and leaving the left lobe;

- left lobectomy involves resection of the left lobe segments II, III and IV; the caudate lobe (segment I) may also be removed;
- trisegmentectomy is a misnomer, but indicates resection of most of the liver but leaving just the left lateral segments (II and III); since this resection removes the most liver, care has to be taken to ensure that sufficient viable liver remains to sustain life.

31

The gallbladder and bile ducts

Learning objective

✓ To know the causes of gallstones, their varying presentations and treatment.

Congenital anomalies

Developmentally, a diverticulum grows out from the ventral wall of the foregut (primitive duodenum), which differentiates into the hepatic ducts and the liver. A lateral bud from this diverticulum becomes the gallbladder and cystic duct (Figure 31.1).

Anomalies are found in 10% of subjects and these are of importance to the surgeon during cholecystectomy.

The principal developmental abnormalities include the following:

- A long cystic duct travelling alongside the common hepatic duct to open near the duodenal orifice. This occurs in 10% of cases.
- Congenital absence (agenesis) of the gallbladder: one in 10 000, often associated with other congenital anomalies.
- Duplication of the gallbladder: one in 5000.
- Congenital obliteration of the ducts (biliary atresia, one of the causes of neonatal jaundice): one in 10 000.
- Absence of the cystic duct, the gallbladder opening directly into the side of the common bile duct.

Lecture Notes: General Surgery, 12th edition. © Harold Ellis, Sir Roy Y. Calne and Christopher J. E. Watson. Published 2011 by Blackwell Publishing Ltd.

- A long mesentery to the gallbladder, which allows acute torsion of the gallbladder to occur with consequent gangrene and rupture.
- Anomalies of the arrangement of the blood vessels supplying the gallbladder are common; for example, the right hepatic artery crosses in front of the common hepatic duct instead of behind it in 25% of subjects.
- Cystic dilatation of the main bile ducts (choledochal cyst): one in 200 000, but more common in people of Asian descent (one in 1000 Japanese).

Cholelithiasis (gallstones)

Gallstones are rare in children (although they should still be considered in the differential diagnosis of abdominal pain in children if the diagnosis is not to be overlooked, and should always be considered in children with spherocytosis or elliptocytosis), the incidence increasing with each decade. In the UK, they are found in approximately 10% of women in their forties, increasing to 30% after the age of 60 years. They are about half as common in men. Stones are particularly common in the Mediterranean races, and the highest incidence is found among the Indians of New Mexico.

The aphorism that gallstones occur in fair, fat, fertile women of 40 is only a distant approxima-

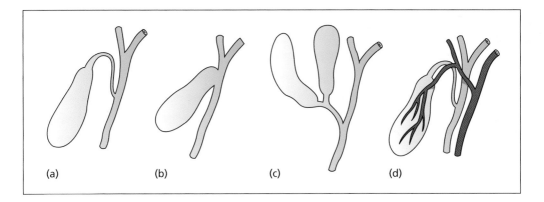

Figure 31.1 Developmental anomalies of the gallbladder. (a) A long cystic duct joining the hepatic duct low down behind the duodenum. (b) Absence of the cystic duct – the gallbladder opens directly into the common hepatic duct. (c) A double gallbladder, the result of a rare bifid embryonic diverticulum from the hepatic duct. (d) The right hepatic artery crosses in front of the common hepatic duct; this occurs in 25% of cases. (Reproduced from Ellis H, Mahadevan V. (2010) *Clinical Anatomy*, 12th edn. Oxford: Wiley-Blackwell.)

tion to the truth; people of either gender, and any age, colour, shape or fecundity may have gallstones, but certainly the incidence is higher in overweight, middle-aged women. To understand gallstones, it is first necessary to understand bile.

Bile composition and function

Bile is a combination of cholesterol, phospholipids (principally lecithin), bile salts (chenodeoxycholic acid and cholic acid) and water. Bile also contains conjugated bilirubin, the breakdown product of haemoglobin, which is quite distinct from bile salts. Cholesterol is not water soluble and is carried in the bile in water-soluble micelles, in which the hydrophobic cholesterol is carried within a 'shell' of phospholipid and bile salts. Once in the gut, bile salts act as a detergent, breaking up and emulsifying fats to facilitate their absorption. The bile salts themselves are resorbed in the distal small bowel, pass back via the portal venous system to the liver, from where they are once again secreted in the bile. This circulation of bile salts is termed the *enterohepatic circulation*, permitting a relatively small pool of bile salts to circulate up to 10 times a day. Diversion or absence of bile from the gut, as may occur in obstructive jaundice, results in a malabsorption of fat and the fat-soluble vitamins (A, D, E and K).

Gallstone types

There are three common varieties of stone (Figure 31.2).

1 *Cholesterol* (20%): these occur either as a solitary, oval stone (the cholesterol solitaire) or as two stones, one indenting the other, or as multiple mulberry stones associated with a strawberry gallbladder (see below). A cut section shows crystals radiating from the centre of the stone; the surface is yellow and greasy to the touch.
2 *Bile pigment* (5%): small, black, irregular, multiple, gritty and fragile.
3 *Mixed* (75%): multiple, faceted one against the other, and can often be grouped into two or more series, each of the same size, suggesting 'generations' of stones. The cut surface is laminated with alternate dark and light zones of pigment and cholesterol respectively.

This traditional classification into three groups is an oversimplification; calculi with widely different appearances simply represent different combinations of the same ingredients.

Cholesterol stones

These may be associated with elevated blood cholesterol, but there is little evidence to suggest this as a cause. There is a definite correlation between

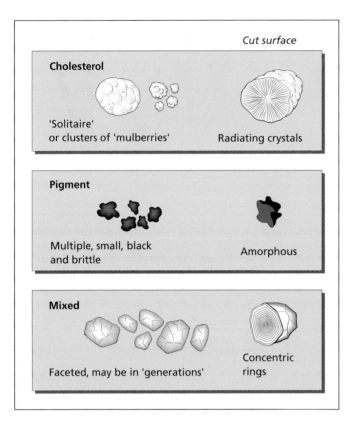

Figure 31.2 The varieties of gallstones.

cholesterol stones and the contraceptive pill and pregnancy, as well as an increase with age. Family history, obesity and low dietary fibre are also risk factors. The supersaturated bile from such patients is termed 'lithogenic' (stone-forming) bile. Bile may also become supersaturated with cholesterol owing to a deficiency of bile salts, which may occur as a result of interruption of the enterohepatic circulation after removal of the terminal ileum, which, for example, may occur following resection in the treatment of Crohn's disease.

Cholesterol stones form in the gallbladder when supersaturated bile is further concentrated. It may be that an excess of mucus production by the gallbladder wall is an important factor in forming calculi. In other cases, clumps of bacteria or desquamated mucosa, perhaps resulting from an episode of infection, may form the nucleus on which crystals may deposit. One rather picturesque view of the aetiology of gallstones states that every gallstone is the tombstone of a dead bacterium. When cholesterol precipitates on the gallbladder wall (cholesterosis), it forms yellow submucous aggregations of cholesterol with an appearance similar to a strawberry skin ('*strawberry gallbladder*').

Pigment stones

Pigment stones are composed of calcium bilirubinate, with some calcium carbonate. They occur in the haemolytic anaemias, e.g. spherocytosis and sickle-cell disease, in which excess of circulating bile pigment is deposited in the biliary tract. If such stones are found in the gallbladder of children or adolescents, haemolytic anaemia should be suspected, particularly if there is a family history of calculus.

Mixed stones

It is now considered that the majority of mixed stones have the same metabolic origin as cholesterol stones, i.e. some slight alteration in the composition of bile enabling precipitation of cholesterol together with bile pigment.

The pathological effects of gallstones

- *Silent*: gallstones lying free in the lumen of the gallbladder produce no pathological disturbance of the wall and the patient is symptom free.
- *Impaction in gallbladder*, either in Hartmann's pouch[1] or in the cystic duct. Water is absorbed from the contained bile, which becomes concentrated and produces a chemical cholecystitis. This is usually at first sterile, but may then become secondarily infected. If a stone impacts in Hartmann's pouch when the gallbladder is empty, the wall of the gallbladder may continue to secrete mucus and the gallbladder distends to form a mucocele.
- *Choledocholithiasis*: gallstones may migrate into the common bile duct. These may be silent, or produce an intermittent or complete obstruction of the common bile duct with pain and jaundice.
- *Gallstone ileus*: this is uncommon, and occurs when a large gallstone ulcerates through the wall of the gallbladder into the adjacent duodenum. The gallstone may pass per rectum or produce a gallstone ileus – this is impaction of the stone in the narrowest part of the small bowel (the distal ileum) with resulting intestinal obstruction. (Note that gallstone ileus is thus a misnomer and is in fact mechanical obstruction by an intraluminal stone, and not a paralytic ileus.) A key feature in such cases is the presence of air in the biliary tree that has entered the bile ducts via the fistula created when the gallstone ulcerates through into the gut and which can be readily seen on a plain abdominal radiograph provided the clinician looks closely in the appropriate area.

In addition, the presence of gallstones in the biliary tree is associated with the following:

- *acute and chronic pancreatitis*;
- *carcinoma of the gallbladder*.

Clinical features

The following syndromes can be recognized:

- biliary colic;
- acute cholecystitis;
- chronic cholecystitis;
- obstruction and/or infection of the common bile duct.

Two or more of these syndromes may occur in the same patient.

Biliary colic

The gallbladder contracts following stimulation by the hormone cholecystokinin, which is produced from the duodenum and small intestine in response to fat in the lumen of the bowel. Physiologically this delivers bile salts to aid the absorption of dietary fat, and the hormone also stimulates secretion of enzymes from the pancreas to aid digestion.

Biliary colic occurs when the gallbladder contracts against an obstruction, such as a stone impacted in either Hartmann's pouch or the cystic duct, producing severe pain, which usually comes on 2–3 hours after eating and often wakes the patient. It is a continuous pain, usually rising to a plateau, and may last for many hours. The pain is usually situated in the right subcostal region but may be epigastric, or it may spread as a band across the upper abdomen and be accompanied by vomiting and sweating. Radiation of the pain to the inferior angle of the right scapula is common. Characteristically, the patient tends to lie still. In contrast to acute cholecystitis the patient is usually not systemically unwell.

A variant of biliary colic occurs when a stone impacts in the sphincter of Oddi, in which case the patient is mildly jaundiced, the pain is colicky, and the patient is restless and rolls about in agony. Relief may be sudden as the stone passes into the duodenum.

Differential diagnosis is from the other acute colics, especially ureteric colic (Box 31.1).

Acute cholecystitis

If the stone remains impacted in the gallbladder outlet, the gallbladder wall becomes inflamed owing to the irritation of the concentrated bile contained within it producing a chemical cholecystitis. The gallbladder fills with pus, which is frequently sterile on culture. In these instances, the pain persists and progressively intensifies. There is a fever in the range of 38–39°C with marked toxaemia and leucocytosis. The upper

---

[1]Henri Hartmann (1860–1952), Professor of Surgery, Hôtel Dieu, Paris, France.

Box 31.1 Abdominal colic

Colicky pain is the result of smooth muscle contraction against a resistance. The common causes of colic occur in the uterus and tubes, renal tract, intestinal tract and biliary tract.

Biliary tract

- Stone in Hartmann's pouch
- Stone in cystic duct
- Stone in sphincter of Oddi

Renal tract

- Ureteric colic due to stone, blood clot or tumour
- Bladder colic in acute retention owing to enlarged prostate

Intestinal tract

- Mechanical obstruction
- Appendicular colic as appendix lumen occludes

Uterus and fallopian tubes

- Parturition
- Menstruation
- Ectopic pregnancy in a fallopian tube

abdomen is extremely tender, and often a palpable mass develops in the region of the gallbladder. This represents the distended, inflamed gallbladder wrapped in inflammatory adhesions to adjacent organs, especially the omentum. Occasionally, an empyema of the gallbladder develops or, rarely, gallbladder perforation into the general peritoneal cavity takes place. The swollen gallbladder may press against the adjacent common bile duct and produce a tinge of jaundice, even though stones may be absent from the duct system.

Ninety-five per cent of cases of acute cholecystitis are associated with gallstones. Occasionally, fulminating acalculous cholecystitis may occur and this may be associated with typhoid fever or gas gangrene.

The *differential diagnosis* is from acute appendicitis, perforated duodenal ulcer, acute pancreatitis, right-sided basal pneumonia and coronary thrombosis.

Chronic cholecystitis

This is almost invariably associated with the presence of gallstones. Repeated episodes of inflam-

mation result in chronic fibrosis and thickening of the entire gallbladder wall, which may contain thick, sometimes infected, bile.

There are recurrent bouts of abdominal pain owing to mild cholecystitis, which may or may not be accompanied by fever. Discomfort is experienced after fatty meals as the gallbladder contracts onto the stones; there is often flatulence. The picture may be complicated by episodes of acute cholecystitis or symptoms produced by stones passing into the common bile duct.

The *differential diagnosis* is from other causes of chronic dyspepsia, including peptic ulceration and hiatus hernia. Occasionally, the symptoms closely mimic coronary insufficiency. It is as well to remain clinically suspicious – any or all of these common diseases may well occur in association with gallstones.

Stones in the common bile duct (choledocholithiasis)

This may be symptomless. More often, there are attacks of biliary colic accompanied by obstructive jaundice with clay-coloured stools and dark urine, the attacks lasting for hours or several days. The attack ceases either when a small stone is passed through the sphincter of Oddi or when it disimpacts and falls back into the dilated common duct. Above the impacted stone, other stones or biliary sludge may deposit. Occasionally, the jaundice is progressive and, rarely, it is painless.

If the obstruction is not relieved either spontaneously or by operation, the chronic back-pressure in the biliary system may result in secondary biliary cirrhosis and liver failure.

The *differential diagnosis* of stones in the common bile duct is as follows:

1 With jaundice (75% of cases):
   a carcinoma of the pancreas or other malignant obstructions of the common bile duct;
   b acute hepatitis;
   c other causes of jaundice (Chapter 30, p. 252).
2 Without jaundice (25% of cases):
   a renal colic;
   b intestinal obstruction;
   c angina pectoris.

Ascending cholangitis

Infection of the common bile duct, which occurs in the presence of an obstruction to the normal biliary drainage, usually as a complication of

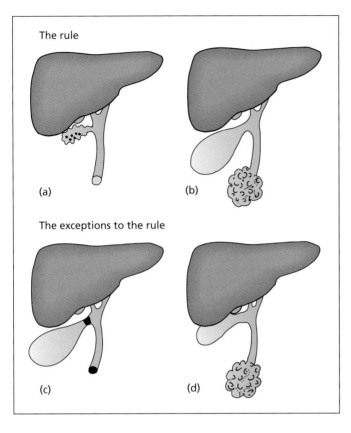

The rule

(a)   (b)

The exceptions to the rule

(c)   (d)

Figure 31.3 Obstructive jaundice due to stone is usually associated with a small, contracted gallbladder (a). Therefore, in the presence of jaundice, a palpable gallbladder indicates that the obstruction is probably due to some other cause – the most common being carcinoma of the pancreas (b). Exceptions are a palpable gallbladder produced by one stone impacted in Hartmann's pouch resulting in a mucocele, another in the common duct causing obstruction (c), which is very rare, or, more commonly, the gallbladder is indeed distended but is clinically impalpable (d).

stones in the duct. Jaundice and pain are accompanied by rigors, a high intermittent fever and severe toxaemia (the intermittent hepatic fever of Charcot[2]). In these instances, the duct system is severely inflamed and filled with pus, and the liver may be dotted with multiple small abscesses. Treatment is with appropriate antibiotics and urgent biliary drainage (e.g. endoscopic sphincterotomy).

Courvoisier's law[3] (Figure 31.3)

'If in the presence of jaundice the gallbladder is palpable, then the jaundice is unlikely to be due to stone.' This is an extremely useful rule provided it is quoted correctly. The principle on which it is based is that, if the obstruction is due to stone, the gallbladder is usually thickened and fibrotic and therefore does not distend. Moreover, unlike obstruction due to malignant disease, calculus

obstruction is not usually complete. This allows some escape of bile into the duodenum, with decompression of the gallbladder. Obstruction of the common bile duct due to other causes (e.g. carcinoma of the head of the pancreas) is usually associated with a normal gallbladder, which can dilate. However, in carcinoma of the bile ducts arising above the origin of the cystic duct, the gallbladder, distal to the obstruction, will be collapsed and empty.

Note that the law is not phrased the other way round – 'If the gallbladder is *not* palpable, the jaundice is due to stone' – as 50% of dilated gallbladders cannot be palpated on clinical examination, owing to either the patient's obesity or overlap by the liver, which itself is usually enlarged as a result of bile engorgement.

Only rarely is the gallbladder dilated when jaundice is due to stone. These circumstances occur when a stone impacts in Hartmann's pouch to produce a mucocele while at the same time jaundice is produced by a second stone in the common duct, or when a stone forms *in situ* in the common

[2]Jean Charcot (1825–1893), Neurologist, Paris, France.
[3]Ludwig Courvoisier (1843–1918), Professor of Surgery, Basle, Switzerland.

bile duct, the gallbladder itself being normal and therefore distensible.

Special investigations

- *Ultrasound*: this non-invasive technique gives three pieces of information:
  - the presence of gallstones within the gallbladder, revealed as intensely echogenic foci, which cast a clear acoustic shadow beyond them;
  - the thickened wall of the gallbladder in acute or chronic inflammation;
  - the diameter of the common bile duct which, if over 7 mm, is suggestive of the presence of stones within.

  Unfortunately, ultrasound, like computed tomography (CT), is unreliable in detecting stones in the bile ducts, especially at the lower end where they are obscured by the overlying duodenal gas.
- *Plain abdominal X-ray* reveals radio-opaque gallstones in only 10% of cases. These usually appear as rings due to calcium deposited on a central translucent organic core. Occasionally, the gallbladder may be seen to be calcified ('porcelain gallbladder').
- *Upper gastrointestinal endoscopy* may be advisable to exclude an associated peptic ulcer or hiatus hernia when there is any degree of uncertainty in the clinical picture, even though gallstones have been noted on ultrasound.
- *Liver function tests* are performed whenever jaundice, present or past, is a feature. Persistently raised alkaline phosphatase is suspicious of choledocholithiasis. Prothrombin time should also be checked in the presence of jaundice lest any invasive procedure be required.
- *Magnetic resonance cholangiopancreatography (MRCP)* permits visualization of the biliary tree and contained calculi can be detected. This non-invasive procedure provides the same diagnostic information as can be obtained with ERCP but without the small but important risk of complications (perforation, bleeding, pancreatitis) associated with ERCP.
- *Endoscopic retrograde cholangiopancreatography (ERCP)*: endoscopic intubation of the bile ducts through the ampulla of Vater is more invasive than MRCP, but in addition to visualizing the ducts and contained stones it also permits their extraction, often after first carrying out a diathermy sphincterotomy opening up the sphincter of Oddi[4] to facilitate instrumentation of the bile duct. ERCP has been largely replaced by MRCP for diagnosis but remains an essential part of hepatobiliary management in offering endoscopic therapeutic options and removing the reliance on open surgical procedures.

Treatment

Acute cholecystitis

At least 90% resolve on bed rest with antibiotics and pain relief. Elective cholecystectomy is commonly performed about 6 weeks later because of the undoubted danger of further attacks although early urgent cholecystectomy during the first 72 hours of admission offers an excellent alternative to the patient, optimizing recovery and minimizing the disruption to their normal lifestyle. Cholecystectomy is routinely performed laparoscopically, with the advantages of minimal scarring of the abdominal wall and rapid convalescence compared with an open procedure. Nevertheless, operative difficulties, anatomical aberrations and equipment failures may necessitate conversion to an open operation in approximately 2–5% of cases.

An *empyema of the gallbladder* usually requires more active intervention, with emergency drainage (cholecystostomy), either percutaneously under ultrasound guidance or at cholecystectomy.

Perforation of the acutely inflamed gallbladder is rare and requires urgent surgery. This complication carries a high mortality.

If diagnosis is in doubt in the early stages of acute cholecystitis, laparoscopy is performed. Cholecystectomy is comparatively easy in the first 24–48 hours of the illness; dissection is facilitated by the oedema of adjacent tissues, although after this time operation becomes difficult because of the inflammatory adhesions. Many surgeons advise early surgical intervention in acute cholecystitis with early resolution of the presenting illness and its underlying cause.

---

[4]Ruggero Oddi (1864–1913), Surgeon, Genoa, Italy. The sphincter was first described in 1654 by Francis Glisson (1597–1677), Regius Professor of Physic, Cambridge, UK.

Chronic cholecystitis

Cholecystectomy is performed, usually laparoscopically. The cystic duct is intubated and an operative cholangiogram performed by injecting radio-opaque contrast medium into the common duct. If stones are demonstrated at laparoscopic operation an MRCP is performed following recovery; many will have passed spontaneously. If they are still present they are removed at ERCP. If an open cholecystectomy has been performed, the common bile duct is explored, the stones removed and the bile duct drained using a latex T-tube inserted into the common duct. The T-tube is removed 10 days postoperatively, provided a check cholangiogram taken through the tube confirms that the ducts are clear and that there is free flow of contrast into the duodenum. Alternatively, at laparoscopic cholecystectomy, the surgeon may perform a laparoscopic exploration of the bile ducts, but this is uncommon and most small stones seem to pass spontaneously following cholecystectomy.

Obstructive jaundice due to stones

Impacted stones are removed using a balloon or Dormia[5] basket at ERCP. Subsequent cholecystectomy is performed as soon as possible lest new stones pass into the ducts. The presence of high fever makes removal of the impacted stones and drainage of the obstructed common bile duct imperative as an emergency procedure. Any intervention is preceded by giving intravenous vitamin K, since a lack of bile salts in the gut reduces absorption of this fat-soluble vitamin; hence, serum prothrombin is lowered with consequent bleeding tendency.

Non-surgical treatment of gallstones

- *Gallstone dissolution.* Because cholesterol is held in solution by bile salts, dissolution of small cholesterol stones is possible by administering bile salts orally in the form of chenodeoxycholic or ursodeoxycholic acid. This therapy may be used for small, non-calcified stones in a functioning gallbladder. Treatment must be continued for many months and may be interrupted by attacks of biliary colic as small fragments of calculus pass through the bile ducts. Moreover, recurrences commonly occur after therapy is discontinued since an abnormal gallbladder remains. The indications for this treatment are limited and may be appropriate in less than 10% of cases. It is largely reserved as an option in elderly medically unfit patients in whom there is a strong contraindication to laparoscopic cholecystectomy.
- *Lithotripsy.* Ultrasonic destruction of small stones as used in the renal tract appeared to be an attractive option, but there is the problem of the passage of small fragments of stone through the duct system that may cause biliary colic, biliary obstruction and pancreatitis. Additionally, the residual fragments in the gallbladder appeared to provide a nidus for further stone formation. Lithotripsy has thus been abandoned in routine practice.

The symptomless gallstone

The incidental diagnosis of gallstones is becoming increasingly common during routine ultrasound examination of the abdomen for a variety of non-biliary reasons. Cholecystectomy may be recommended when the patient is at significantly increased risk of complications owing to concomitant comorbidities such as diabetes or chronic renal failure, but will not normally prompt surgical intervention unless they become symptomatic; the risks (albeit low) of elective cholecystectomy need to be balanced against the long-term risks of complications of cholelithiasis (acute cholecystitis, obstructive jaundice, pancreatitis and gallbladder cancer). In younger patients, in whom the likelihood of complications over time is high and the risks of surgery low, cholecystectomy is advised; in older patients with asymptomatic stones and a shorter life expectancy, it is often unwise to intervene.

Complications of cholecystectomy

There are two special dangers after cholecystectomy, whether performed by laparotomy or laparoscopy.

1 *Leakage of bile.* This may result from the following:
  a injury to bile canaliculi in the gallbladder bed of the liver;

[5]Enrico Dormia (1928-2009), Professor of Urology, Milan, Italy.

b injury to the common hepatic or common bile duct;

c slipping of the ligature or clip from the cystic duct;

d leakage from the common bile duct after exploration.

ERCP may identify the site of the leak, and temporary stenting[6] will ensure adequate biliary drainage, thus allowing the bile fistula to close spontaneously; if this does not occur, further exploration may be required. A percutaneous drain is usually placed to prevent generalized biliary peritonitis.

2 *Jaundice.* This may be due to the following:

a missed stones in the common bile duct;

b inadvertent injury to the common bile duct;

c cholangitis or associated pancreatitis.

Residual stones in the common duct can usually be removed by ERCP; if a T tube is still present in the common duct they can be removed by means of a Burhenne basket[7] passed along the track formed by the tube under X-ray control.

Gallbladder polyps

Pathology

Gallbladder polyps may be single or multiple and are increasingly being detected by ultrasound examination. They appear as lesions within the gallbladder which do not cast an acoustic shadow (as stones do) and which do not move when the patient rolls onto one side, indicating that they are attached to the gallbladder wall. When multiple, they represent the ultrasonographic appearance of cholesterosis of the gallbladder wall and are of no other significance. When a single polyp is present, it may represent a premalignant lesion, the risk of malignancy rising with increasing size of polyp, becoming significant when the size reaches 1 cm and probable when the size reaches 1.5 cm.

Clinical features

Gallbladder polyps may be entirely asymptomatic and simply represent an incidental finding on an ultrasound examination performed for reasons other than biliary symptoms; if they are situated distally in the gallbladder close to Hartmann's pouch they may produce symptoms identical to those of gallstones.

Treatment

Polyps causing symptoms similar to those of cholelithiasis are appropriately managed by cholecystectomy. If there are three or fewer polyps detected in an otherwise asymptomatic patient, then the possible malignant potential is the key management issue. In these cases, 6 monthly surveillance using ultrasound is recommended with cholecystectomy being indicated if the polyps are increasing in size and particularly when they reach or exceed 1 cm in diameter. The management of multiple polyps is more controversial and, since they usually represent cholesterosis, it can be argued that intensive follow-up is therefore unnecessary. When the gallbladder is removed it is common to find that the polyps were in fact small gallstones adherent to the gallbladder wall.

Carcinoma of the gallbladder

Pathology

This is a relatively uncommon tumour, but it is associated in about 85% of cases with the presence of gallstones. It is debatable whether this is due to chronic irritation or to the carcinogenic effect of cholic acid derivatives. Fifty per cent of 'porcelain' gallbladders are associated with carcinoma. As gallstones are commoner in women, carcinoma of the gallbladder is, not surprisingly, four times commoner in women than men. Ninety per cent are adenocarcinoma and 10% squamous carcinoma.

There is local invasion of the liver and its ducts and lymphatic spread to the nodes in the porta hepatis; portal vein dissemination to the liver may occur.

Clinical features

Carcinoma of the gallbladder usually presents with a picture closely resembling chronic cholecystitis, with right upper quadrant pain, nausea

---

[6]Charles Stent (1845–1901), English Dentist.
[7]H. Joachim Burhenne (1925–1996), Radiologist, Vancouver, Canada.

and vomiting, in addition to weight loss and, later, progressing to obstructive jaundice. At this stage, a palpable mass may be present in the gallbladder region.

Treatment

Occasionally, cholecystectomy performed for stones reveals the presence of an unexpected tumour. Under these circumstances, long-term survival may follow. Sadly, most cases present late with liver involvement and nodal spread leaving few surgical options. If direct infiltration into the liver has already occurred, as is common, local excision or radical liver resection is only rarely possible and the prognosis is therefore usually poor, with death within months.

Cholangiocarcinoma

Pathology

The incidence of carcinoma of the bile ducts, cholangiocarcinoma, is increasing. The disease commonly occurs after 50 years of age and is more common in men. It is associated with inflammatory bowel disease, particularly in the presence of sclerosing cholangitis. Congenital hepatic fibrosis, choledochal cysts and polycystic liver are all associations.

Macroscopically, cholangiocarcinomas may occur within the liver substance, or in the larger extrahepatic bile ducts. The confluence of the left and right hepatic ducts, or the common hepatic duct with the cystic duct, are common sites.

Microscopically, they are mucin-secreting adenocarcinomas.

Clinical features

The usual presentation is with painless progressive jaundice, with dark urine and pale stools. Epigastric pain, steatorrhoea and weight loss are common. There may be hepatomegaly, usually without a palpable gallbladder because the tumour is proximal to, or at, the cystic duct confluence. Confirmation is by MRCP, ERCP or percutaneous transhepatic cholangiography and brush cytology (poor sensitivity), and CT-guided needle biopsy if possible.

Treatment

The tumours are slow growing, and palliation is often achieved by endoluminal stenting at ERCP, or surgical bypass. The prognosis is poor, and curative resection is seldom possible, although, in a small percentage of cases with early presentation of hilar tumours (Klatskin tumour[8]), good results have been reported with extended right hepatectomy together with excision of the adjacent portal vein and venous reconstruction. In the rarer cases in which the tumour is located distally in the common bile duct, a Whipple's resection (see Figure 32.2) may be possible.

[8]Gerald Klatskin (1910–1986), Liver Physician, Yale, New Haven, CT, USA; pioneered the liver biopsy and was considered to be one of the fathers of hepatology.

32

The pancreas

Learning objectives
- ✓ To know the causes and management of acute pancreatitis, and the factors that predict its severity.
- ✓ To have knowledge of pancreatic cancer, its presentation and the surgical approach to treatment of carcinoma of the head of the pancreas.

Congenital anomalies

The pancreas develops as a dorsal and a ventral bud from the duodenum (Figure 32.1). The ventral bud rotates posteriorly, thus enclosing the superior mesenteric vessels; it forms the major part of the head of the pancreas and its duct becomes the main duct of Wirsung,[1] which in the great majority of cases has a shared opening with the common bile duct in the ampulla of Vater.[2] The larger dorsal bud becomes the body and tail and its duct becomes the accessory duct of Santorini.[3]

Annular pancreas

The two developmental buds may envelop the second part of the duodenum, producing this rare form of extrinsic duodenal obstruction.

Heterotopic pancreas

This is produced occasionally by an accessory budding from the primitive foregut. A nodule of

[1]Johann Georg Wirsung (1589–1643), Professor of Anatomy, University of Padua, Italy, where he was murdered.
[2]Abraham Vater (1684–1751), Professor of Anatomy, Wittenberg, Germany.
[3]Giovanni Domenico Santorini (1681–1737), Professor of Anatomy and Medicine, Venice, Italy.

Lecture Notes: General Surgery, 12th edition. © Harold Ellis, Sir Roy Y. Calne and Christopher J. E. Watson. Published 2011 by Blackwell Publishing Ltd.

pancreatic tissue may be found in the stomach, duodenum or jejunum. This may produce obstructive or dyspeptic symptoms.

Acute pancreatitis

Acute inflammation of the pancreas is a common cause of acute abdominal pain, with significant morbidity and mortality.

Aetiology

Most cases of acute pancreatitis are associated with either gallstones or alcohol, although a number of less common causes have been identified.

- *Gallstones* are present in half of the cases in the UK, and, indeed, small gallstones can be recovered from the faeces of many patients with acute pancreatitis.
- *Alcohol*: the majority of cases of non-gallstone pancreatitis are alcohol related. This is particularly common in France and North America. Alcohol is also the most common cause of recurrent pancreatitis. The mechanism is unclear, and it may follow either chronic alcohol abuse or binge drinking.

Other less common causes of pancreatitis include the following:

- *Postoperative*: particularly after cardiopulmonary bypass or damage to the

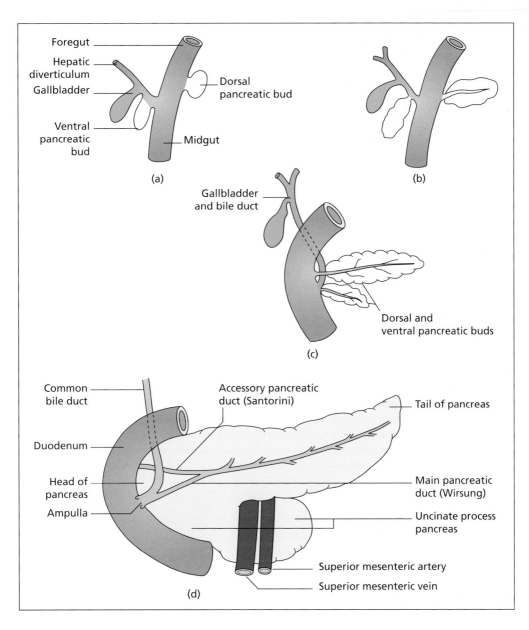

Figure 32.1 (a–d) The development of the pancreas and biliary tree. (Reproduced from Ellis H, Mahadevan V. (2010) *Clinical Anatomy*, 12th edn. Oxford: Wiley-Blackwell.)

pancreas during mobilization of the duodenum at partial gastrectomy or splenectomy.

- *After endoscopic retrograde cholangiopancreatography (ERCP)*: particularly if pancreatography was performed or there was difficulty cannulating the papilla with subsequent oedema and obstruction.

- *Carcinoma of the pancreas.*
- *Infection*, e.g. mumps, cytomegalovirus or coxsackie infection.
- *Trauma*: particularly blunt trauma or crush injury.
- *Drugs*, e.g. corticosteroids, sodium valproate.
- *Hypothermia.*
- *Hypercalcaemia.*

- *Hyperlipidaemia.*
- *Vascular*: pancreatitis may occur in malignant hypertension, cholesterol emboli and polyarteritis nodosa, probably as a result of local infarction causing enzyme liberation.

Pathology

Acute pancreatitis differs from other inflammatory conditions because of the autodigestion that may result from liberation of digestive enzymes. The pancreas is normally protected from autodigestion by storing its enzymes in intracellular zymogen granules before secreting them as proenzymes. Trypsin, for example, is secreted as trypsinogen and converted to trypsin by the action of enterokinase in the gut. Trypsin itself then cleaves other proenzymes, thus activating them. One such enzyme is phospholipase A which, in pancreatitis, is involved in cell wall damage and fat necrosis along with pancreatic lipase.

The mechanisms initiating autodigestion are multiple. Duodenopancreatic reflux is an important factor that may occur as a result of injury to the papilla following endoscopic cannulation, trauma or surgery in this region, or as a result of damage to the sphincter owing to the recent passage of a stone (hence the strong association of pancreatitis and biliary calculi). Duodenal fluid containing enterokinase then refluxes into the duct, activating the pancreatic proenzymes. Duodenal reflux can be shown experimentally to produce pancreatitis, and may be a common factor that underlies many of the aetiological associations mentioned above. As inflammation proceeds, local infarction may occur as arterioles thrombose, and more proenzymes leak out of the necrotic cells to be activated. Once started, pancreatitis can be rapidly progressive, with widespread autodigestion not only confined to the pancreas.

As inflammation and autodigestion progress, liquefying necrotic material and inflammatory exudate collect in the lesser sac. This fluid, walled off by the stomach in front and necrotic pancreas behind, is the pancreas pseudocyst, and commonly appears from day 10 onwards.

Macroscopic pathology

At operation, the appearances are quite typical. There is a blood-stained peritoneal effusion. White spots of fat necrosis are scattered throughout the peritoneal cavity; these are produced by lipase released from the pancreas, which liberates fatty acids and glycerol from fat; these acids combine with calcium to produce insoluble calcium soaps. The pancreas is swollen, haemorrhagic or, in severe cases, actually necrotic. Occasionally, suppurative pancreatitis may occur.

Clinical features

The condition can present at any age but is uncommon in childhood and in young adults. The patient presenting with gallstone pancreatitis is commonly middle aged or elderly. By contrast, the alcohol-related form commonly first presents in patients who are younger than 40. Pain is of rapid onset, is severe, constant, usually epigastric and often radiates into the back. The patient typically sits forward, and repeated retching is common. Vomiting is early and profuse. The patient may be shocked with a rapid pulse, cyanosis (indicating circulatory collapse) and a temperature that may be either subnormal or raised up to 39.5°C (103°F). The abdomen reveals generalized tenderness and guarding. About 30% of patients are jaundiced owing to oedema of the pancreatic head obstructing the common bile duct.

On rare occasions, a few days after a severe attack, the patient may develop a bluish discoloration in the loins from extravasation of blood-stained pancreatic juice into the retroperitoneal tissues (Grey Turner's sign[4]). The tracking of fluid that results in this sign can often be seen on computed tomography (CT) imaging of patients with acute pancreatitis even when it is not clinically apparent.

Differential diagnosis

The less severe episode of acute pancreatitis simulates acute cholecystitis; the more severe attack, with a marked degree of shock, is usually mistaken for a perforated peptic ulcer or coronary thrombosis. Differentiation must also be made from high intestinal obstruction and from other causes of peritonitis.

Special investigations

The investigation comprises tests to confirm the diagnosis and tests to assess the severity of the disease (i.e. diagnostic and prognostic).

---

[4]George Grey Turner (1877–1951), Professor of Surgery, University of Durham, then Foundation Professor of Surgery at the Royal Postgraduate Medical School, London, UK.

- *Serum amylase.* Amylase is liberated into the circulation by the damaged pancreas, and exceeds the kidney's ability to excrete it, so the serum concentration rises. It is usually significantly raised (fivefold or more) in the acute phase, but returns to normal within 2–3 days; the urinary amylase is elevated for a longer period and may be useful in the diagnosis of cases presenting late. Occasionally, an overwhelming attack of pancreatitis with extensive destruction of the gland, or an attack occurring as an acute exacerbation of chronic pancreatitis, is associated with a normal serum amylase. Other causes of raised serum amylase need to be borne in mind before assuming a diagnosis of pancreatitis (Box 32.1).
- *Full blood count*: there is a moderate leucocytosis, and anaemia in severe cases.
- *Blood glucose* is often raised, with glycosuria in 15% of cases.
- *Serum bilirubin* is often raised.
- *Arterial blood gases*: hypoxia occurs in severe cases.
- *Serum calcium* may be lowered, partly as a result of fat saponification; tetany may occur. The prognosis is bad in such cases.
- *CT* may confirm pancreatitis if the amylase is normal or the diagnosis otherwise unclear. At a later stage, necrotic pancreas, abscess or pseudocyst may be visualized.
- *Electrocardiography (ECG)* may show diminished T waves, or arrhythmia, and can cause confusion with cardiac ischaemia.
- *Abdominal X-rays* often give no direct help. The absence of free gas or of localized fluid levels assists in the differential diagnosis of perforated duodenal ulcer or high intestinal obstruction. In some cases, a solitary dilated loop of proximal jejunum may be seen (the 'sentinel loop sign'). Radio-opaque pancreatic calculi may be present in cases of chronic pancreatitis.
- *Ultrasound* will demonstrate associated gallstones and dilatation of the common bile duct suggestive of choledocholithiasis. It may also show enlargement of the pancreas, although overlying bowel gas often prevents a good view of the pancreas.

Note that each of the three enzymes liberated by the pancreas plays a part in the overall picture of acute pancreatitis:

Box 32.1 Raised serum amylase

The causes of raised serum amylase are listed below. Only those marked with an asterisk cause a marked increase in amylase (fivefold or more).

Impaired renal excretion

- Renal failure*
- Macroamylasaemia (amylase not cleared by kidneys owing to complexing or protein binding)

Salivary gland disease

- Salivary calculi
- Parotitis

Metabolic causes

- Severe diabetic ketoacidosis*
- Acute alcoholic intoxication
- Morphine administration (causing sphincter of Oddi spasm[5])

Abdominal causes

- Acute pancreatitis*
- Perforated peptic ulcer
- Acute cholecystitis
- Intestinal obstruction
- Afferent loop obstruction following partial gastrectomy
- Ruptured abdominal aortic aneurysm
- Ruptured ectopic pregnancy
- Mesenteric infarction
- Trauma, open or blunt

---

1 *Trypsin* produces the autodigestion of the pancreas.
2 *Lipase* results in the typical fat necrosis.
3 *Amylase* absorbed from the peritoneal cavity produces a rise in the serum level and is thus a helpful test in diagnosis.

Management

The management of a patient with suspected pancreatitis involves first confirming the diagnosis (serum amylase and/or CT) and determining the

---

[5]Ruggero Oddi (1864–1913). Identified the sphincter while a medical student in Perugia, Italy.

severity of the attack. Mortality in severe pancreatitis is high, so severe cases should be managed in an intensive care environment where pulmonary, renal and abdominal complications can be promptly diagnosed and treated.

Severe acute pancreatitis

Severe pancreatitis is associated with haemorrhagic necrosis of the pancreas and systemic release of many vasoactive peptides and enzymes, as well as sequestration of large volumes of fluid within the abdomen. Acute lung failure occurs, characterized by increased capillary permeability and reduced oxygen transfer, and the combination of toxins and loss of circulating fluid results in acute renal failure. Several criteria predictive of the development of severe pancreatitis have been identified (Box 32.2); the presence of three or more is predictive of severe pancreatitis. Both a raised C-reactive protein (>140 mg/L) and non-perfusion of areas of the pancreas on a contrast-enhanced CT also predict a poor prognosis. Identification of such high-risk cases enables aggressive intensive management to be instituted at an early stage. Nevertheless, severe acute pancreatitis has a mortality of over 25%.

Box 32.2 Glasgow criteria for severe acute pancreatitis

The factors are assessed over the first 48 hours. Presence of three or more factors indicates severe pancreatitis with a high mortality.

- Age over 55 years
- Hyperglycaemia (glucose >10 mmol/L in the absence of a history of diabetes)
- Leucocytosis (>15 × 10^9/L)
- Urea >16 mmol/L (no response to intravenous fluids)
- PO_2 <8 kPa (60 mmHg)
- Calcium <2.0 mmol/L
- Albumin <32 g/L
- Lactate dehydrogenase >600 IU/L
- Raised liver transaminases (aspartate transaminase >100 IU/L)

Supportive treatment

In the established case, treatment is initially non-operative and consists of the following:

- *Analgesia*: relief of pain, traditionally with pethidine to avoid the sphincter spasm associated with morphine.
- *Fluid replacement* with colloid or blood transfusion, to treat shock and establish a diuresis. In less severe cases, electrolyte and water replacement alone may suffice.
- *Resting the pancreas* by removing stimuli for secretion: the patient is not allowed to take fluid or food by mouth, and nasogastric aspiration is started if the patient is vomiting.
- *Nutrition*: total parenteral nutrition (TPN) may be instituted early in severe cases. There is good evidence that nasojejunal feeding may be superior to TPN in the absence of an ileus probably because of improved maintenance of the gut mucosal integrity decreasing bacterial translocation and reducing septic complications.
- *Antibiotics* (e.g. co-amoxiclav) are commenced in severe cases and if the pancreatitis is associated with gallstones.
- *Prophylaxis against gastric erosions* with sucralfate or an H$_2$-receptor antagonist (e.g. ranitidine) or proton pump inhibitor (e.g. omeprazole).
- *Endoscopic sphincterotomy* performed early in the admission may be indicated in severe gallstone pancreatitis; a dilated common bile duct on ultrasound associated with deranged liver function tests also represents an indication for urgent ERCP and sphincterotomy.

Attempts at treatment with drugs that reduce pancreatic enzyme activation (e.g. aprotonin) or secretion (e.g. probanthine or atropine) are of no proven benefit.

Surgery

Surgery should be avoided early in the acute attack when possible. Later in the disease percutaneous drainage of collections or abscesses may be indicated, often requiring multiple drains; failure to resolve in spite of adequate drainage may be an indication for operative debridement of the necrotic pancreas (necrosectomy). Operative drainage of a pseudocyst may also be required at a later stage (peripancreatic collections in the lesser sac are common in the early stages but usually resolve without intervention). In the case of gallstone pancreatitis, cholecystectomy should be performed as soon as the patient recovers from the acute attack, preferably during the same admission.

Prognosis

Mortality is in the region of 10% and is directly proportional to the severity of the attack.

Complications

- *Abscess formation* with pancreatic necrosis, characterized by pyrexia and persistent leucocytosis.
- *Peripancreatic collections and pseudocyst formation*, characterized by symptoms attributable to the pressure effect on the stomach with fullness and discomfort commonly associated with a palpable epigastric mass.
- *Gastrointestinal bleeding* from acute gastric erosions or peptic ulceration.
- *Renal failure* associated with shock and pancreatic necrosis.
- *Pulmonary insufficiency*: acute lung injury.
- *Further attacks* (relapsing pancreatitis).
- *Diabetes mellitus*, resulting from a severe attack with pancreatic necrosis, or chronic relapsing pancreatitis.

Chronic pancreatitis

Chronic and acute pancreatitis are clinically distinct entities, although bouts of acute pancreatitis may occur in the course of the development of chronic pancreatitis, and the pathogenesis of chronic pancreatitis has much in common with alcoholic acute pancreatitis. In acute pancreatitis the gland is normal before the attack; chronic pancreatitis is characterized by gradual destruction of the functional pancreatic tissue.

Aetiology

In the Western world, alcoholism is the main cause of chronic pancreatitis. In parts of Asia and Africa, chronic pancreatitis is associated with malnutrition; hereditary pancreatitis and hypercalcaemia are uncommon causes.

Clinical features

The patient may present with one or more of the following:

- *asymptomatic* (X-ray diagnosis only from pancreatic calcification);
- *recurrent abdominal pain* radiating through to the upper lumbar region, relieved by sitting forward;
- *steatorrhoea* due to pancreatic insufficiency, resulting in malabsorption and weight loss;
- *diabetes* due to β-cell damage;
- *obstructive jaundice*, which even at operation can be very difficult to differentiate from carcinoma of the head of the pancreas.

Special investigations

- *Serum amylase* estimations performed during attacks of pain may be elevated, but in long-standing disease are often normal, there being insufficient pancreatic tissue remaining to cause a large rise.
- *Abdominal X-ray* may show evidence of calcification or calculi.
- *CT* may demonstrate enlargement and irregular consistency of the gland together with calcification and ductal changes, although the latter may be better appreciated by the use of magnetic resonance cholangiopancreatography (MRCP).
- *ERCP* may show dilatation and irregularity of the pancreatic duct and compression of the bile duct by the inflamed pancreatic head.
- *Endoscopic ultrasound* has become the standard technique for examining the head of the pancreas, and aspiration cytology can be carried out from any suspicious areas to help differentiate chronic pancreatitis or areas of focal pancreatitis from carcinoma.
- *Exocrine function tests*, such as the faecal elastase test, have largely replaced older techniques such as faecal fat estimation.

However, despite preoperative investigation, it is still true that at times the differential diagnosis from a pancreatic carcinoma may only be established following laparotomy and resection when formal histology is obtained.

Treatment

The principal treatment is to remove causative factors such as alcohol consumption. Alcohol should be avoided by anyone with pancreatitis.

- *Analgesics*: the pain is often sufficient to warrant opiate analgesia, but long-term use may result in addiction. Getting the analgesia right is often one of the most difficult aspects of management.
- *Diet*: a low-fat diet with pancreatic enzyme supplements (pancreatin) by mouth.
- *Insulin* when diabetes mellitus occurs.
- *Surgery* if attacks are very frequent or if there is severe pain. Partial pancreatectomy or, in patients in whom the pancreatic duct is grossly dilated, drainage of the whole length of the pancreatic duct into a loop of intestine may be required (Puestow procedure[6]). Occasionally, total pancreatectomy is required, with consequent diabetes and steatorrhoea. In these patients, the diabetes may be very difficult to control partly because of their poor compliance and partly because of the loss of the glucagon-secreting function when the whole pancreas has been removed.
- *Painless obstructive jaundice* may be relieved by a bypass using a Roux-en-Y reconstruction, usually to the common hepatic duct. However, if diagnostic uncertainty remains or if there is a coincident problem with gastric emptying, a Whipple's operation (pancreaticodoudenectomy) may be appropriate.

Pancreatic cysts

Classification

True (20%)

- Congenital polycystic disease of pancreas.
- Retention.
- Hydatid.
- Neoplastic: cystadenoma or cystadenocarcinoma.

False

A collection of fluid in the lesser sac (80%):

- after trauma to the pancreas;
- following acute pancreatitis;
- owing to perforation of a posterior gastric ulcer (rare).

Clinical features

A pancreatic cyst presents as a firm, large, rounded, upper abdominal swelling. Initially, the cyst is apparently resonant because of loops of gas-filled bowel in front of it, but as it increases in size the intestine is pushed away and the mass becomes dull to percussion.

Treatment

True cysts require surgical excision; false cysts are drained. This may be performed internally (by anastomosis either into the stomach or into the small intestine), or percutaneously, under ultrasound control.

Pancreatic tumours

Classification

Benign

1 Adenoma.
2 Cystadenoma.
3 Islet cell tumour (see Box 38.1, p. 324):
   a Zollinger–Ellison tumour;
   b insulinoma (β-cell tumour);
   c glucagonoma (α-cell tumour).

Malignant

1 *Primary*:
   a adenocarcinoma;
   b cystadenocarcinoma;
   c malignant islet cell tumour.
2 *Secondary*: invasion from carcinoma of the stomach or bile duct.

[6]Charles Puestow (1902–73), Professor of Surgery, College of Medicine, University of Illinois, Chicago, IL, USA.

Pancreatic neuroendocrine tumours

These tumours arise from cell types within the islets of Langerhans and, although rare (less than 2% of pancreatic neoplasms), are of great interest because of their metabolic effects, even from small lesions, which may be difficult to localize even with CT and magnetic resonance (MR) imaging or selective angiography.

Types of tumours

Pancreatic neuroendocrine tumours are derived from amine precursor uptake and decarboxylation (APUD) cells, and are thus sometimes termed APUD-omas. They secrete a number of polypeptides according to the cell type of origin. These may be active hormones and present relatively early, or polypeptides for which no function has been identified; often, more than one polypeptide is secreted. A pancreatic islet contains many cell types of which the alpha (α) cells (producing glucagon), beta (β) cells (insulin) and delta (δ) cells (somatostatin) are best known. In addition, interacinar cells produce pancreatic polypeptide (F cells) and serotonin (enterochromaffin cells). The islet cells may also produce hormones not normally found in the pancreas, such as gastrin (gastrinoma), vasoactive intestinal polypeptide (VIP-oma), and adrenocorticotrophic hormone (ACTH) (Cushing's syndrome[7]).

The islet cell tumours may be associated with other endocrine tumours elsewhere as part of a multiple endocrine neoplasia (MEN) syndrome, often involving the parathyroid and the anterior pituitary gland (see Box 38.1, p. 324).

Insulinoma (β-cell tumour)

Ninety per cent are benign, 10% malignant and about 10% are multiple tumours. Because of the high production of insulin by the tumour, two groups of hypoglycaemic symptoms may be produced.

1 *Central nervous system phenomena*: weakness, sweating, trembling, epilepsy, confusion, hemiplegia and eventually coma, which may be fatal.
2 *Gastrointestinal phenomena*: hunger, abdominal pain and diarrhoea.

These symptoms appear particularly when the patient is hungry, or during physical exercise. They are often present early in the morning before breakfast and are relieved by eating. Often, there is excessive appetite with gross weight gain. Although once the diagnosis has been made the cause of the symptomatology is clear, it is not uncommon for diagnosis to be delayed, and psychiatric diagnoses and referrals being made during the course of the illness is common.

Diagnosis: Whipple's triad[8]

The main diagnostic characteristics of the syndrome are as follows:

- The attacks are induced by starvation or exercise.
- During the attack, hypoglycaemia is present.
- Symptoms are relieved by sugar given orally or intravenously.

Differential diagnosis of spontaneous hypoglycaemia in adults includes self-administration of insulin or alcohol, and suprarenal, pituitary or hepatic insufficiency.

Special investigations

- *Insulin levels*: raised insulin levels in the presence of hypoglycaemia. The hypoglycaemia can be prompted by a period of prolonged fasting (14–16 hours).
- *C-peptide levels* may be measured to rule out exogenous insulin administration, as these will be high with insulinoma and low when exogenous insulin is administered.
- *Localization tests* include CT, MR, endoscopic ultrasound (EUS) and selective angiography. Occasionally, localization is not achieved until laparotomy is performed, when the tumour can usually be located using careful palpation and intraoperative ultrasound.

[7]Harvey Cushing (1869–1939), Professor of Surgery, Harvard Medical School, Boston, MA, USA.

[8]Allen Oldfather Whipple (1881–1963), Professor of Surgery, Columbia University, New York, NY, USA. Also described the operation for carcinoma of the head of the pancreas.

Treatment

Treatment is excision of the tumour. Depending on the site, this may require either a Whipple's procedure or a distal pancreatectomy, but in patients in whom the insulinoma is well defined and superficial, simple enucleation is often possible.

Gastrinoma (Zollinger–Ellison syndrome,[9] non-β-cell islet tumour)

This tumour of non-β-cells may be benign or malignant, solitary or multiple, and a quarter are part of an MEN syndrome. Malignant tumours are less common in sporadic forms (30%) than in those related to MEN syndromes (60%); the malignant tumours are also relatively slow growing, although they eventually produce hepatic metastases. The gastrinoma secretes a gastrin-like substance into the bloodstream, which produces an extremely high gastric secretion of HCl. Many patients also develop oesophagitis owing to the high acid secretion; diarrhoea is common (probably related to the high acid output). The majority of patients develop fulminating peptic ulceration, presenting with bleeding or perforation, and have multiple duodenal ulcers. Symptoms relapse after cessation of medical therapy.

Special investigations

- *Serum gastrin* concentration in the blood is 10 times normal.
- *Basal acid output*, measured by nasogastric aspiration, is very high (>15 mmol/h).
- *Localization*: as for insulinoma.

Treatment

Treatment comprises excision of the tumour or, if this is not possible, control of the high acid secretion by means of proton pump inhibitors (e.g. omeprazole) or high doses of histamine H_2-receptor antagonists (cimetidine, ranitidine).

[9]Robert Milton Zollinger (1903–1992), Professor of Surgery, Ohio State University, Columbus, OH, USA. Edward Horner Ellison (1918–1970), Associate Professor at the same institution.

Modern acid suppression therapy has largely replaced surgical treatment by total gastrectomy.

Pancreatic carcinoma

Pathology

Sixty per cent are situated in the head of the pancreas, 25% in the body and 15% in the tail.

Of the tumours of the head of the pancreas, one-third are periampullary, arising from the ampulla of Vater, the duodenal mucosa or the lower end of the common bile duct.

The incidence in the UK is 10 per 100 000 population, with men and women now almost equally affected. It affects the middle-aged and elderly, and the disease is more common in those who smoke.

Macroscopically, the growth is infiltrating, hard and irregular; rarer types are characterized by cystic lesions near the tail of the pancreas.

Microscopically, the tumours may be

- ductal adenocarcinomas (most common): tumours arising in the cells lining the pancreatic ducts;
- acinar cell carcinoma;
- undifferentiated.

Less common tumours include:

- mucinous cystic neoplasm (MCN): cystic tumours that predominantly affect the tail of the pancreas and occur in middle-aged women;
- intraductal papillary mucinous tumour (IPMN): ductal tumours that are characterized by the production of a large amount of mucus. They are slow-growing tumours that may be benign or malignant, and occur more commonly in older men.

Spread

1 *Direct invasion into*:
   a common bile duct – obstructive jaundice;
   b duodenum – occult or overt intestinal bleeding and duodenal obstruction;
   c portal vein – portal vein thrombosis, portal hypertension and ascites;
   d inferior vena cava – bilateral leg oedema.
2 *Lymphatic*: to adjacent lymph nodes and nodes in the porta hepatis.

3 *Bloodstream*: to the liver and then to the lungs.
4 *Transcoelomic*: with peritoneal seeding and ascites.

Clinical features

Carcinoma of the pancreas may present in a variety of ways:

- *Painless progressive jaundice* is the classical presentation, but this form is rather uncommon and is most often found in the periampullary type of tumour. This is because the bile duct is compressed at an early stage, before extensive painful invasion of surrounding tissues.
- *Pain*: at least 50% of patients present with epigastric pain of a dull, continuous, aching nature, which frequently radiates into the upper lumbar region. This pain often precedes the development of jaundice.
- *Diabetes*: recent-onset diabetes in the elderly is suspicious.
- *Thrombophlebitis migrans* (Trousseau's sign[10]); the pathogenesis of this is unknown.
- *The general features of malignant disease*: anorexia and, in particular, loss of weight.

Examination

The patient is frequently jaundiced, and half have a palpable gallbladder (Courvoisier's law; see Figure 31.3, p. 271). If the tumour is large, an epigastric mass may be palpable. The liver is frequently enlarged, either because of back-pressure from biliary obstruction or because of secondary deposits.

Special investigations

- *Ultrasound* will confirm dilated bile ducts and a distended gallbladder, but should not be relied on to obtain adequate views of the pancreas.
- *CT* may demonstrate the tumour mass and facilitate fine-needle biopsy.
- *Endoscopy* may visualize a periampullary growth, which can then be biopsied.
- *EUS*, in which a specialized endoscope is used to obtain ultrasound images of the pancreatic head from within the duodenum, will give detailed information about the location of the tumour and its relationship to the portal vein and superior mesenteric artery and will demonstrate local extent of spread and also visualize enlarged lymph nodes. EUS is thus a key step in defining the operability of a tumour in terms of local invasion and spread.
  - Needle aspiration under EUS control will allow cytological diagnosis of the tumour itself and lymph node metastases.
  - Needle aspiration of cystic lesions may distinguish between pseudocysts (high amylase content) and mucinous tumours (high Ca 19.9 and CEA; see Chapter 7, Table 7.1, p. 37).
- *MRCP and ERCP* will demonstrate an obstruction in the bile duct.
- *Barium studies* may show widening of the duodenal loop and a filling defect or irregularity of the duodenum resulting from invasion by the tumour, but have largely been replaced by CT imaging with three-dimensional reconstruction when necessary.
- *Occult blood* may be present in the stools, especially from a periampullary tumour ulcerating into the duodenum. The stools are pale in the presence of jaundice, and may have a silvery appearance owing to the periampullary bleeding (the silvery stools of Ogilvie[11]).
- *Serum amylase* is rarely elevated.
- *Biochemical analysis* confirms the changes of obstructive jaundice (high bilirubin and alkaline phosphatase). The tumour marker Ca 19.9 may be elevated.

Differential diagnosis

This is from other causes of obstructive jaundice and from other causes of upper abdominal pain. Carcinoma of the body and tail of the pancreas, in which obstructive jaundice does not occur, is notoriously difficult to diagnose, the diagnosis often only being made at a late stage following many weeks or months of upper abdominal pain when a CT scan is performed. The tumour at this stage is usually inoperable.

Treatment

Treatment of carcinoma of the pancreas is usually symptomatic, and thus applicable to tumours of the head of the pancreas, which present with

---

[10]Armand Trousseau (1801–1867), Physician, Hôpital St. Antoine and Hôpital Dieu, Paris, France.

[11]Sir William Heneage Ogilvie (1887–1971), Surgeon, Guy's Hospital, London, UK.

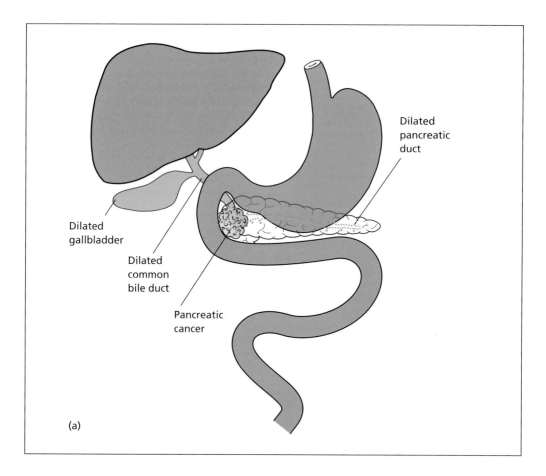

Dilated
pancreatic
duct

Dilated
gallbladder

Dilated
common
bile duct

Pancreatic
cancer

(a)

Figure 32.2 Whipple's pancreaticoduodenectomy. (a) The initial appearance characterized by a distended gallbladder, dilated bile duct and pancreatic duct, and mass in the head of the pancreas. (b) Following resection, the stomach remnant is anastomosed to the proximal jejunum as a gastrojejunostomy; the common hepatic duct is anastomosed to a Roux-en-Y loop of jejunum, the end of which is anastomosed to the pancreatic duct.

obstructive jaundice and duodenal obstruction. In approximately 15% of cases, attempted curative resection may be possible; otherwise, palliation is more appropriate.

- *Curative surgical resection* is possible when disease is confined to the periampullary region. The procedure (Whipple's pancreaticoduodenectomy; Figure 32.2) involves removal of the duodenal 'C' along with the pancreatic head and common bile duct; a gastroenterostomy and biliary drainage using a Roux loop[12] of jejunum are fashioned to restore continuity, together with the implantation of the pancreatic duct into the

jejunal Roux loop. However, most tumours are inoperable and, even among the 15% which are operable, the long-term prognosis is poor except in early periampullary tumours without lymph node involvement.

- *Palliative surgical bypass* comprises a short circuit between the distended bile duct and a loop of jejunum (choledochojejunostomy), together with a duodenal bypass by a gastroenterostomy if duodenal obstruction is present.
- *Palliative intubation*, by passage of a stent across the ampulla and through the obstructed common bile duct, is the other alternative to treat the obstructive jaundice. This may be performed either endoscopically (ERCP) or transhepatically (percutaneous transhepatic

[12]Cesar Roux (1857–1934), Professor of Surgery, Lausanne, Switzerland.

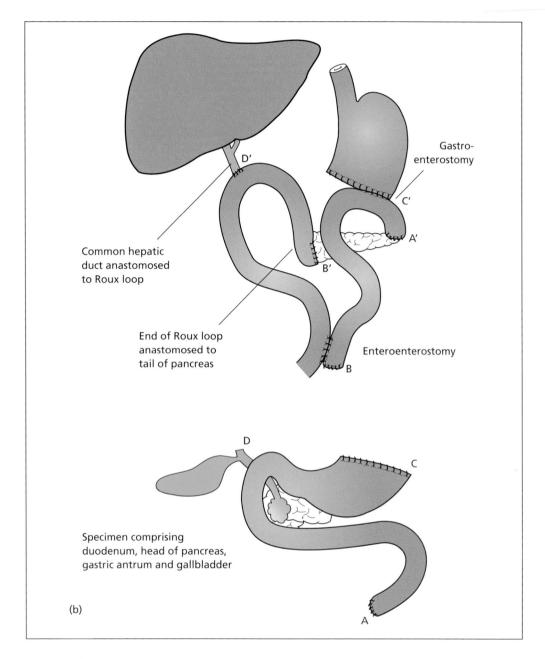

Gastro-
enterostomy

Common hepatic
duct anastomosed
to Roux loop

End of Roux loop
anastomosed to
tail of pancreas

Enteroenterostomy

Specimen comprising
duodenum, head of pancreas,
gastric antrum and gallbladder

(b)

Figure 32.2 *Continued*

cholangiography). Plastic stents are commonly used when the diagnosis has not been established or when operative resection is planned, but expanding metal stents can be used in the palliative situation when the diagnosis is clear because they have better patency rates. Duodenal obstruction can now also be treated by endoscopic stenting, potentially allowing the terminally ill patient to be spared the additional morbidity of a laparotomy and surgical bypass. Alternatively, laparoscopic gastroenterostomy can be used to palliate duodenal obstruction.

- *Severe pain* often requires management with opiates, but coeliac plexus block performed either via the percutaneous approach or under EUS guidance can offer good pain control in some cases.

Prognosis

The outlook for patients with carcinoma of the pancreas itself is gloomy; even if the growth is resectable, the operation has a mortality of about 2–5% and only a small percentage survive for 5 years. Periampullary growths, however, which present relatively early, have a reasonably good prognosis after resection, with about a 25% 5 year survival.

Palliative chemotherapy currently uses protocols based on gemcitabine. The place of radiotherapy is unclear, although some centres do use a combination of radiotherapy and chemotherapy in selected patients. Recent trials have shown a definite survival benefit in patients who have undergone attempted curative resection and who receive postoperative chemotherapy.

Occasionally, a patient has a surprisingly prolonged survival after a palliative bypass operation. In such a case, the diagnosis was more likely to have been chronic pancreatitis mistaken for carcinoma.

33

The spleen

Learning objective

✓ To know the common causes of splenomegaly, the presentations of a ruptured spleen and the prophylaxis and treatment of post-splenectomy syndrome.

Splenomegaly

Physical signs

The spleen must be enlarged to about three times its normal size before it becomes clinically palpable. It then forms a swelling that descends below the left costal margin, moves on respiration and has a firm lower margin, which may or may not be notched. The mass is dull to percussion, the dullness extending above the costal margin.

There are three important differential diagnoses:

1 An enlarged left kidney; unless this is enormous, there is resonance over the swelling anteriorly, as it is covered by the gas-containing colon.
2 Carcinoma of the cardia or upper part of the body of the stomach; by the time such a tumour reaches palpable proportions, there are usually symptoms of gastric obstruction, which suggest the site of the lesion.
3 An enlarged left lobe of liver.

Classification

It is essential to have a working classification of enlargements of the spleen.

1 *Infections.*

  a Viruses: glandular fever.
  b Bacterial: typhus, typhoid, septicaemia ('septic spleen').
  c Protozoal: malaria, kala-azar, Egyptian splenomegaly (schistosomiasis).
  d Parasitic: hydatid.
2 *Haematological diseases.*
  a Leukaemia: chronic myeloid and chronic lymphocytic.
  b Lymphoma: Hodgkin's and non-Hodgkin's lymphoma.
  c Myelofibrosis, idiopathic thrombocytopenia, polycythaemia rubra vera.
  d Haemolytic anaemias, e.g. spherocytosis, β-thalassaemia.
3 *Portal hypertension.* Increased pressure in the portal system causes progressive enlargement of the spleen and may lead to hypersplenism with overactivity of the normal splenic functions such as removal of platelets, resulting in thrombocytopenia.
4 *Metabolic and collagen disease.*
  a Amyloid: secondary to rheumatoid arthritis, collagen diseases, chronic sepsis.
  b Storage diseases, e.g. Gaucher's disease.[1]
5 *Cysts, abscesses and tumours of the spleen*: all uncommon.

Massive splenomegaly in the UK is likely to be due to one of the following: chronic myeloid leukaemia, myelofibrosis, lymphoma, polycythaemia or portal hypertension.

Lecture Notes: General Surgery, 12th edition. © Harold Ellis, Sir Roy Y. Calne and Christopher J. E. Watson. Published 2011 by Blackwell Publishing Ltd.

[1]Phillipe Gaucher (1854–1918), Physician, Hôpital St Louis, Paris, France.

If the spleen is palpable, special attention must be paid to detecting the presence of hepatomegaly and lymphadenopathy (Chapter 34, p. 292).

Splenectomy

Splenectomy is indicated under the following circumstances:

- *Rupture*: either from closed or open trauma or from accidental damage during abdominal surgery.
- *Haematological disease*: haemolytic anaemia, thrombocytopenic purpura.
- *Tumours and cysts*.
- *Part of another operative procedure*, e.g. radical excision of carcinoma of the stomach, distal pancreatectomy, splenorenal anastomosis for portal hypertension.

Complications of splenectomy

Gastric dilatation

Following splenectomy, there may be a gastric ileus. Swallowed air causes rapid dilatation of the stomach, which may tear ligatures on the short gastric vessels on the greater curve of the stomach, which are tied during splenectomy; haemorrhage results. To prevent this, a nasogastric tube is placed and regularly aspirated.

Thrombocytosis

Following splenectomy, the platelet count rises, often to a level of 1000×10^9/L (normal is $<400 \times 10^9$/L). In time, the count falls, but while it is high the patient is at a greater than normal risk of deep vein thrombosis and pulmonary embolus. Antiplatelet agents such as aspirin are given as prophylaxis in addition to low-molecular-weight heparin.

Postsplenectomy sepsis

One of the spleen's functions is to clear capsulated microorganisms (such as *Pneumococcus*, *Meningococcus* and *Haemophilus influenzae*) from the bloodstream after they have been opsonized by the binding of host antibodies to their surface as part of the normal immune response. The spleen also has important phago-cytic properties, as well as being the largest repository of lymphoid tissue in the body.

Removal of the spleen in splenectomy predisposes the patient, especially a child, to infection with organisms such as the *Pneumococcus*. The clinical course is of a fulminant bacterial infection, with shock and circulatory collapse, termed overwhelming postsplenectomy sepsis.

Prophylactic immunization with pneumococcal, meningococcal and *H. influenzae* type B vaccines should be administered, preoperatively when possible. In addition, children should have prophylactic daily low-dose penicillin at least until they reach adulthood. Adults should have penicillin for at least the first 2 years after splenectomy, and longer if immunosuppressed. Annual flu immunizations are also recommended to minimize the additional risk of bacterial superinfection and special care is required if the patient is to travel to malarial areas.

Ruptured spleen

This is the commonest internal injury produced by non-penetrating trauma to the abdominal wall. It usually occurs in isolation, but may coexist with fractures of the ribs, or rupture of the liver, the left kidney, the diaphragm or the tail of the pancreas.

Clinical features

Rupture of the spleen manifests in one of the following ways:

1 *Immediate massive bleeding* with rapid death from shock. This results from a complete shattering of the spleen or its avulsion from the splenic pedicle, and death may occur in a few minutes. Fortunately, this is rare.
2 *Peritonism from progressive blood loss*. Following injury, there are the symptoms and signs of progressive blood loss together with evidence of peritoneal irritation. Over a period of several hours after the accident, the patient becomes increasingly pale, the pulse rises and the blood pressure falls. There is abdominal pain, which is either diffuse or confined to the left flank. The patient may complain of pain referred to the left shoulder tip or admit to this only on direct questioning.

On examination, the abdomen is generally tender, particularly on the left side. There may be marked generalized rigidity, or it may be confined to slight guarding in the left flank. Bruising of the abdominal wall is often absent or only slight.

3 *Delayed rupture*. This may occur from hours up to several days after trauma. Following the initial injury the concomitant pain soon settles. Then, following a completely asymptomatic interval, the signs and symptoms described above become manifest. This picture is produced by a subcapsular haematoma of the spleen, which increases in size and then ruptures the thin overlying peritoneal capsule with a resultant sudden, sharp haemorrhage.

4 *Spontaneous rupture*. A spleen diseased by, for example, malaria, glandular fever or leukaemia may rupture spontaneously or after only trivial trauma.

Special investigations

The diagnosis of a ruptured spleen is a clinical one, and an unstable patient must be resuscitated aggressively and the surgeon proceed at once to laparotomy. In the less acute situation, and only after resuscitation has begun, the following investigations are useful:

- *Chest X-ray* may reveal associated rib fractures, rupture of the diaphragm or injury to the left lung.
- *Abdominal X-ray*: the stomach bubble may be displaced to the right and there may be indentation of its gas shadow. The splenic flexure of the colon, if containing gas, may be seen to be displaced downwards by the haematoma.
- *Ultrasound* may reveal free fluid, an intrasplenic haematoma or a laceration of the capsule, although the last may be overlooked. Ultrasound is increasingly used as a diagnostic tool in the accident and emergency department for such cases.
- *Computed tomography* is the investigation of choice in all cases of abdominal trauma, and will demonstrate the laceration of the spleen, the presence of intra-abdominal fluid and identify traumatic injuries to other organs.
- *Urinalysis for blood*: haematuria will suggest associated coincidental renal damage.

Treatment

Resuscitation with plasma expanders initially and blood replacement as soon as blood is available is commenced, and laparotomy performed. If the spleen is found to be avulsed or hopelessly pulped, emergency splenectomy is required. If there is minor laceration of the spleen, an attempt is made to preserve it, especially in children and young adults, in whom there is a greater risk of postsplenectomy sepsis. This may be carried out by using fine sutures, fibrin glues and haemostatic absorbable gauze.

Having controlled the bleeding at laparotomy, it is important to carry out a full examination to exclude injury to other organs.

34

The lymph nodes and lymphatics

Learning objectives
✓ To know the causes of lymphadenopathy and the appropriate management.
✓ To have knowledge of lymphoedema and its causes.

Enlarged lymph nodes are a common diagnostic problem. It is as well, therefore, to have a simple classification and clinical approach to this topic.

The lymphadenopathies

The lymphadenopathies are conveniently divided into those due to local and those due to generalized disease.

Classification

Localized

1 *Infective*:
   a acute, e.g. a cervical lymphadenopathy secondary to tonsillitis;
   b chronic, e.g. tuberculous nodes of neck.
2 *Neoplastic*: due to secondary spread of tumour.

Generalized

1 *Infective*:
   a acute, e.g. glandular fever (mononucleosis), septicaemia;
   b chronic, e.g. human immunodeficiency virus (HIV), secondary syphilis.

2 *The reticuloses*: Hodgkin's disease,[1] non-Hodgkin's lymphoma, chronic lymphocytic leukaemia.
3 *Sarcoidosis*.

Clinical examination

The clinical examination of any patient with a lymph node enlargement is incomplete unless the following three requirements have been fulfilled:

1 The area drained by the involved lymph nodes has been searched for a possible primary source of infection or malignant disease. There are four important points to remember.
   a *Cervical lymphadenopathy*. In addition to examining the skin of the head and neck, the inside of the oropharynx together with the larynx should be examined for chronic sepsis or malignant disease.
   b *Inguinal lymphadenopathy*. If a patient has an enlarged lymph node in the groin, the skin of the leg, buttock and lower abdominal wall below the level of the umbilicus must be scrutinized, together with the external genitalia and the anal canal.
   c *Testicular tumours* drain along their lymphatics, which pass with the testicular

Lecture Notes: General Surgery, 12th edition. © Harold Ellis, Sir Roy Y. Calne and Christopher J. E. Watson. Published 2011 by Blackwell Publishing Ltd.

[1]Thomas Hodgkin (1798–1866), Curator of Pathology, Guy's Hospital, London, UK.

vessels to the para-aortic lymph nodes, and not to the inguinal lymph nodes.

d *Virchow's node*[2] is a prominent node in the left supraclavicular fossa arising from malignant disease below the diaphragm, e.g. gastric carcinoma, with secondaries ascending the thoracic duct to drain into the left subclavian vein (Troisier's sign[3]). A supraclavicular node may also signify spread from intrathoracic, testicular or breast tumours.

2 The other lymph node areas are examined, as enlarged lymph nodes elsewhere would suggest a generalized lymphadenopathy.

3 The liver and spleen are carefully palpated; their enlargement will suggest a reticulosis, sarcoid or glandular fever.

Special investigations

In many instances, the cause of the lymphadenopathy will by now have become obvious. The following investigations may be required in order to elucidate further the diagnosis:

- *Examination of a blood film* may clinch the diagnosis of glandular fever or leukaemia.
- *Chest X-ray* may show evidence of enlarged mediastinal nodes or may reveal a primary occult tumour of the lung, which is the source of disseminated deposits.
- *Serological tests*: an HIV antibody test is performed if infection is suspected; syphilis may be confirmed by specific treponemal antigen tests.
- *Lymph node biopsy*: ultrasound-guided needle core biopsy, or surgical removal of one of the enlarged lymph nodes, may be necessary for definite histological proof of the diagnosis. This is particularly so in Hodgkin's disease and non-Hodgkin's lymphoma.
- *Computed tomography* of chest, abdomen and pelvis to define the stage of any lymphoma, or to identify the primary tumour
- *X-ray of cervical nodes*: enlarged painless cervical lymph nodes may be X-rayed; tuberculous nodes often show typical spotty calcification.

> ### Box 34.1 **A swollen leg**
>
> **Generalized disease**
>
> - Cardiac failure
> - Nephrotic syndrome
> - Liver failure
>
> **Venous disease**
>
> - Venous thrombosis*
> - Deep venous insufficiency
> - Arteriovenous fistula,* e.g. Klippel–Trénaunay syndrome[4]
>
> **Lymphatic disease**
>
> - Primary lymphoedema*
> - Secondary lymphoedema,* e.g. filariasis, malignant infiltration, following surgery or irradiation to lymphatics
>
> *Also may cause unilateral upper limb swelling.

Lymphoedema

Lymphoedema results from the obstruction of lymphatic flow, owing to inherited abnormalities of the lymphatics, their obliteration by disease or their operative removal. It is characterized by an excessive accumulation of interstitial fluid. The causes of lymphoedema may be divided into congenital and acquired (Box 34.1).

Inherited lymphoedema

There are two autosomal dominant inherited forms of lymphoedema. Both are more common in women.

- *Type 1* (also known as Milroy's disease,[5] Nonne–Milroy[6] disease and primary congenital lymphoedema) is very uncommon and is caused by a mutation in the *FLT4* gene, which encodes vascular endothelial growth factor receptor 3, itself involved in

---

[2]Rudolf Ludwig Karl Virchow (1821–1902), Professor of Pathology in Würzburg and later Berlin, Germany.
[3]Charles Émile Troisier (1844–1919), Professor of Pathology, Paris, France.

[4]Maurice Klippel (1858–1942), French Neurologist, Salpêtrière Hospital, Paris, France. Paul Trénaunay (b. 1875), French Neurologist. The syndrome involves multiple congenital venous malformations producing varicose veins together with hypertrophy of bones and soft tissues and extensive cutaneous haemangiomas, usually affecting the lower limbs.
[5]William Forsyth Milroy (1855–1942), Professor of Medicine, University of Nebraska, Omaha, NE, USA.
[6]Max Nonne (1861–1959), Neurologist, Hamburg, Germany.

lymphangiogenesis. It is characterized by onset soon after birth with lower limb swelling.

- *Type 2* (also known as Meige's syndrome[7]) is associated with mutations in *FOXC2*, a forkhead family transcription factor gene. It is characterized by lymphoedema that is particularly severe below the waist. It has been arbitrarily divided into *lymphoedema praecox*, which develops between puberty and the age of 35, and the less common *lymphoedema tarda*, which develops in adult life.

There are three principal pathological processes affecting the lymphatic channels in congenital lymphoedema: aplasia, hypoplasia and varicose dilatation (megalymphatics).

Acquired lymphoedema

- *Post-inflammatory*: the result of fibrosis obliterating the lymphatics following repeated attacks of streptococcal cellulitis, particularly when the lymphatic drainage is already compromised.
- *Filariasis: Filaria bancrofti[8]* infects lymphatics; a chronic inflammatory reaction is set up with consequent lymphatic obstruction. There is gross lymphoedema, especially of the lower limbs and genitalia, often called elephantiasis.
- *Following radical surgery*, particularly after block dissection of the axilla, groin or neck in which extensive removal of lymphatics is performed.
- *Post-irradiation fibrosis*.
- *Malignant disease*: late oedema of the arm after axillary clearance and radical mastectomy is often indicative of massive recurrence of tumour in the axilla occluding the residual lymphatic pathways.

Special investigations

- *Lymphoscintigraphy* involves injecting a radiolabelled protein subcutaneously and monitoring its movement through the lymphatics. It will confirm lymphatic obstruction.

- *Magnetic resonance imaging* may be used to confirm the cause of obstruction in secondary cases.

Differential diagnosis

The diagnosis of lymphoedema depends first of all on the exclusion of other causes of oedema, for instance venous obstruction, cardiac failure or renal disease, and, second, on demonstration of one of the causes mentioned above. It was previously taught that lymphoedema could readily be differentiated from other forms of oedema on the simple physical sign of absence of pitting in the lymphoedematous limb. However, lymphoedema of acute onset will initially pit on pressure, although it is true that, when it becomes chronic; the subcutaneous tissues become indurated from fibrous tissue replacement, and pitting will not then occur. However, oedema of any nature, if chronic, will have this characteristic.

Treatment of congenital lymphoedema

Conservative

Mild cases will respond to elevation and graduated elastic compression stockings.

Surgery

In severe cases, surgery may be appropriate. Two approaches are possible. The first is to remove all the oedematous subcutaneous tissue down to the deep fascia with removal of the overlying skin as a split-skin graft and its reapplication directly to the deep fascia. This leaves considerable scarring. The second approach is to provide alternative lymphatic drainage bypassing obstructions, such as by tunnelling a tongue of omentum down to the inguinal nodes, to provide drainage along mesenteric lymphatics to the thoracic duct, bypassing obstructed iliac nodes. Unfortunately, the results are poor.

---

[7]Henri Meige (1866–1940), Professor of Medicine, Hôpital de Salpêtrière, Paris, France.
[8]Joseph Bancroft (1836–1894), Physician and Public Health Officer, Brisbane, Australia.

The breast

Developmental anomalies

Accessory nipples and breasts

Extra nipples or breasts may develop along the primitive milk line. Accessory nipples are usually found just below the normal breast, while the axilla is the commonest site for accessory breast tissue. They are influenced by circulating hormones, and the nipples may discharge during lactation.

Hypoplasia or absence of the breast

Although asymmetry of the breasts is normal, complete failure of development of the breast may occur and is often associated with chest wall defects. Bilateral developmental failure may be associated with ovarian failure or Turner's syndrome.[1] Asymmetry can be treated by a combination of ipsilateral breast augmentation and contralateral breast reduction.

[1]Henry Hubert Turner (1892–1970), Endocrinologist and Professor of Medicine, University of Oklahoma, Norman, OK, USA.

Lecture Notes: General Surgery, 12th edition. © Harold Ellis, Sir Roy Y. Calne and Christopher J. E. Watson. Published 2011 by Blackwell Publishing Ltd.

Symptoms of breast disease

There are five common symptoms of breast disease that warrant urgent attention:

- a new, discrete lump;
- nipple discharge – blood stained or persistent;
- nipple retraction or distortion of recent onset;
- altered breast contour or dimpling;
- suspected Paget's disease.

Other common symptoms that require further investigation include persistent asymmetrical nodularity, pain (mastalgia) that interferes with a patient's lifestyle and a family history of breast cancer.

A lump in the breast

Ninety-five per cent of all lumps in the breast will be one of:

1 *Carcinoma of the breast.*
2 *Cyst.*
3 *Fibroadenoma.*
4 *Fibroadenosis.*

In addition, the following less common causes need to be considered:

1 *Trauma*: fat necrosis.
2 *Other cysts*:
  a galactocele;
  b abscess;

c cystadenoma;
d retention cyst of the glands of Montgomery.[2]
3 *Other tumours*:
   a duct papilloma;
   b sarcoma (extremely rare);
   c hamartoma;
   d lipoma.

Uncommon chest wall swellings may rarely be confused with breast swellings. Examples of such are rib swellings (e.g. tumour, Tietze's syndrome or tuberculosis), superficial venous thrombosis (Mondor's disease[3]), eroding aortic aneurysm (syphilitic) and cold abscess (empyema necessitans).

Management

The diagnosis of discrete breast lumps is based on a triple assessment that comprises the following:

1 Clinical examination.
2 Radiological imaging:
   a *mammography*, usually in older patients (over 35 years);
   b *ultrasound*, both diagnostic and to guide biopsy;
   c *magnetic resonance*, useful in symptomatic patients with breast implants in whom ultrasound is not diagnostic. It is also used to detect local recurrence when ultrasound and mammography are unhelpful.
3 Biopsy, usually ultrasound guided:
   a fine-needle aspiration cytology;
   b core biopsy.

The predictive value for benign disease when all three components of the triple assessment are benign is 99%. If there is discordance between any of the three tests, open biopsy is considered.

Discharge from the nipple

1 *Blood-stained*:
   a duct papilloma, when blood arises from a single duct;
   b intraduct carcinoma;
   c Paget's disease;
   d invasive carcinoma (rare).
2 *Clear*: intraduct papilloma.

3 *Multicoloured (often multiduct)*: duct ectasia (discharge commonly yellow, brown or green).
4 *Milky*: galactorrhoea: may follow lactation but can also be drug-induced or a manifestation of hyperprolactinaemia (or, occasionally, hypothyroidism).
5 *Purulent*: breast abscess.

Management

The majority of cases of nipple discharge are benign, and this symptom is rarely a presenting feature of breast cancer, even when blood stained. Clear, single-duct or blood-stained discharge requires further investigation; if a lump is present, it should be managed by triple assessment (above). In the absence of a lump, the management of discharge is as follows.

Multicoloured, multiduct discharge

If clinical examination and mammography are normal, a diagnosis of duct ectasia is likely and no further treatment is required.

Clear single-duct discharge

If mammography is normal, the diagnosis is likely to be an intraduct papilloma and excision of the affected duct (a microdochectomy) is indicated.

Bloody nipple discharge

The presence of blood in the discharge should be confirmed by cytology. If blood is present, a mammogram (for women over 35 years) is performed with a biopsy of any abnormal tissue. If mammography is normal, a microdochectomy is performed if a single duct can be identified; a total duct clearance (Hadfield's procedure[4]) is performed if a single duct cannot be clearly identified.

Pain in the breast (mastalgia)

Breast pain (mastalgia) can be separated into cyclical and non-cyclical mastalgia, of which cyclical mastalgia is the most common and is best considered as an alteration of the normal cyclical pattern that occurs during the reproductive years.

Cyclical mastalgia

Cyclical mastalgia is breast pain that is usually bilateral, worse premenstrually and relieved fol-

---

[2]William Featherstone Montgomery (1797–1859), Professor of Midwifery, Dublin, Ireland.
[3]Henri Mondor (1885–1962), Professor of Surgery, Hôpital Salpêtrière, Paris, France.

[4]Geoffrey John Hadfield (1923–2006), Surgeon, Stoke Mandeville Hospital, Aylesbury, UK.

lowing menstruation. It usually occurs in young women (under 35), and other potential risk factors for the development of breast pain include diet (caffeine, dietary fat intake), hormone preparations (the oral contraceptive pill (OCP) and hormone replacement therapy (HRT)) and other medications. In addition to a careful clinical examination, patients over 35 years should also have mammography; as with all mammograms, suspicious areas should be subjected to core biopsy.

Management

Initial therapy comprises gamma-linolenic acid (GLA), which can take 4–6 weeks to have an effect. In addition, the patient is advised to reduce her intake of caffeine and animal fats. An alteration to, or introduction of, the OCP or HRT should be considered. If the patient remains symptomatic despite GLA, the following may be considered:

- *danazol*, an anti-gonadotrophin that binds to oestrogen and progesterone receptors in the breast;
- *tamoxifen*, an oestrogen receptor inhibitor;
- *luteinizing hormone-releasing hormone (LHRH) analogues*, to inhibit ovarian hormone production.

Non-cyclical mastalgia

Causes of non-cyclical mastalgia include the following:

- *breast abscess*;
- *carcinoma of the breast*: uncommon presenting symptom, this may give rise to heaviness or a 'pricking' sensation;
- *Tietze's syndrome*,[5] chondritis of the costal cartilage, is of unknown aetiology, affects one or more of the second, third or fourth costochondral junctions and, left alone, resolves over a number of months;
- *chest wall lesions*, e.g. herpes zoster.

Duct ectasia

This is an involutional change in the ducts associated with the menopause. The terminal ducts behind the nipple become dilated (ectasia) and engorged with secretions. Secondary infection may lead to retroareolar abscess, and fibrosis may result in nipple retraction.

[5]Alexander Tietze (1864–1927), Surgeon, Breslau, Germany.

Nipple inversion

This may be primary (present since birth) or secondary to duct ectasia or a carcinoma of the breast and of recent onset, when the process is more appropriately called nipple retraction. Primary indrawn nipples may cause problems during lactation but are of no other significance.

Traumatic fat necrosis

Aetiology

Fat necrosis may be associated with a history of trauma and is a common result of seat belt injury or surgical trauma. Its importance lies in its ability to mimic breast carcinoma, and the fact that many women presenting with a lump in the breast attribute this to injury.

Clinical features

Fat necrosis commonly presents with a painless, irregular, firm lump in the breast and there may be a previous history of trauma. It is often associated with skin thickening or retraction and as a result is often difficult to distinguish from carcinoma on clinical examination. The lump usually decreases in size with time, but following resolution may leave a fat cyst within the breast.

Treatment

Although mammography may demonstrate non-specific changes, or mimic carcinoma, ultrasound will often reveal characteristic features. The diagnosis can be confirmed by core biopsy and the palpable mass should resolve. In the absence of a firm diagnosis, an open biopsy is recommended.

Acute inflammation of the breast (mastitis)

There are three causes of acute breast inflammation:

- *mastitis neonatorum*: erythema of a breast bud, or abscess formation, secondary to *Staphylococcus aureus* or *Escherichia coli*;

- *acute bacterial mastitis*: may be lactational or non-lactational;
- *periductal mastitis*.

Acute bacterial mastitis

The most common and most important acute inflammation of the breast; the majority occur during lactation. It presents as cellulitis or abscess formation secondary to *S. aureus*.

Non-lactational breast abscesses may be associated with systemic conditions such as diabetes, steroid therapy and rheumatoid arthritis. The common organisms include α-haemolytic streptococci, enterococci and *Bacteroides*.

Clinical features

Common symptoms include pain, swelling and tenderness of the breast. The inflammation may be localized, with erythema and tenderness of a segment of the breast, or may spread to involve the entire breast. In the later stages, there may be a fluctuant mass and patients may have a pyrexia, tachycardia and leucocytosis.

Treatment

Cellulitis

In the early phase of mastitis, appropriate antibiotics can prevent abscess formation. In lactational mastitis, breast-feeding should be continued as it may speed up recovery. It is rarely necessary to suppress lactation.

Abscess

Patients with clinical or radiological evidence of pus should have aspiration performed in addition to appropriate antibiotic therapy. Repeat aspiration may be necessary and resolution of the abscess can be monitored with sequential ultrasound examinations. If the abscess fails to resolve, or the overlying skin is thin or necrotic, incision and drainage should be performed.

Periductal mastitis

This is an inflammatory process that occurs around dilated milk ducts near the nipple; hence, the alternative name periareolar mastitis. It is linked to smoking, and nipple rings may increase the risk of infection. It occurs in premenopausal women, in contrast to duct ectasia.

Clinical features

Common features include pain and nipple discharge. There may be cellulitis, nipple retraction or a mass deep to the nipple. An associated mammary duct fistula may be present in the periareolar region. Ultrasound may confirm a thickened or dilated duct or abscess formation.

Treatment

Initial treatment is with appropriate antibiotics (usually flucloxacillin) and advice to stop smoking. Remove the ring if present. Patients with recurrent periareolar inflammation and duct discharge should be treated with total duct excision. A mammary duct fistula is treated by total duct excision combined with excision of the fistulous track between the duct and the skin.

Chronic inflammatory conditions of the breast

There are two uncommon chronic inflammatory conditions of the breast:

1 *Lymphocytic lobulitis* occurs in patients with autoimmune diseases, particularly type 1 diabetes mellitus, and usually presents with a firm, irregular lump. The diagnosis is made on core biopsy, with fibrosis and lymphoid infiltrate on microscopy. No further treatment is required.
2 *Granulomatous mastitis* may be secondary to systemic conditions (sarcoidosis), infections (tuberculosis, fungal) or foreign material (silicone). Management includes treatment of any organisms cultured and exclusion of malignancy.

Benign breast disease

From the fourth decade onwards, the breast undergoes a process termed involution. This process includes microcyst formation and an increase in fibrous tissue within the breast. Aberrations of this process include the formation of large cysts, which may present as palpable masses, and the formation of radial scars and sclerosing lesions.

Cystic disease

Cysts are common in the perimenopausal age group but uncommon after the menopause. This, together with an association with HRT, suggests an underlying hormonal aetiology.

Clinical features

Cysts often present with a short history as a painful, tender swelling in the breast. The lump may be fluctuant, but tense cysts may mimic a solid lump. Cysts may be multiple and bilateral. They appear as well-defined, rounded opacities on mammography, and are clearly differentiated from a solid lump by ultrasound.

Treatment

Newly diagnosed or symptomatic cysts should be aspirated to dryness. Uniformly blood-stained fluid should be sent for cytology. If a palpable mass remains following aspiration, or if there is evidence of a solid area in the cyst wall on ultrasound, further investigation is necessary, either by fine-needle aspiration cytology or by core biopsy. Patients with cystic disease may have an increased risk of breast cancer.

Radial scars

Radial scars are radiological findings, appearing as an area of distortion on screening mammography. The mammographic and ultrasound appearance is often difficult to distinguish from carcinoma with lines radiating out from a central scar; hence, excision biopsy is essential. A number of radial scars will be associated with atypical hyperplasia or carcinoma *in situ*.

Sclerosing adenosis

Patients may present with pain or lumpiness in the breast, or there may be areas of increased density or microcalcification on screening mammography which may be indistinguishable from *in situ* carcinoma. Definitive diagnosis will only be made following stereotactic core biopsy. Characteristic microscopic features include proliferation of lobular epithelial, myoepithelial and stromal cells with dense hyaline sclerosis and apocrine metaplasia. Once the diagnosis has been confirmed, no further treatment or follow-up is required.

Non-neoplastic breast lumps

Fibroadenoma

Previously classified as a benign neoplasm, but now considered as an aberration of normal development. They arise from an entire lobule and have both stromal and epithelial components. There is no increased risk of malignancy and the majority will resolve over a period of several years.

Clinical features

Fibroadenomas affect women of all ages, but the peak incidence is in the third decade. It is usually presents as a discrete, firm, mobile lump usually under 3 cm in diameter; some patients present with multiple lumps. They are highly mobile 'breast mice' which are not attached to the skin.

Treatment

Like all solid breast lumps fibroadenomas must be investigated by *triple assessment*. In those patients with multiple fibroadenomas, the largest lump should undergo core biopsy. Surgery should be avoidable in the majority of cases but should be considered in the following circumstances:

- *lump increasing in size* (clinically and/or at ultrasound);
- *symptomatic lump* – pain or tenderness;
- *patient preference*.

Hamartoma

These rare lesions may present clinically as a breast lump or may be incidental findings on screening mammography, when they have the appearance of a 'breast within a breast'. They have a well-defined capsule and comprise a variable mixture of breast lobules, stroma and fat. Once the diagnosis has been confirmed no further treatment is necessary.

Gynaecomastia

A benign condition arising from proliferation of male breast tissue in neonates, at puberty and in adults. It is thought to be due to an imbalance of oestrogens and androgens and must be excluded from carcinoma of the male breast. Causes include the following:

- *drugs*: digoxin, spironolactone, cimetidine, oestrogens or androgens;
- *cirrhosis of the liver*;
- *renal failure*;
- *hypogonadism*;
- *suprarenal tumours*;
- *testicular tumours*;
- *idiopathic*.

Clinical features

Gynaecomastia presents as a diffuse, bilateral soft swelling but may be unilateral. In patients with any suspicious features (firm or eccentric lump or skin changes), carcinoma must be excluded.

Treatment

The majority of cases will resolve with no intervention. Patients with gynaecomastia that does not settle, is symptomatic or which causes embarrassment may be offered surgery. Current surgical practice favours liposuction and/or excision biopsy.

Tumours

Classification

Benign

- Intraduct papilloma.
- Phyllodes tumour.

Malignant

1 *Primary*:
   a duct carcinoma *in situ*;
   b invasive duct carcinoma;
   c lobular carcinoma *in situ*;
   d invasive lobular carcinoma;
   e inflammatory carcinoma;
   f Paget's disease of the nipple;
   g sarcoma.
2 *Secondary*:
   a direct invasion from tumours of the chest wall;
   b metastatic deposits, e.g. from melanoma.

Intraduct papilloma

A benign neoplasm which may be single or multiple and which usually arises in the subareolar ducts. It presents with watery-clear or blood-stained nipple discharge from a single duct. If the papilloma is large, there may be a palpable mass in the periareolar area.

Treatment involves excision of the affected duct (microdochectomy) through a circumareolar incision.

Phyllodes tumour

Although phyllodes[6] tumours have many of the clinical features of fibroadenomas, they are true neoplasms with a wide range of characteristics from benign to malignant. They arise from stromal cells in the breast and are classified as low, intermediate or high grade depending on their microscopic features. They rarely metastasize but can recur locally if inadequately excised.

Clinical features

These lesions usually present as a firm, discrete lump and patients may note a recent increase in size. They should be investigated by triple assessment to confirm the diagnosis.

Treatment

All phyllodes tumours should be treated by wide excision to achieve a clear margin around the tumour. In large lesions, this may require mastectomy with immediate reconstruction.

Carcinoma

This is an immensely important subject – the commonest malignant disease in the UK, with 45000 new cases and about 12000 deaths annually; one in nine women will develop breast cancer during their lifetime. One in 10 breast lumps referred to a breast clinic will prove to be malignant.

Aetiology

There is an increased incidence of breast cancer with age, and, although any age may be affected, it is rare below the age of 30 years and 80% of cases

[6]Phyllodes means 'leaf-like', a reference to the lobulated appearance of the cut surface of the tumour.

occur in women aged 50 and over. In addition, the following have been identified as important risk factors.

Genetic factors

The majority of breast cancers are sporadic in nature, with up to 10% due to genetic predisposition.

- *Family history.* A premenopausal first-degree relative (mother or sister) with breast cancer confers a lifetime risk of 25%, which reduces to 14% if the same relative is postmenopausal. If both mother and sister develop premenopausal breast cancer, the risk is 33%.
- *Gene carriage.* Two inherited susceptibility genes have been identified, *BRCA1* and *BRCA2*. These are autosomal dominant genes with variable penetrance of 80–90%. An individual whose mother carries a mutation in one of these genes has a 50% chance of inheriting that mutation, which will confer a lifetime risk of 80–90%. The presence of a mutation in *BRCA1* also confers an increased risk of ovarian cancer. The carriage rate for the *BRCA1* mutation is 1 in 300 women.

Hormonal factors

A number of hormonal factors lead to minor increases in breast cancer risk; most correlate with increased exposure to oestrogens.

- *Gender*: women are 100 times more likely to have a breast carcinoma than men.
- *Menarche and menopause*: early age at menarche (under 12 years) and late menopause (over 50 years) are associated with a twofold higher risk.
- *Parity*: nulliparous women have a higher risk than multiparous women; later age at first pregnancy increases risk compared with younger age. Breast-feeding may contribute to reducing overall risk.
- *HRT* may slightly increase the incidence of breast cancer, with the risk proportional to the length of treatment.
- *Oral contraceptive users* have a small (1.25 times) increased risk, which returns to normal over time after stopping the pill.
- *Obesity* confers a 30% increase in risk in postmenopausal women.

Benign breast disease

A number of benign breast conditions are known to carry an increased risk of breast cancer. The presence of atypical lobular or ductal hyperplasia confers a four- to fivefold increased risk.

Radiation exposure

Exposure to ionizing radiation in adolescence or early adulthood can cause marked increases in breast cancer risk. Young women treated with mantle radiotherapy for lymphoma may have a substantial increased risk, especially if they were under the age of 20 during treatment.

Pathology

Breast cancers arise in the terminal duct lobular unit, either from the ductal epithelium or from the lobular epithelium (Figure 35.1). Carcinomas

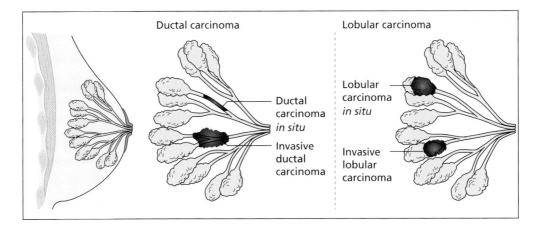

Figure 35.1 The different origins of *in situ* and invasive ductal and lobular carcinomas.

which have not penetrated through the basement membrane are known as carcinoma *in situ*.

Ductal carcinoma *in situ*

Ductal carcinoma *in situ* (DCIS) arises in the duct epithelium and is completely retained within the ducts; it is the most common type of non-invasive breast cancer. It usually occurs in localized areas of the breast, but may be extensive; untreated it will become invasive. DCIS is generally asymptomatic, appearing as a mammogram finding, sometimes with microcalcification. Because of its malignant potential, treatment is complete excision of the disease, and extensive disease (≥4 cm) may necessitate mastectomy.

Lobular carcinoma *in situ*

Lobular carcinoma *in situ* (LCIS) arises in the lobular epithelium. It is a marker of increased risk of breast cancer (approximately 20% over a 20 year period). An incidental finding of LCIS on diagnostic biopsy requires no surgery. However, when LCIS is found on core biopsy of an area of mammographic calcification, it may be associated with invasive lobular carcinoma and therefore formal diagnostic excision biopsy should be considered.

Invasive ductal carcinoma

This is the most common type of breast cancer, accounting for about 85% of all breast cancers. It is often described as being of 'no special type' (NST) to distinguish it from 'special types' of cancer such as invasive lobular cancer or rarer tumours such as tubular, cribriform, mucinous and medullary carcinomas.

Invasive lobular carcinoma

Invasive lobular carcinoma accounts for about 10% of breast cancers and is most common between the ages of 45 and 55. It does not always form a firm lump but rather an area of thickening, so tends to present late.

Spread

- *Direct extension.* Involvement of skin and subcutaneous tissues leads to skin dimpling, retraction of the nipple and eventually ulceration. Extension deeply involves pectoralis major, serratus anterior and, eventually, the chest wall.
- *Lymphatic.* Blockage of dermal lymphatics leads to cutaneous oedema pitted by the orifices of the sweat ducts, giving the appearance of *peau d'orange* (orange peel). Dermal lymphatic invasion produces daughter skin nodules and eventually 'cancer *en cuirasse*', the whole chest wall becoming a firm mass of tumour tissue (a cuirasse was an armour breastplate made of leather). The main lymph channels pass directly to the axillary and internal thoracic lymph nodes (Figure 35.2). Later, spread occurs to the supraclavicular, abdominal, mediastinal, groin and contralateral axillary nodes.
- *Bloodstream.* Blood-borne spread is most commonly to lungs, liver and bones (at the sites of red bone marrow, i.e. skull, vertebrae, pelvis, ribs, sternum, upper end of femur and upper end of humerus). The brain, ovaries and suprarenals are also frequent foci of deposits.

Prognostic factors

A number of prognostic factors are routinely determined following breast cancer surgery to help predict the outcome of an individual patient and help plan adjuvant systemic therapy.

- *Axillary node spread.* The best single determinant of prognosis; the greater the number of ipsilateral nodes involved, the worse the prognosis.
- *Tumour size.* The size of a tumour has a positive correlation with the metastatic potential. Larger tumours are therefore more likely to be lymph node positive and to have a worse survival.
- *Tumour grade.* Breast carcinoma is graded according to the level of differentiation. Histological grading is classified as I, II or III based on a scoring system comprising three components: tubular differentiation, nuclear pleomorphism and mitotic rate. Grade I tumours (well differentiated) have a better prognosis than grade III tumours (poorly differentiated), the latter being associated with a 5 year survival of approximately 45%.
- *Nottingham Prognostic Index (NPI).* Nodal status, tumour size and histological grade can be combined to form a prognostic index estimating long-term (10 year) survival. The NPI is calculated as follows:

$$NPI = 0.2 \times \text{tumour diameter (cm)} + \text{grade} + \text{nodal status}$$

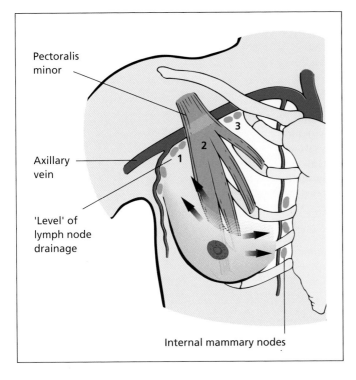

Figure 35.2 The lymphatic drainage of the breast.

Table 35.1 Nottingham Prognostic Index (NPI) and 10 year survival

NPI	Prognostic group	10 year survival (surgery alone) (%)	10 year survival (surgery and adjuvant therapy) (%)
<2.4	Excellent	95	95
2.41–3.4	Good	85	90
3.41–4.4	Moderate 1	70	79
4.41–5.4	Moderate 2	50	71
>5.4	Poor	20	41

where tumour grade is scored between 1 and 3, and nodal status between 1 (no affected nodes) and 3 (more than three nodes affected).

Table 35.1 describes 10 year survival data, in five prognostic groups according to NPI, for patients treated by surgery alone and shows the improvement with adjuvant therapy particularly in the poor prognosis (higher NPI) group.

Additional prognostic factors in invasive breast cancer include:

- *vascular invasion* by the tumour signifies a poor prognosis, even in the absence of nodal involvement;

- *hormone (oestrogen and/or progesterone) receptor expression* implies a less aggressive hormone-responsive tumour;
- *human epidermal growth factor receptor 2 (HER2) overexpression* signifies a more aggressive tumour;
- *histological type*: mucinous, tubular and cribriform tumours have a better prognosis.

Clinical features

The majority of patients with invasive carcinoma will present with a lump in the breast. Other features that warrant urgent investigation include altered breast contour, recent nipple inversion, blood-stained nipple discharge and unilateral nipple eczema (Paget's disease).

The breasts are inspected with the patient both lying supine and sitting with the arms elevated. The latter often accentuates any skin tethering or dimpling. Any evidence of nipple inversion or eczema should be noted.

Palpation should be with the flat of the hand with the patient lying flat and the head supported. Both breasts and both axillae should be examined as well as the supraclavicular fossae. Any lump should be carefully examined for evidence of skin or muscle fixation and the clinical size and position in relation to the nipple noted. Large, firm nodes in the axilla may suggest metastatic disease. In patients with suspected tumours, liver palpation and chest auscultation should be performed.

Special investigations

Diagnostic investigations

The diagnosis of breast carcinoma is made by triple assessment comprising clinical examination, imaging (mammography and/or ultrasound) and biopsy (see p. 296). In the vast majority of cases the diagnosis has been confirmed prior to surgery.

Staging investigations

Depending on the size of the tumour, and the presence of other symptoms, the following investigations may be indicated to assess the extent of spread when it may affect management:

- *full blood count*: anaemia and leucopenia suggest widespread bone marrow involvement;
- liver function tests;
- chest X-ray;
- isotope bone scan;
- liver ultrasound. The liver and chest imaging may alternatively be performed by computed tomography.

Staging

Cancers should be staged using the TNM classification. It should be noted that the TNM classification was originally based on clinical examination. As clinical staging can be inaccurate, a 'pathological TNM' classification is now used. The TNM staging for breast cancer is shown in Table 35.2.

Table 35.2 TNM staging for breast cancer.

TNM staging

T	Primary tumour
TX	Primary tumour cannot be assessed
T0	No evidence of primary tumour
Tis	Carcinoma *in situ* (DCIS, LCIS or Paget's disease with no invasive tumour)
T1	Tumour 2 cm or less in greatest dimension
T2	Tumour >2 cm and <5 cm in greatest dimension
T3	Tumour >5 cm in greatest dimension
T4	Tumour of any size with skin or chest wall involvement
N	**Regional lymph nodes**
NX	Regional lymph nodes cannot be assessed (e.g. previously removed)
N0	No regional lymph node metastasis
N1	Metastasis to movable ipsilateral axillary nodes
N2	Metastasis to fixed ipsilateral axillary lymph nodes
N3	Metastasis to ipsilateral internal thoracic (mammary) nodes
M	**Distant metastasis**
MX	Distant metastasis cannot be assessed
M0	No distant metastasis
M1	Distant metastasis

Treatment

The treatment of breast cancer involves a multidisciplinary approach comprising the following elements:

1 Surgery.
   a *Tumour excision.* Surgery depends on the pathological type of the tumour, so that surgery for lobular carcinoma *in situ*, ductal carcinoma *in situ* and invasive cancer all differ.
   b *Surgery to the axilla* also varies according to histological type.
   c *Breast reconstruction.*
2 Adjuvant systemic therapy.
   a *Hormonal therapy.*
   b *Chemotherapy.*
3 Adjuvant radiotherapy.

Tumour excision

- *Wide local excision.* A cylinder of breast tissue is excised down to the pectoral muscle in order to achieve complete excision ('clear resection margins'). Postoperative radiotherapy to the breast is routine after such a procedure. For lumps of 4 cm or less, there is good evidence that such an approach is equally as effective as mastectomy with regard both to local control and to survival.
- *Mastectomy.* A simple mastectomy involves excising the breast tissue. It is usually combined with reconstructive surgery to restore the breast contour. Axillary surgery is performed at the same time. The combination of mastectomy and axillary clearance avoids the need for postoperative radiotherapy in most cases, although this depends on axillary node status and tumour size and grade.

Surgical treatment of invasive ductal or lobular carcinoma

The aims of surgery are to remove the primary tumour and involved lymph nodes, to determine prognosis and to plan systemic therapy. Small tumours (<3 cm) may be suitable for breast-conserving surgery (wide local excision). Larger tumours (>3 cm), central tumours or multifocal tumours require mastectomy with or without breast reconstruction (see below). Other indications for mastectomy include patient preference and local recurrence following breast-conserving surgery.

Surgical management of the axilla

Axillary node status is the most important prognostic indicator in the treatment of invasive breast cancer. As a result, axillary surgery should be performed on all patients with invasive operable breast cancer, but is not generally required for *in situ* disease. There are two surgical options:

- *Sentinel lymph node (SLN) biopsy*, in which the first axillary lymph node(s) draining the cancer field is identified, excised and examined for metastatic tumour. An intradermal, periareolar injection of blue dye and radioisotope has been shown to be the most sensitive method for identifying the sentinel node(s) with the fewest false-negative results. Patients with a negative SLN require no further axillary surgery.
- *Axillary sampling.* A minimum of four nodes should be removed for histological analysis. If any of the four nodes are positive for tumour, then further treatment is necessary by axillary radiotherapy or surgical 'clearance' of the axilla, removing all nodes lateral and deep to pectoralis minor (level II) (Figure 35.2). The use of blue dye (as for SLN) may increase the sensitivity of axillary sampling (blue dye-assisted sampling).

Breast reconstruction

Breast reconstruction does not appear to impede the ability to detect local recurrence and may be of psychological benefit. It may be performed either at the time of mastectomy or as a delayed procedure. The combination of skin-sparing mastectomy and immediate breast reconstruction has been reported to produce better cosmetic results.

The possibility of immediate breast reconstruction should be discussed with suitable patients prior to mastectomy. The choice of reconstruction for an individual patient will depend on several factors, including breast size, the adequacy of skin flaps, whether radiotherapy is planned or has previously been used, abdominal size and previous abdominal operations, the patient's concern about silicone and the patient's preference. Typical reconstructions involve the use of myocutaneous flaps of latissimus dorsi or rectus abdominis, augmented when necessary with a silicone implant.

Adjuvant systemic therapy

Adjuvant systemic therapy using cytotoxic agents and/or endocrine therapy improves survival, with greatest benefit in those women at greatest risk of relapse.

The choice of adjuvant systemic therapy will be based on known prognostic factors that predict relapse and survival, including node status, histological grade and tumour size, oestrogen receptor (ER) status and menopausal status. The NPI may help to categorize this risk and select appropriate adjuvant therapy (see p. 303).

- *Endocrine therapy.* Tamoxifen, an oestrogen receptor antagonist, reduces the incidence of recurrence and is particularly effective in women in whom nodal spread was present and in women with ER-positive tumours. Ovarian ablation (by radiotherapy, surgery or drug therapy) is indicated in premenopausal women with ER-positive tumours.

- *Combination chemotherapy (e.g. anthracyclines and taxanes)* also reduces the probability of recurrence.
- *Trastuzumab (Herceptin),* a monoclonal antibody to HER2, has been shown to be an effective therapy in HER2-positive metastatic disease. HER2 is overexpressed in 15–20% of all breast cancers and is associated with a more aggressive breast cancer with a worse prognosis.

A suggested outline for adjuvant systemic therapy is as follows:

1 Premenopausal women.
   a *Low-risk disease*: tamoxifen if ER positive.
   b *Intermediate/high-risk disease and ER-positive tumours*: chemotherapy and tamoxifen possibly with ovarian ablation. Trastuzumab if HER2 positive.
   c *Intermediate/high-risk disease which is ER negative*: chemotherapy.
2 Postmenopausal women.
   a *Low-risk disease*: tamoxifen if ER positive.
   b *Intermediate/high-risk disease*: chemotherapy, with tamoxifen if ER positive. Trastuzumab if HER2 positive.

Adjuvant radiotherapy

- *Following wide local excision.* Following breast-conserving surgery, such as wide local incision for invasive cancer, radiotherapy significantly reduces the risk of recurrence within the breast.
- *Following mastectomy.* Radiotherapy after mastectomy reduces the risk of local recurrence. In premenopausal women receiving adjuvant chemotherapy, postmastectomy radiotherapy may also improve survival. The factors associated with a high risk of local recurrence are tumour size, high grade, nodal involvement, lymphatic invasion and involvement of deep margins.
- *Following axillary surgery.* After all forms of axillary surgery, the decision as to whether the axilla should be irradiated represents a balance between the risks of recurrence and the risk of morbidity. After axillary sampling, the axilla should be irradiated only if node positive or inadequately sampled. After axillary clearance, the axilla is not normally irradiated. If there is doubt about residual disease in the axilla

following axillary clearance, then radiotherapy should be considered.

Survival

Several factors are thought to have contributed to increased survival rates for breast cancer, including breast screening, specialist multidisciplinary teams and more individualized treatment plans that optimize each aspect of patient treatment. The 10 year survival is now 72%, with 64% of all women surviving for 20 years as compared with 44% in the 1980s. These figures are likely to improve with recent advances in hormone therapy, chemotherapy and targeted therapies such as trastuzumab.

Inoperable and locally advanced tumours

Locally advanced breast cancers are usually defined as tumours greater than 5 cm with or without involved axillary lymph nodes or skin involvement. For the majority of these patients, the initial management will be non-surgical. In patients with locally advanced breast cancer, the overall response rates to chemotherapy are good, although the rate of complete pathological response is rarely more than 15%. As a result, the majority of these patients subsequently proceed to surgery and/or radiotherapy. Radiotherapy is not recommended as sole treatment for local control of advanced disease but may be an option in those patients unfit for chemotherapy or surgery, for ulcerating tumours or for ER-negative tumours.

Inflammatory breast cancer

Inflammatory breast cancer is rare, representing only 2% of breast cancers. The breast appears swollen, red, firm and warm to touch, all cardinal features of inflammation. Symptoms can appear quite quickly as cancer cells block the small lymphatics in the breast, and mastectomy is usually required. It is an aggressive disease associated with 5 and 10 year survival rates of the order of 50% and 30%, respectively. The combination of chemotherapy, surgery and chest wall radiotherapy is accepted as achieving the highest local control and survival. The majority of these tumours will be ER negative; tamoxifen is indicated if they are ER positive.

Patients unfit for surgery

These will usually be elderly patients, and some may have locally advanced tumours. The principles of management are closer to those for metastatic disease, the aim of therapy being to control the primary tumour while maintaining the best quality of life. Many patients will respond to tamoxifen or other hormonal therapy.

Metastatic disease

The aim of treatment is to relieve symptoms while maintaining the highest quality of life. All patients with metastatic disease should be considered for some form of systemic therapy. Hormone therapy is less toxic than chemotherapy and is therefore often used as the first line of treatment. Patients who have had a long disease-free interval and/or soft tissue or bony metastases will often respond to hormone therapy, as will ER-positive tumours.

For patients with advanced visceral disease (e.g. liver metastases), the response to hormone therapy is low and these patients should be considered for chemotherapy. As the disease progresses patients may require referral to palliative care specialists for control of symptoms and to augment support for patients and carers.

Carcinoma of the male breast

This accounts for less than 1% of all cases of breast cancer. In men, breast cancer affects an older age group, with a peak incidence at 60 years.

Clinically, it usually presents as a firm, painless, subareolar lump, although gynaecomastia, breast tenderness and nipple discharge may also be present. Microscopically, it is usually a ductal carcinoma, and is quite advanced at presentation.

Treatment consists of an extended mastectomy with lymph node clearance. As so little skin is available, it may be necessary to perform reconstruction with a latissimus dorsi flap to cover the resulting cutaneous defect. For *in situ* disease, simple mastectomy will suffice.

The prognosis for men is worse than for women, probably because of the sparse amount of breast tissue present, which allows rapid dissemination of the growth into the regional lymphatics.

Postoperative radiotherapy reduces the incidence of local recurrence, but does not affect overall survival; most tumours respond to tamoxifen, which is therefore given as adjuvant therapy. For advanced disseminated disease, chemotherapy can produce reasonable palliation.

Paget's disease of the nipple

Presentation

Paget's[7] disease of the nipple occurs in middle-aged and elderly women. It presents as a unilateral red, bleeding, eczematous lesion of the nipple and areolar epithelium. Histologically, the epithelium of the nipple is thickened, with multiple clear malignant 'Paget cells' with small dark-staining nuclei; these are hydropic malignant cells. It is associated with an intraduct carcinoma of the underlying breast in 50% of cases, which may or may not form a palpable mass. Diagnosis is confirmed by biopsy.

Treatment

Treatment will be determined by any underlying breast carcinoma detected on clinical or radiological investigation. Surgical management includes mastectomy and axillary surgery for lesions associated with invasive disease. In the absence of invasive disease, or if a small central tumour lies close to the nipple, cone excision of the nipple and underlying tissue followed by breast radiotherapy may be considered.

Breast screening

A number of trials have demonstrated a reduction in breast cancer mortality for women aged 50–70 who undergo breast screening. Screen-detected cancers tend to be smaller and node negative with an increasing detection rate of *in situ* disease. As a result, women aged 50–70 in the UK are offered 3 yearly mammographic screening and there are plans to extend this further to cover the age range from 47 to 73 years. Recent evidence suggests that the screening programme is now contributing to reductions in breast cancer mortality rates in the UK.

[7]Sir James Paget (1814–1899), Surgeon, St Bartholomew's Hospital, London, UK. He also described diseases of the bone and penis, and discovered the parasite of trichinosis in humans while a first-year medical student.

36

The neck

Learning objectives

✓ To know the different causes of neck lumps.

✓ To know about the origin, presentation and management of branchial cysts.

The thyroid gland is considered separately in Chapter 37, and the parathyroids in Chapter 38. A summary of the possible causes of a lump in the neck is given in Box 36.1.

Branchial cyst and sinus

Anatomy

There are six arches and five clefts in the branchial system (Figure 36.1). The first arch forms the lower face, its external cleft the external auditory meatus, and its internal cleft the eustachian tube. The second arch grows down over the third and fourth arches to form the skin of the neck. Normally, there is no external cleft, while the internal cleft forms the tonsillar fossa.

Aetiology

Persistence of remnants of the second branchial arch may lead to formation of a branchial cyst, sinus or fistula. The external cleft remnants open just anterior to the sternocleidomastoid, at the junction of the upper one-third and lower two-thirds. A sinus or fistula represents a patent second branchial arch sinus, which passes between the internal and external carotid artery to the tonsillar

Lecture Notes: General Surgery, 12th edition. © Harold Ellis, Sir Roy Y. Calne and Christopher J. E. Watson. Published 2011 by Blackwell Publishing Ltd.

fossa. That a branchial cyst is a remnant of the second branchial arch has been questioned, based on the observation that the cysts are lined with stratified squamous epithelium rich in lymphatic tissue. This countertheory suggests that the cyst arises from cystic degeneration of lymphoid tissue in the neck and is thus better termed a lateral cervical cyst.

Clinical features

A *branchial cyst* usually presents in early adult life and forms a soft swelling 'like a half-filled hot water bottle', which bulges forward from beneath the anterior border of the sternocleidomastoid. It is lined by squamous epithelium and contains pus-like material, which is in fact cholesterol. It often presents following an upper respiratory tract infection. Clinical diagnosis can be clinched by aspirating a few drops of this fluid from the cyst and demonstrating cholesterol crystals under the microscope. Occasionally, the cyst may become infected.

Differential diagnosis is from a tuberculous gland of the neck or from an acute lymphadenitis.

The rare *first branchial arch cyst* may present just below the external auditory meatus at the angle of the jaw, with extension closely related to the VII nerve.

A *branchial sinus* presents as a small orifice, discharging mucus, which opens over the anterior border of the sternocleidomastoid in the lower part of the neck. The majority are present at birth but a secondary branchial sinus may form

Box 36.1 **A lump in the side of the neck**

When considering the swellings that may arise in any anatomical region, one enumerates the anatomical structures lying therein and then the pathological swellings that may arise from them. The side of the neck is an excellent example of this exercise.

Skin and superficial fascia

- Sebaceous cyst
- Lipoma

Lymph nodes

- Infective
- Malignant
- The lymphomas, lymphatic leukaemia (Chapter 34, p. 292).

Lymphatics

- Cystic hygroma

Artery

- Carotid body tumour
- Carotid artery aneurysm

Salivary glands

- Submandibular salivary tumours or sialectasis
- Tumour in the lower pole of the parotid gland

Pharynx

- Pharyngeal pouch

Branchial arch remnant

- Branchial cyst

Bone

- Cervical rib

if an infected branchial cyst ruptures, or if part of the cyst is left behind at operation. The sinus extends upwards between the internal and external carotid arteries to the sidewall of the pharynx. It may open into the tonsillar fossa (which represents the second internal cleft) to form a branchial fistula.

Treatment

Surgical excision is required.

Tuberculous cervical adenitis

With a general decline in tuberculosis, this once common lesion (mainly of children) is now relatively rarely seen in the UK, except in the aged, those with acquired immune deficiency syndrome (AIDS) and immigrants from developing countries. Cervical nodes are usually secondarily involved from a tonsillar primary focus, although the adenoids or even the dental roots may occasionally be the primary source of infection. The organisms may be human or bovine, and occasionally the disease is secondary to active pulmonary infection. The upper jugular chain of nodes is most commonly affected.

Clinical features

At first, the nodes are small and discrete; then, as they enlarge, they become matted together and caseate, and the abscess so formed eventually bursts through the deep fascia into the subcutaneous tissues. This results in one pocket of pus deep to and one superficial to the deep fascia, both connected by a small track: a 'collar stud' abscess. Left untreated, this discharges onto the skin, resulting in a chronic tuberculous sinus.

Differential diagnosis

Solid nodes must be differentiated from acute lymphadenitis, one of the lymphomas or secondary deposits. The breaking down abscess must be differentiated from a branchial cyst (see above).

Diagnosis may be assisted by an X-ray of the neck; usually, the chronic tuberculous nodes show flecks of calcification.

Treatment

A full course of antituberculous chemotherapy is given. Small nodes are treated conservatively and the patient is kept under observation. If the nodes enlarge, e.g. to 1 cm or more in diameter, they should be excised. If the patient presents with a 'collar stud' abscess, the pus is evacuated, a search made for the hole penetrating through the deep fascia, and the underlying caseating node evacuated by curettage.

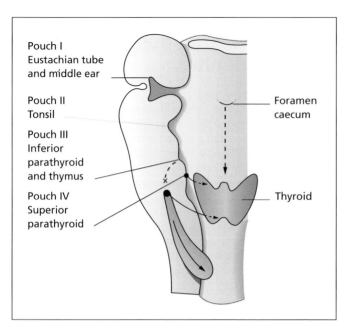

Pouch I
Eustachian tube
and middle ear

Pouch II
Tonsil

Pouch III
Inferior
parathyroid
and thymus

Pouch IV
Superior
parathyroid

Foramen
caecum

Thyroid

Figure 36.1 The derivatives of the branchial pouches and clefts. (Reproduced from Ellis H, Mahadevan V. (2010) *Clinical Anatomy*, 12th edn. Oxford: Wiley-Blackwell.)

It is not usually necessary to treat the infected tonsils or adenoids, as the infection resolves with the chemotherapy.

Carotid body tumour (chemodectoma)

Pathology

Also called carotid glomus tumours or paraganglionomas, these are slow-growing tumours that arise from the chemoreceptor cells in the carotid body at the carotid bifurcation. Most behave in a benign fashion; in a few patients, the tumour becomes locally invasive and may metastasize. There is a familial tendency to development of the tumour.

Macroscopically, it is a lobulated, yellowish tumour closely adherent to the internal and external carotid arteries at the bifurcation.

Microscopically, it is made up of large chromaffin polyhedral cells in a vascular fibrous stroma.

Clinical features

The tumour presents as a slowly enlarging mass in a patient over the age of 30 years, which transmits the carotid pulsation. The mass itself may be so highly vascular that it too demonstrates pulsation with a bruit on auscultation. Occasionally, pressure on the carotid sinus from the tumour produces attacks of faintness. Extension of the tumour may lead to cranial nerve palsies (VII, IX, X, XI and XII), resulting in dysphagia and hoarseness.

Special investigations

- *Duplex ultrasound* gives precise localization of the tumour and its relation to the carotid and its bifurcation.
- *Arteriography* shows the carotid bifurcation to be splayed open by the mass and the rich vascularity of the tumour is demonstrated.
- *Magnetic resonance imaging and computed tomography* show the tumour and its relation to the carotid artery, and have replaced arteriography in the assessment of the tumour.

Treatment

It is often possible to dissect the tumour away from the carotid sheath. If the carotid vessels are firmly involved, resection can be performed with graft replacement of the artery.

In the elderly, these slow-growing tumours can be left untreated, or treated with local radiotherapy (the 'Gamma knife').

37

The thyroid

Learning objectives
✓ To know the embryological course of the thyroid and related remnants.
✓ To know the causes of goitres and their treatments, and to have knowledge of thyroid cancers and their management.

Congenital anomalies

Embryology

The thyroid gland forms as a diverticulum originating in the floor of the pharynx, and descends through the tongue, past the hyoid, to its position in the neck. The diverticulum usually closes, leaving a pit at the base of the tongue (the foramen caecum, which lies in the midline at the junction of the anterior two-thirds and the posterior third of the tongue). Failure of the thyroid to descend or incomplete descent of the track may result in ectopic thyroid tissue (Figure 37.1). Incomplete obliteration of the track may result in fistula or sinus formation. In all cases of unexplained midline nodules in the neck, thyroid tissue should be suspected. A radioiodine scan should be performed to ensure that there is normal thyroid tissue present in the correct place before the lump is removed.

Lingual thyroid

Rarely, the thyroid fails to descend into the neck. Such a patient presents with a lump at the foramen caecum of the tongue. This is termed a lingual

Lecture Notes: General Surgery, 12th edition. © Harold Ellis, Sir Roy Y. Calne and Christopher J. E. Watson. Published 2011 by Blackwell Publishing Ltd.

thyroid, and may represent the sum total of thyroid tissue, or may be just a remnant that failed to descend.

Thyroglossal cyst

A thyroglossal cyst forms in the embryological remnants of the thyroid and presents as a fluctuant swelling in or near the midline of the neck. It is diagnosed by its characteristic physical signs.

1 It moves upwards when the patient protrudes the tongue, because of its attachment to the tract of the thyroid descent.
2 It moves on swallowing, because of its attachment to the larynx by the pretracheal fascia.

Treatment

Such cysts should be removed surgically, together with remnants of the thyroglossal tract and the body of the hyoid bone, to which the tract is closely related.

Thyroglossal fistula

This presents as an opening onto the skin in the line of the thyroid descent, in the midline of the neck. It may discharge thin, glairy fluid and attacks of infection can occur.

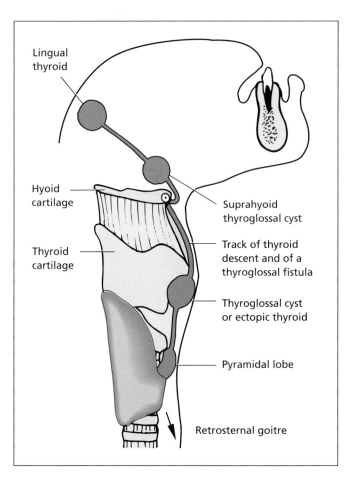

Lingual thyroid

Hyoid cartilage

Suprahyoid thyroglossal cyst

Track of thyroid descent and of a thyroglossal fistula

Thyroid cartilage

Thyroglossal cyst or ectopic thyroid

Pyramidal lobe

Retrosternal goitre

Figure 37.1 The descent of the thyroid, showing possible sites of ectopic thyroid tissue or thyroglossal cysts, and also the course of a thyroglossal fistula. (The arrow shows the further descent of the thyroid that may take place retrosternally into the superior mediastinum.)

Treatment

The treatment is to excise the fistula, and this excision must be complete. The track runs in close relationship to the body of the hyoid; therefore, this should be removed in addition to the fistula. Dissection is continued up to the region of the foramen caecum of the tongue.

Thyroid physiology

The thyroid gland is concerned with the synthesis of the iodine-containing hormones thyroxine (tetra-iodothyronine, T4) and tri-iodothyronine (T3), which control the metabolic rate of the body; T3 is the active hormone, and T4 is converted to T3 in the periphery. The thyroid gland also secretes calcitonin from the parafollicular C cells, which reduces the level of serum calcium and is therefore antagonistic to parathormone.

Iodine in the diet is absorbed into the bloodstream as iodide, which is taken up by the thyroid gland. After entering the follicle, the iodide is converted into organic iodine, which is then bound with the tyrosine radicals of thyroglobulin to form the precursors of the thyroid hormones. The colloid within the thyroid vesicles is composed of thyroglobulin, which is synthesized in the follicular cells, and T3 and T4. These hormones are released into the bloodstream after being separated from thyroglobulin within the follicular cells. In the general circulation, about 99% of T3 and T4 is bound to protein, and it is the minute amount of unbound 'free' thyroid hormones in the circulating blood that produces the endocrine effects of the thyroid gland.

Physiological control of secretion

The immediate control of synthesis and liberation of T3 and T4 is by thyroid-stimulating hormone (TSH) produced by the anterior pituitary. TSH is secreted in response to the level of thyroid hormones in the blood by a negative feedback mechanism. The secretion of TSH is also under the influence of the hypothalamic thyrotrophin-releasing hormone.

Pharmacological control of secretion

The production of thyroid hormones can be inhibited by the thiouracils and carbimazole, which block the binding of iodine but do not interfere with the uptake of iodide by the gland. Although less T3 and T4 is produced, the thyroid gland tends to become large and vascular with treatment by these drugs.

High doses of iodide given to patients with excessive thyroid hormone production result in an increase in the amount of iodine-rich colloid, and a diminished liberation of thyroid hormones; the gland also becomes less vascular. The effects of iodide treatment are maximal after 2 weeks of treatment and then diminish.

Lack of iodine in the diet prevents the formation of thyroid hormones, and excess pituitary TSH is produced, which may result in an iodine-deficient goitre. Thiocyanates prevent the thyroid gland from taking up iodide.

Pathology of goitre

The term 'goitre' is used to describe any enlargement of the thyroid gland irrespective of the underlying pathology. It includes colloid goitre (see below) and the hyperplasia of Graves' disease but the commonest cause is multinodular goitre.

Multinodular goitre

The aetiology of multinodular goitre is unclear. One hypothesis for its development is the presence of less differentiated cells in the adult thyroid gland that have a higher growth potential than normal follicular cells, some of which may replicate even in the absence of TSH. There is an excessive degree of activity and regression resulting in a varied appearance of the gland. Some follicles are lined with hyperactive epithelium and others with flattened atrophic cells. Some contain no colloid, others an excessive amount. The thyroid interstitium is excessive, with a certain amount of fibrosis and mononuclear cell infiltration. Nodular goitres may produce a normal amount of T4, but sometimes excessive T4 production results in hyperthyroidism in this condition ('secondary hyperthyroidism'). Radioactive iodine-131 is the treatment of choice in such cases.

The thyroid is usually enlarged, irregular and nodular and, although one lobe often predominates at presentation, the condition does affect the entire gland.

Symptoms

The enlarging thyroid can produce a number of 'pressure' symptoms including dysphagia, breathlessness, orthopnoea, hoarseness and facial swelling.

Investigation of multinodular goitre

Patients require two specific investigations:

- *TSH concentration* is low in the few patients with hyperthyroidism in association with multinodular goitre.
- *Computed tomography (CT) scan of the neck and thoracic inlet* to define the size of the goitre, the extent of the goitre including retrosternal extension, and to identify the presence of tracheal compression (Box 37.1).

Box 37.1 Symptoms of multinodular goitre

- *Dysphagia*: usually of solids, worse with certain food, e.g. meat

- *Breathlessness*: worse on exertion, bending forward (especially retrosternal extension)

- *Orthopnoea*: owing to the weight of the gland pressing on the trachea when lying flat

- *Hoarseness*: from pressure on one recurrent laryngeal nerve

- *Stridor*: from pressure on both recurrent laryngeal nerves or significant tracheal compression

- *Facial congestion*: venous engorgement especially on raising arms (Pemberton's sign[1])

---

[1]Hugh Spear Pemberton (1890–1956), Physician, Liverpool, UK.

Complications

- Tracheal displacement or compression.
- Haemorrhage into a cyst, producing pain and increased swelling (which may produce sudden tracheal compression).
- Toxic change.
- Malignant change (rare).

Colloid goitre (endemic goitre)

All diseases of the thyroid are more common in geographical locations in which the water and diet are low in iodine. In the UK, the most notorious district was Derbyshire, and the frequency of goitres in this region gave rise to the term 'Derbyshire neck'. Iodination of table salt has all but abolished this state of affairs. Switzerland, Nepal, Ethiopia and Peru are also areas where natural iodine is very scarce in the diet and water, and thyroid disease is common. The most common lesion of the thyroid gland due to iodine deficiency is the colloid goitre, in which the gland is enlarged and the acini are atrophic with a large amount of colloid. As has been mentioned, this accumulation of colloid is probably due to oversecretion of TSH from the anterior pituitary, acting on the thyroid, which is unable to produce T4.

Hyperplasia

In primary hyperthyroidism (Graves' disease[2]), the thyroid is uniformly enlarged and there is hyperactivity of the acinar cells with reduplication and infolding of the epithelium. The gland is very vascular and there is little colloid to be seen. Lymphocyte infiltration is usually a predominant feature.

Clinical features in thyroid disease

Patients may present complaining of a lump in the neck and/or with symptoms due to excessive or diminished amounts of circulating thyroxine.

[2]Robert Graves (1796–1853), Physician, Meath Hospital, Dublin, Ireland.

The thyroid swelling

The characteristics of an enlarged thyroid are a mass in the neck on one or both sides of the trachea, which moves on swallowing, since it is attached to the larynx by the pretracheal fascia.

Retrosternal goitre

Evidence of retrosternal enlargement of the thyroid should be sought by palpation and percussion with the neck fully extended. A retrosternal thyroid can block the venous return to the superior vena cava and result in engorgement of the jugular veins and their tributaries and in oedema of the upper part of the body – a cause of the superior mediastinal syndrome. In such cases, CT imaging of the thoracic inlet should be performed to assess its extent.

Tracheal displacement

The trachea should be examined to determine displacement or compression by the thyroid enlargement; the patient should be asked to take a deep breath with the mouth open, when stridor may become apparent.

Vocal cord integrity

The vocal cords should be examined by indirect laryngoscopy, as thyroid carcinoma may infiltrate the recurrent laryngeal nerves and cause vocal cord paralysis. If surgery is contemplated, it is important to know whether or not the cords are functioning normally before operation.

Regional nodes

As with any other lump, the regional lymph nodes must be examined in any case of thyroid swelling. The draining nodes of the thyroid lie along the carotid sheath on each side. Hard enlarged nodes strongly suggest malignant disease of the thyroid.

The physiological state of the patient

Determine whether the patient is euthyroid, hyperthyroid or hypothyroid. In the majority of patients, this can be determined from the clinical features.

Hyperthyroidism

Clinical features of hyperthyroidism are determined by examination of the eyes and the hands, as well as from the history and examination of the neck. Thyroxine potentiates the actions of adrenaline (epinephrine), and many of the features of hyperthyroidism represent increased activity of the sympathetic nervous system.

History

The patient is irritable and nervous, and cannot keep still. The appetite is increased and yet there is loss of weight; diabetes mellitus is the other condition in which this paradox occurs. Diarrhoea is occasionally a feature. The patient prefers cold environments rather than warm. Palpitations due to tachycardia or atrial fibrillation may occur.

Examination

The thyroid gland

The thyroid itself is usually smoothly enlarged but not invariably so. It may be highly vascular and demonstrate a bruit and thrill.

Eye signs

- *Exophthalmos* is present in most patients with hyperthyroidism of Graves' disease, owing to oedema and infiltration by mononuclear cells of the orbital fat and extrinsic muscles of the eye.
- *Lid retraction*: the innervation of the levator palpebrae superioris is partly under sympathetic control. In hyperthyroidism, it is tonically active, retracting the upper lid, giving the appearance that the patient is staring.
- *Lid lag*: ask the patient to follow your finger as you move it from over the head downwards – the upper lid does not immediately drop, revealing the white sclera above the cornea.
- *Dilated pupils* owing to increased sympathetic pupil dilator tone.
- *Double vision* following the examiner's finger to the upper outer quadrant. This is due to infiltration of the extrinsic muscles of the eye, which causes exophthalmic ophthalmoplegia.

Exophthalmos is an extremely distressing condition for the patient and, if severe, the patient is unable to close the eyelids; the eyes are then liable to corneal ulceration and eventual blindness. This condition is difficult to treat, but may respond to high-dosage corticosteroids; surgical decompression of the orbit with suture of the eyelids across the eyeball (tarsorrhaphy) may be required.

The hands

- *Sweating*: the hands are warm and moist.
- *Tachycardia*: a rapid pulse is almost invariable and typically the sleeping pulse is also raised. There may be atrial fibrillation and indeed the patient may present with heart failure. A rapid sleeping pulse rate permits differentiation of hyperthyroidism from an acute anxiety state; such patients when sleeping will have a normal pulse rate, whereas, in patients with hyperthyroidism, the sleeping pulse will remain elevated.
- *Fine tremor* of the outstretched hands is present and reflects the increased sympathetic activity.
- *Finger clubbing*, more accurately termed thyroid acropachy.
- *Onycholysis*: the nail lifts off the nail bed, a condition also seen in psoriasis and with some fungal infections.
- *Pretibial myxoedema*, thickening of the subcutaneous tissues in front of the tibia, is a rare feature.

Aetiology

Patients with hyperthyroidism fall into two groups, primary (Graves' disease) and secondary.

Primary hyperthyroidism (Graves' disease)

This occurs usually in young women with no preceding history of goitre. The gland is smoothly enlarged and exophthalmos common. Symptoms are primarily those of irritability and tremor; exophthalmos and ophthalmoplegia are often quite marked. Primary hyperthyroidism is due to the action of autoantibodies which bind to, and stimulate, the TSH receptor. These thyroid-stimulating antibodies have a prolonged stimulatory effect compared with TSH; hence, the traditional name of 'long-acting thyroid stimulators'.

Secondary hyperthyroidism

Secondary hyperthyroidism is overactivity developing in an already diseased and hyperplastic gland. It is a disease of middle age, occurring in patients with a pre-existing non-toxic (euthyroid) goitre. The gland is nodular and there are no eye changes. Symptoms fall more on the cardiovascular system, the patient often presenting in heart failure with atrial fibrillation, although nervousness, irritability and tremor may also be present.

Hypothyroidism

Congenital hypothyroidism

Congenital hypothyroidism or cretinism is a condition in which the child is born with little or no functioning thyroid. The infant is stunted and mentally subnormal, with puffy lips, a large tongue and protuberant abdomen, often surmounted by an umbilical hernia.

Adult hypothyroidism

In adults, hypothyroidism (or myxoedema) usually affects women, and most often occurs in the middle-aged or elderly. These patients have a slow, deep voice and are usually overweight and apathetic, with a dry, coarse skin and thin hair, especially in the lateral third of the eyebrows. In contrast with hyperthyroidism, myxoedematous patients usually feel cold in hot weather, have a bradycardia and are constipated. They are often anaemic and may suffer from heart failure owing to myxoedematous infiltration of the heart.

Investigations in thyroid disease

- *Serum free T4 and free T3*. Measurement of the biologically active unbound fraction is more accurate than measurement of total T3 and T4; elevation suggests hyperthyroidism.
- *TSH level*: raised in myxoedema; suppressed in hyperthyroidism, in which the gland secretes T4 autonomously.

- *Thyroid scintogram*: radioiodine studies of the thyroid gland provide very useful information. A small tracer dose of γ-ray-emitting iodine-131 is injected intravenously and the gland scanned with a γ-ray detector to map areas of high uptake reflecting high activity. A nodule in the thyroid gland that is hyperactive can be pinpointed by this method, a so-called 'hot nodule'. Similarly, a nodule that is not producing T4 will not take up the radioiodine, e.g. a cyst or tumour ('cold nodule').
- *Thyroid antibodies*, against thyroglobulin or the 'microsomal' antigen (now identified as thyroid peroxidase), indicate an autoimmune pathology such as Hashimoto's thyroiditis, or Graves' disease; other autoantibodies are often present.
- *Ultrasound* of the thyroid gives valuable information as to whether a mass is solid or cystic, unifocal or multifocal, and can be used to direct needle biopsy.
- *Fine-needle aspiration and core biopsy* allow material to be obtained for cytological and histological examination. It is now the principal investigation for all solitary nodules, often under ultrasound guidance.
- *Serum cholesterol* is usually raised in myxoedema and may be normal or a little low in hyperthyroidism.
- *Electrocardiogram (ECG)*: in myxoedema, cardiac involvement will show low electrical activity with small complexes. Atrial fibrillation complicating hyperthyroidism will be confirmed.
- *CT scan*: allows definition of size and extent of goitre and presence of tracheal compression.

Clinical classification of thyroid swellings

The clinical assessment of a patient with a thyroid swelling has two components:

1 The physical characteristics of the gland itself. Is it smoothly enlarged? Is there a single nodule present? Is it multinodular?
2 The endocrine state of the patient. Is the patient euthyroid, hyperthyroid or hypothyroid?

A synthesis of these two observations gives a simple clinical classification of the vast majority of thyroid swellings, as follows:

- *Smooth, euthyroid enlargement of the thyroid gland*: this is the 'physiological' goitre, which tends to occur at puberty and pregnancy.
- *Nodular, euthyroid gland*: this is the common nodular goitre, there being either a solitary nodule or multiple nodules.
- *Smooth, hyperthyroid goitre*: primary hyperthyroidism or Graves' disease.
- *Nodular hyperthyroid goitre*: secondary hyperthyroidism.

The less common findings are as follows:

- *Smooth, firm enlargement with myxoedema*: Hashimoto's disease (see p. 321). Usually in a middle-aged woman, and the gland is sometimes asymmetrical and irregular.
- *Invasive enlargement, hard*: carcinoma.

Riedel's thyroiditis and acute thyroiditis are uncommon (see p. 322).

Outline of treatment of goitre

Euthyroid nodular enlargement

Multinodular goitre

Thyroidectomy is advised in patients with an enlarged, euthyroid, nodular goitre when there are symptoms of tracheal compression and dyspnoea. In addition, in younger patients, it is reasonable to advise operation because of the danger of haemorrhage into a thyroid cyst with the risks of acute tracheal compression, and because of the small risk of toxic or malignant change in the gland. The patient may also be concerned with the cosmetic appearance of the swollen neck.

In elderly patients with a long-standing goitre that is symptomless, it is good practice to leave well alone.

T4 replacement may be effective by reducing TSH secretion, and so suppressing further enlargement. It is best given following thyroidectomy to suppress enlargement of the remaining gland tissue.

Single euthyroid nodule

In the patient with a single nodule in the thyroid, this may be a solitary benign adenoma, a malignant tumour or, most likely of all, a cyst in a thyroid showing the histological changes of a nodular goitre. Half of all solitary nodules are in fact prominent areas of multinodular goitres.

Traditionally, all solitary nodules were excised to make a diagnosis. Nowadays, fine-needle aspiration combined with isotope and ultrasound scans can usually differentiate nodules that should be excised from benign cysts. Cysts are aspirated, and checked at an interval to ensure that they do not re-collect. Cytology cannot distinguish benign adenomas from carcinomas, so these should all be excised.

Hyperthyroidism

The available therapy comprises the following:

- antithyroid drugs, of which carbimazole is the drug of choice;
- β-adrenergic blocking drugs;
- antithyroid drugs combined with subsequent thyroidectomy;
- radioactive iodine-131.

Carbimazole

This is given in a dosage of 10 mg 8 hourly, and is combined with sedation and bed rest in the acute phase of hyperthyroidism. There is rapid regression of symptoms, the patient beginning to feel better and to gain weight with reduction of tachycardia within 1–2 weeks. Treatment is continued for 12 months. If symptoms recur, a further 6 months' treatment is given, after which surgery is advised. Unfortunately, a high relapse rate (up to 60%) occurs after terminating the treatment, even if this is prolonged for 2 or more years. Medical treatment alone is therefore usually confined to the treatment of primary hyperthyroidism in children and adolescents.

The toxic effects of carbimazole include a drug rash, fever, arthropathy, lymphadenopathy and agranulocytosis; the last is a dangerous and potentially lethal complication, but occurs in well under 1% of patients. The first symptom is a sore throat and patients on carbimazole must be warned to discontinue treatment immediately if this occurs and to report to hospital. Granulocyte colony-stimulating factor may be required.

β-Adrenergic blocking drugs

In patients with severe hyperthyroidism, propranolol induces rapid symptomatic improvement of the cardiovascular features by blocking sympathetic overactivity, while the hyperthyroidism comes under control with specific antithyroid therapy.

Drugs and surgery combined

The majority of adult patients in the UK are treated with preliminary carbimazole until euthyroid; relapse after medical therapy is an indication for subtotal thyroidectomy. Most patients will be euthyroid following a course of drug therapy although 50% will relapse and require further drug treatment at a later stage. At that stage, the treatment options are either radioiodine or surgery. Radioiodine has a higher relapse rate than surgery, and a high incidence of late-onset hypothyroidism, but may be more suitable for treating older patients. It is not associated with increased malignancy.

The surgical management of primary hyperthyroidism (Graves' disease) is now usually limited to younger patients in their late teens or early twenties who have relapsed following their second course of drug treatment and who are looking for a long-term cure for their disease. The traditional operation for primary hyperthyroidism has been subtotal thyroidectomy in an attempt to render the patient euthyroid with no need for exogenous thyroxine. Unfortunately, most patients will require thyroxine replacement in time, and, by leaving too much thyroid tissue *in situ*, there is a risk of recurrence. As a result, total thyroidectomy is becoming the operation of choice for these patients in the same way as for patients with multinodular goitre.

Radioactive iodine

From the patient's point of view, this is the most pleasant treatment, as all the patient has to do is swallow a glass of water containing the radioiodine. There is no need for prolonged treatment with drugs or the risk of operation; it is particularly useful in recurrence of hyperthyroidism after thyroidectomy. It usually takes 2–3 months before the patient is rendered euthyroid. Antithyroid drugs,

with or without a beta-blocker, may be used to control symptoms during this time.

There is a theoretical risk of malignant change in the irradiated gland, although it is very uncommon. Nevertheless it is current practice not to use radioiodine in patients under the age 45 and, in addition, not to use it in young women who may become pregnant during treatment, as there is a very real danger of affecting the infant's thyroid. Another disadvantage of this treatment is the high incidence of late hypothyroidism, which rises to near 30% after 10 years and which requires replacement therapy with T4.

Complications of thyroidectomy

In addition to the hazards of any surgical operation, there are special complications to consider following thyroidectomy. These can be divided into hormonal disturbances (the thyroid itself and the adjacent parathyroid glands) and injury to closely related anatomical structures.

1 *Hormonal*:
   a paraesthesiae, owing to coincidental parathyroid removal or bruising;
   b tetany (parathyroid removal or bruising);
   c thyroid crisis;
   d hypothyroidism, owing to extensive removal of thyroid tissue;
   e late recurrence of hyperthyroidism owing to inadequate excision of the hyperthyroid gland.
2 *Damage to related anatomical structures*:
   a recurrent laryngeal nerve;
   b injury to trachea;
   c pneumothorax.
3 *The complications of any operation, especially*:
   a haemorrhage;
   b sepsis;
   c postoperative chest infection;
   d hypertrophic scarring (keloid).

Some of these complications require further consideration here.

Hypoparathyroidism

This may result from inadvertent removal of the parathyroids or their injury during operation. The patient may develop paraesthesia or tetany (Chapter 38, p. 323) a few days postoperatively with typical carpopedal spasms, which may be induced by tourniquet around the arm (Trousseau's sign, Chapter 38, p. 324), and a positive Chvostek's sign (Chapter 38, p. 324); this is elicited by tapping lightly over the zygoma, when the facial muscles will be seen to contract. The serum calcium falls to below 1.5 mmol/L.

Treatment

Treatment consists of giving 10 mL of 10% calcium gluconate intravenously followed by oral calcium together with vitamin D derivatives (ergocalciferol or alfacalcidol). Often, the tetany is transient and the injured parathyroids recover; in other cases, permanent treatment with alfacalcidol is required. Parathormone is not used.

In addition to frank tetany, which occurs in about 1% of cases, milder degrees of hypoparathyroidism may occur and may present with mental changes (depression or anxiety neurosis), skin rashes and bilateral cataracts. A low postoperative calcium is treated by the administration of oral calcium and/or vitamin D daily by mouth.

Thyroid crisis

An acute exacerbation of hyperthyroidism seen immediately postoperatively is now extremely rare because of the careful preoperative preparation of these patients. It is, however, a frightening phenomenon with mania, hyperpyrexia and marked tachycardia, which may lead to death from heart failure. The cause is not fully understood, but it may be due to a massive release of thyroxine from the hyperactive gland during the operation.

Treatment

Treatment comprises heavy sedation with barbiturates, propranolol, intravenous iodine and cooling by means of ice packs.

Recurrent laryngeal nerve injury

The recurrent laryngeal nerve lies in the groove between the oesophagus and trachea in close relationship to the inferior thyroid artery. Here it is at risk of division, injury from stretching or compression by oedema or blood clot.

If one nerve alone is damaged, the patient may have little in the way of symptoms apart from slight hoarseness because the opposite vocal cord compensates by passing across the midline during phonation. However, if both recurrent nerves are damaged there is almost complete loss of voice and serious narrowing of the airway; a permanent tracheostomy may be required, although an incomplete injury may recover in time. It is estimated that the nerve is injured in about 2–3% of thyroidectomies.

Vocal cord assessment by indirect laryngoscopy should be performed prior to thyroid surgery, and is essential for patients with known malignancy, previous neck surgery and for patients with hoarseness or stridor.

Haemorrhage

If this occurs shortly after thyroidectomy it is a dangerous condition, as bleeding into the thyroid bed may compress the trachea, which is already softened by pressure from the thyroid swelling. The neck becomes distended with blood; there is acute dyspnoea and stridor, as well as shock from blood loss.

Treatment

This may be an extreme emergency and must be dealt with at once by decompressing the neck in the ward. The skin and the subcutaneous sutures are removed, the wound is opened and the blood clot expressed. The patient can then be transferred to theatre, anaesthetized, bleeding points secured and the wound resutured.

Thyroid tumours

Classification

Benign

- Follicular adenoma.

Malignant

1 *Primary* (five main types):
   a papillary adenocarcinoma;
   b follicular adenocarcinoma;
   c anaplastic;
   d medullary carcinoma;
   e lymphoma (rare).
2 *Secondary*
   a direct invasion from adjacent structures, e.g. oesophagus;
   b very rare site for blood-borne deposits.

Benign adenoma

Although benign encapsulated nodules in the thyroid gland are common, the majority are part of a nodular colloid goitre. A small percentage represent true benign adenomas, of which 10% are 'hot nodules', i.e. they produce excess thyroxine. Thyroid adenomas are four times more common in women.

Thyroid carcinoma

Thyroid carcinoma affects women twice as often as men, often arising in pre-existing goitres, and has been reported following radiation of the neck in childhood. It has an incidence of around 2 in 100 000 and long-term survival rates following treatment are excellent. Forty year survival rates for papillary and follicular cancer are 94% and 84%, respectively. Papillary and follicular cancer, together referred to as differentiated thyroid cancer, account for approximately 90% of all thyroid cancers.

Differentiated thyroid cancer is usually curable when detected at an early stage. The high cure rate can be attributed to a multidisciplinary approach, including specialist surgery, radioiodine ablation, TSH suppression and, finally, the use of thyroglobulin as a thyroid-specific tumour marker. Despite this management strategy, a small number of patients will develop recurrence and 50% of thyroid cancer deaths will be due to respiratory failure secondary to either pulmonary metastasis or airway obstruction.

Pathology

Papillary carcinoma

This is the most common type of thyroid cancer, constituting 60% of thyroid cancers. It occurs in young adults, adolescents or even children. It is a slow-growing tumour and lymphatic spread occurs late. Deposits in the regional lymph nodes may be solitary and in the past have been mistakenly regarded as lateral aberrant thyroid tissue. However, a careful search of the thyroid gland will reveal a well-differentiated tumour in the ipsilateral lobe.

Follicular carcinoma

This occurs in young and middle-aged adults, the incidence peaking in the fifth decade. It is more common in areas where endemic goitres are common. It has a tendency to bloodstream spread and therefore a worsened prognosis; lymph node spread is uncommon.

Medullary carcinoma

This arises from the parafollicular C cells and may secrete calcitonin. It may occur at any age and, unlike other thyroid tumours, has a roughly equal sex distribution. It may be familial and may be associated with other cancers in the multiple endocrine neoplasia syndrome (type II, associated with phaeochromocytoma and either parathyroid tumours or neurofibromas; Chapter 38, p. 324). The characteristic finding is deposits of amyloid between the nests of tumour cells.

The disease is multicentric in all familial forms, usually affects both thyroid lobes and is associated with C cell hyperplasia. In contrast, the sporadic form is usually unifocal with no associated hyperplasia. The tumour cells produce calcitonin, which acts as a tumour marker and can be used as a screening test in syndromic families or to detect recurrence in follow-up of operated patients. Fine-needle aspiration cytology of medullary thyroid carcinoma may be diagnostic.

Anaplastic carcinoma

This occurs in the elderly, thus reversing the usual state of affairs, in that the more malignant tumours of the thyroid occur in the older age group. Rapid local spread takes place with compression and invasion of the trachea. There is early dissemination to the regional lymphatics and bloodstream spread to the lungs, skeleton and brain.

Clinical features

Tumours may present like other goitres as a lump in the neck, often more rapidly growing. Dysphagia is uncommon, and suggestive of an anaplastic tumour; more common is the complaint that swallowing is uncomfortable. Pain may occur with local infiltration, and hoarseness is suggestive of infiltration of the recurrent laryngeal nerve. Deep cervical lymph nodes may be palpably enlarged. The patients are usually euthyroid. Ultrasound-guided core needle biopsy or fine-needle aspiration cytology are used to confirm the diagnosis.

Treatment of differentiated thyroid cancer

Surgery

Well-differentiated tumours can be treated by a combination of surgery, thyroid suppression by thyroxine and radioiodine.

Total thyroidectomy should be considered for patients at high risk of recurrence according to prognostic scoring systems. Adverse prognostic factors, which increase risk of recurrence, include tumour size, presence of lymph node metastasis and older age (>45 years) at presentation. Furthermore, radioiodine ablation is facilitated by total thyroidectomy.

Thyroid lobectomy is therefore appropriate surgery for unifocal, papillary tumours less than 1 cm in diameter in the absence of lymph node metastasis. In addition, it may also be adequate for follicular tumours with minimal capsular invasion, small tumour size and no metastatic disease. Most other patients with differentiated thyroid cancer will require total thyroidectomy and possible radioiodine therapy.

Radioiodine ablation

Iodine-131 ablation of the thyroid bed and remnant has become an essential component of the treatment of differentiated thyroid cancer. First, a large remnant may obscure the presence of metastatic disease and, second, the high TSH levels required to enhance ^{131}I tumour uptake are not possible if a large remnant persists. Finally, ^{131}I will be taken up by any remaining thyroid tissue, either in the thyroid bed or in occult metastasis, thereby reducing the risk of tumour recurrence. In general, those patients who require total thyroidectomy may also require ^{131}I therapy.

Complications of ^{131}I therapy include oedema and swelling, or thyroiditis, in those patients with a large thyroid remnant. In addition, radiation sialadenitis affecting the parotid or submandibular glands may present with painful swelling of the gland(s) after eating. There are few long-term sequelae from radioiodine providing that the cumulative dose is kept to a minimum.

TSH suppression

Recurrence rates are reduced by postoperative thyroxine therapy although there is uncertainty about the optimal dose. At present, the minimum thyroxine dose to keep the serum TSH <0.03 U/L should be given. In general, this dose will be approximately double the normal replacement dose of thyroxine.

Thyroglobulin

Serum thyroglobulin is the best way of detecting the presence of normal or malignant thyroid tissue and most patients who are free of disease will have undetectable levels. In patients in whom the thyroglobulin rises during follow-up, careful clinical examination and whole body scanning should be performed to look for local or systemic recurrence.

Medullary carcinoma

Phaeochromocytoma and hyperparathyroidism should be excluded in the relevant syndromes. All patients with medullary carcinoma require total thyroidectomy and central lymph node dissection. Radical neck dissection may be required when cervical lymphadenopathy is present.

Prophylactic thyroidectomy is indicated in unaffected kindred members with the germline *RET* mutation. At present, this is often carried out in patients as young as 5–7 years old.

Anaplastic carcinoma

This condition has a very poor prognosis with a 1 year survival of <15%. The main aim of treatment following diagnosis is local control of the disease. Useful palliation may be achieved with external beam radiotherapy, and tracheostomy should be avoided if at all possible.

Hashimoto's disease

Hashimoto's disease[3] is an uncommon thyroid disease that has received considerable attention, as it was the first of the autoimmune diseases to be elucidated. The patient is usually a middle-aged woman with clinical evidence of hypothyroidism. The gland is uniformly enlarged and firm, although it may occasionally be asymmetrical and irregular.

Macroscopically, its cut surface is lobulated and greyish yellow. Microscopically, there is diffuse

[3]Hakaru Hashimoto (1881–1934), Surgeon, Kyushu University, Kyushu, Japan.

infiltration with lymphocytes, increased fibrous tissue and diminished colloid. It is an autoimmune disease in which the patient has developed both a humoral and cell-mediated autoimmune reaction to elements within her own thyroid. Thyroglobulin and microsomal antibodies can be demonstrated in about 90% of patients.

It is important to diagnose the condition correctly by demonstrating the presence of thyroid antibodies and, if necessary, by biopsy, because thyroidectomy will precipitate severe hypothyroidism in these cases. Occasionally, lymphoma occurs in such glands.

Treatment

Thyroxine replacement therapy of up to 300 μg/day will shrink the gland and the symptoms of myxoedema should disappear.

Riedel's thyroiditis

Riedel's thyroiditis[4] is an extremely rare disease of the thyroid in which the gland may be only slightly enlarged, but is woody hard with infiltration of adjacent tissues. The cause of this condition is not known, but it may represent a late stage of Hashimoto's disease or possibly be inflammatory in origin.

It is mistaken clinically for a thyroid carcinoma, but histologically the gland is replaced by fibrous tissue containing chronic inflammatory cells. It is associated with other conditions such as retroperitoneal fibrosis, sclerosing cholangitis and fibrosing mediastinitis.

A wedge resection of a portion of the gland may be required if symptoms of tracheal compression develop.

de Quervain's thyroiditis

de Quervain's thyroiditis[5] is a rare condition usually affecting young women. It often follows a viral infection of the upper respiratory tract. The gland is slightly enlarged, firm and tender. It is generally self-limiting, and rarely leads to hypothyroidism.

---

[4]Bernhard Riedel (1846–1916), Professor of Surgery, Jena, Germany.

[5]Fritz de Quervain (1868–1940), Professor of Surgery, Bern, Switzerland.

38

The parathyroids

Learning objective

✓ To know the presentations of both hypoparathyroidism and hyperparathyroidism and their management.

Anatomy and development

The parathyroids are four endocrine glands (sometimes three or five) about the size of split peas, which usually lie in two pairs behind the lateral lobes of the thyroid gland. The superior parathyroids arise from the fourth branchial pouch and owing to their short migration can usually be found posterior to the upper two-thirds of the thyroid. The inferior glands arise from the third pouch in association with the developing thymus (Figure 36.1, p. 310). The inferior parathyroids may lie almost anywhere in the neck or superior mediastinum although the majority lie within 1 cm of the lower thyroid pole.

Physiology

The parathyroids produce parathormone (PTH), which has profound influence on calcium and phosphate metabolism. The exact mechanisms of its action are not known, but there appear to be three main effects.

1 It increases the excretion of phosphate from the kidney by inhibiting its tubular reabsorption (phosphaturic effect); tubular reabsorption of calcium is reciprocally increased.

Lecture Notes: General Surgery, 12th edition. © Harold Ellis, Sir Roy Y. Calne and Christopher J. E. Watson. Published 2011 by Blackwell Publishing Ltd.

2 It stimulates osteoclastic activity in the bones, resulting in the decalcification and liberation of excessive amounts of calcium and phosphorus in the blood.
3 It activates the 1α-hydroxylase enzyme in the kidney, which converts the inactive 25-hydroxycholecalciferol (25-hydroxy-vitamin D) into 1,25-dihydoxycholecalciferol. The resultant activated 1,25 form of vitamin D facilitates intestinal absorption of calcium.

Effects of increased PTH production

- A raised serum calcium and a lowered serum phosphate, as these substances are related reciprocally.
- An increased excretion of phosphate in the urine (phosphaturic effect of PTH).
- An increased excretion of calcium in the urine. The large amount of calcium filtered (owing to the hypercalcaemia) exceeds the capacity of the tubules to reabsorb it all, so increased calcium excretion occurs.
- Increased osteoclastic activity, with a raised serum alkaline phosphatase associated with decalcification of the bones.

Hypoparathyroidism

Lack of PTH results in low serum calcium. This leads initially to paraesthesia (perioral and fingertips) then hyperirritability of skeletal muscle with carpopedal spasms, the syndrome being called *tetany*. The most common cause of this is removal or bruising of the parathyroids in thyroidectomy (Chapter 37, p. 318). Tetany is liable to occur if the serum calcium falls below 1.5 mmol/L.

Clinical features

Spasms may affect any part of the body, but typically the hands and feet. The wrists flex and the fingers are drawn together in extension, the so-called '*main d'accoucheur*'. This spasm may be induced by placing a tourniquet around the arm for a few minutes (Trousseau's sign[1]). Hyperirritability of the facial muscles may be demonstrated by tapping over the facial nerve, which results in spasm (Chvostek's sign[2]).

Note that clinical tetany may occur with a normal level of serum calcium in alkalosis (e.g. overbreathing, excessive prolonged vomiting) because of a compensatory shift of ionized calcium to the unionized form in the serum.

Hyperparathyroidism

There are four distinct types of pathologically increased PTH secretion: primary, secondary, tertiary and that due to ectopic PTH production by tumours.

Primary hyperparathyroidism

The diagnosis of primary hyperparathyroidism is made following the detection of hypercalcaemia in the presence of inappropriately normal or elevated circulating PTH levels; the PTH should be low if calcium is raised. The hypercalcaemia is usually discovered on routine screening of patients who have general symptoms including fatigue, depression and weakness or less commonly during the investigation of osteopenia or nephrolithiasis, the two main complications of hyperparathyroidism. The annual incidence is highest among middle-aged and elderly women (two per 1000 population).

---

[1]Armand Trousseau (1801–1867), Physician, Hôpital Necker, Paris, France. Also described thrombophlebitis migrans associated with cancer.
[2]Frantisek Chvostek (1835–1884), Physician, Josefs-Akademie, Vienna, Austria.

> **Box 38.1 Multiple endocrine neoplasia (MEN) syndromes**
>
> These syndromes are characterized by the development of a number of endocrine adenomas, or adenocarcinomas, in the same patient. Some, such as medullary carcinoma of the thyroid, may be familial, with autosomal dominant inheritance.
>
> **MEN type I**
> - Pancreatic tumour: islet cell tumours except beta-cell tumours (insulinoma)
> - Hyperparathyroidism
> - Pituitary tumour, e.g. prolactinoma
> - Adrenocortical tumour
>
> **MEN type II**
> - Medullary carcinoma of the thyroid
> - Phaeochromocytoma
> - Hyperparathyroidism – only in type IIA
> - Neurofibromas of tongue, lips and eyelids – only in type IIB

Pathology

In 85–90% of patients, primary hyperparathyroidism is due to a solitary parathyroid adenoma. The lower glands are affected more commonly than the upper ones. The tumours are soft, encapsulated and brownish grey in colour. In 10% of cases, multiglandular hyperplasia is present, which may be associated with multiple endocrine neoplasia (MEN) type I (pancreatic tumours, pituitary tumours, parathyroid tumours) (Box 38.1) or may be sporadic or induced by long-term lithium intake.

Parathyroid carcinoma

Parathyroid carcinoma is a very rare condition and accounts for less than 1% of all cases of primary hyperparathyroidism. Patients often have higher serum calcium and PTH levels, and are more likely to have a palpable neck mass than those with benign hyperparathyroidism.

Surgery is the only effective treatment. Malignancy should be considered with any gland that is firm, has a grey appearance, or that is adherent to surrounding structures. If malignancy is confirmed surgery may involve simple excision or *en bloc* resection, including excision of local structures such as ipsilateral thyroid, thymus, strap muscles and recurrent laryngeal nerve. Approximately 30% of tumours will metastasize, but death from the disease is usually attributable to hypercalcaemia, and its effects on the heart, pancreas and kidney, rather than metastatic tumour burden.

Secondary hyperparathyroidism

In some 10% of patients with hyperparathyroidism, the condition is found to be due to a hyperplasia of all four parathyroid glands. This occurs most commonly in patients with renal failure maintained by dialysis, in whom renal conversion of 25-hydroxycholecalciferol (calcidiol) to 1,25-dihydroxycholecalciferol (calcitriol) is impaired. This active form of vitamin D is required for absorption of calcium from the gut; deficiency results in hypocalcaemia, which chronically stimulates PTH production. The parathyroid glands undergo hyperplasia in response. To prevent this, dialysis patients are routinely given 1α-hydroxycholecalciferol (alphacalcidol), so bypassing renal 1α-hydroxylase.

Tertiary hyperparathyroidism

Prolonged secondary hyperparathyroidism leads to autonomous PTH production, which continues even after renal transplantation replaces the previously deficient renal 1α-hydroxylase conversion step. Total parathyroidectomy is required.

Ectopic PTH production

Hyperparathyroidism is occasionally due to ectopic PTH production by tumours, such as squamous carcinoma of the bronchus.

Clinical features of hyperparathyroidism

These depend on the results of excessive production of PTH by the tumour (see above). Presenting symptoms may include the following:

- *Renal effects*: renal stones, infection associated with renal calculi, calcification in the renal substance (nephrocalcinosis) or uraemia. Urinary tract calculi are the most common clinical manifestation of hyperparathyroidism. It is important to remember that chronic renal disease with impaired excretion of phosphate may result in secondary hyperplasia of the parathyroid glands with features similar to those of a primary adenoma of the parathyroid.
- *Bone changes*: spontaneous fractures or pain in the bones. X-ray will show decalcification of the bones with cyst formation. The weakened bones may be deformed; this condition is known as osteitis fibrosa cystica or von Recklinghausen's disease[3] of bone. There may be metastatic calcification in soft tissues, arterial walls and the kidneys.
- *Abdominal pain*: constipation is common. Dyspepsia or frank duodenal ulceration is also sometimes associated with parathyroid adenoma, as is pancreatitis. If ulcer symptoms persist after treatment of the adenoma, the presence of a gastrinoma should be excluded by serum gastrin assay (MEN syndrome association).
- *Vague ill-health associated with high serum calcium*: the patient very often complains of lassitude, mental disturbances, weakness, anorexia and loss of weight. Thirst and polyuria are common.
- *Cardiovascular*: hypertension may be noted at the initial diagnosis and is often associated with left ventricular hypertrophy. Although serum PTH correlates strongly with left ventricular mass, the reduction in left ventricular mass following parathyroidectomy is not associated with a similar reduction in mean blood pressure. Primary hyperparathyroidism appears to be associated with an increased rate of premature death owing to cardiovascular disease, although early surgical intervention may result in improved survival.
- *Asymptomatic*: an increasing number of patients with very few or no symptoms are now being diagnosed on routine biochemical screening. Despite this, the majority of these patients feel better following parathyroidectomy and this, combined with a recognition that up to 25% of patients will have progressive disease, has led to support for early surgical intervention following initial diagnosis.

[3]Friederich von Recklinghausen (1833–1910), Professor of Pathology, Strasbourg, France. He also described neurofibromatosis.

A careful family history should also be taken to exclude MEN and this, or presentation of primary hyperparathyroidism at an early age, should raise the suspicion of hyperplasia rather than an adenoma.

The main effects may be summarized as: 'stones, bones, abdominal groans, mental moans'.

Special investigations

Diagnostic investigations include the following:

- *Serum calcium and PTH.* A high serum calcium, corrected for plasma albumin, in the presence of detectable serum PTH should raise a strong suspicion of primary hyperparathyroidism. The PTH may be normal or elevated but in either case is *inappropriately elevated* for the level of serum calcium.
- *Serum phosphate* may be low (hypophosphataemia) and *phosphaturia* may also be present.
- *24 hour urine collection* should be taken to exclude familial hypocalciuric hypercalcaemia.
- *Serum urea and creatinine* should be measured to assess renal function.
- *Sestamibi* scanning will identify a solitary parathyroid adenoma, and highlight an ectopic retrosternal location. Sestamibi is technetium-99-labelled *methoxyisobutylisonitrile* and, following injection, is taken up by parathyroid glands and retained at 2 hours by adenomas.

Indications for surgery

Surgery should be considered in any patient once a diagnosis of primary hyperparathyroidism has been confirmed and even patients with mild hypercalcaemia get symptomatic benefit following surgery. When surgery is contraindicated in primary hyperparathyroidism, and in difficult to manage cases of secondary hyperparathyroidism, the calcimimetic drug cinacalcet may be used. Cinacalcet binds to the calcium-sensing receptor on the parathyroid chief cells, causing a reduction in PTH concentration.

Bilateral neck exploration

This procedure is normally carried out using endotracheal intubation and neck extension to facilitate access to the neck. Bilateral neck exploration is carried out through a transverse (Kocher's[4]) incision just above the clavicle to provide access to both retrothyroid spaces to detect and remove one or more enlarged glands.

If a single gland is enlarged, it is likely to be an adenoma and is removed once the remaining glands have been visualized and confirmed to be normal. Frozen section of the gland, or urgent 'near patient' estimation of PTH levels, will confirm the identity of the adenoma.

Unilateral neck exploration

Most (85–90%) patients with primary hyperparathyroidism have a single affected gland. Preoperative localization of the adenoma by sestamibi scanning enables unilateral neck exploration. Patients with multigland disease, MEN-related hyperplasia, familial hypocalciuric hypercalcaemia and renal disease are not suitable for this approach. In addition, patients with a short neck and previous neck surgery or irradiation may also not be suitable.

Focused parathyroidectomy

Following accurate preoperative localization of uniglandular disease, exploration is carried out through a small incision lateral in the neck. The patient is supine with the head in a neutral position. The technique develops the space between the lateral border of the strap muscles and sternomastoid to reach the retrothyroid space. This operation is suitable for day-case surgery and can be performed under either general anaesthesia or cervical local anaesthetic block.

This technique can be combined with intraoperative PTH measurement, a fall of at least 50% indicating removal of all hyperfunctioning parathyroid tissue. This technique has fewer overall complications, a shorter operating time and a substantially reduced postoperative stay compared with the traditional bilateral neck exploration.

Complications of parathyroid surgery

The main complications of parathyroid surgery include:

- *recurrent laryngeal nerve palsy*: occurs in under 1% of patients;

[4]Theodore Kocher (1841–1917), Professor of Surgery, Bern, Switzerland. Won a Nobel Prize in 1909 for work on the thyroid gland.

- *hypocalcaemia*: the remaining parathyroid glands are suppressed by the high PTH levels and may take some time to recover;
- *persistent hypercalcaemia*: residual parathyroid tissue remains, possibly a fifth gland or an ectopic gland within the anterior mediastinum.

Management of persistent or recurrent primary hyperparathyroidism

Despite careful initial surgery, a number of patients will not be cured following initial surgery or will relapse at a later stage. This is most often due to a failure to diagnose multigland disease or the presence of an ectopic parathyroid gland. These patients require extensive imaging (sestamibi, computed tomography and magnetic resonance imaging) prior to surgery to localize and remove the abnormal gland(s). Selective venous sampling, with PTH measurement by catheterization of the venous tributaries in the neck, may also help localization and is often combined with arteriography.

39

The thymus

Learning objective
✓ To have knowledge of the tumours of the thymus and their association with myasthenia gravis.

The thymus gland controls the development of T lymphocytes in the embryo and neonate and lies in the anterior mediastinum between the sternum in front and great vessels and pericardium posteriorly.

In adult life, the thymus is a fat-infiltrated remnant, but to the surgeon it is of importance in having an ill-understood connection with myasthenia gravis and in being a rather rare site of mediastinal tumour.

Tumours

Tumours of the thymus are of complex pathology; they may arise from either the epithelium (Hassall's corpuscles[1]) or lymphoid tissue, or a mixture of both. They may be benign (occasionally cystic) or malignant and rapidly invasive. Peak incidence is in the sixth and seventh decades. The thymus may also be involved in cases of lymphoma, particularly Hodgkin's disease.

Clinical features

There are three modes of presentation:

1 a mediastinal mass;
2 associated with myasthenia gravis;
3 associated with immune deficiency states.

[1]Arthur Hassall (1817–1894), Physician, Royal Free Hospital, London, UK. Published the first textbook on histology in English.

Lecture Notes: General Surgery, 12th edition. © Harold Ellis, Sir Roy Y. Calne and Christopher J. E. Watson. Published 2011 by Blackwell Publishing Ltd.

Treatment

Treatment is by thymectomy via median sternotomy, combined with radiotherapy if malignant, to prevent mediastinal recurrence.

Early invasion, with no more than pleural and mediastinal fat involvement, carries a good prognosis (90% at 5 years); involvement of the pericardium, great vessels or lung has a poor prognosis.

Myasthenia gravis

This condition is characterized by weakness of skeletal muscle caused by autoantibodies directed against the postsynaptic nicotinic acetylcholine receptors at the neuromuscular junction, as a consequence of which the motor endplate becomes refractory to the action of acetylcholine. About 15% of cases are associated with a tumour of the thymus, whereas thymic hyperplasia is present in most of the remaining cases.

Clinical features

Women are twice as commonly affected as men, and the disease usually commences in early adult life. The extrinsic ocular muscles are most often affected and may indeed be the only ones involved, with ptosis, diplopia and squint. The affected muscles become weak with use and recover, partially or completely, after rest. The voice is weak and death may eventually occur from respiratory muscle failure.

Treatment

The majority of cases are controlled by choline esterase inhibitors, e.g. pyridostigmine.

If a thymoma is present, it is excised, although such tumours are often locally invasive.

Thymectomy is otherwise indicated if the disease is progressive and the prognosis is best in young women (under the age of 40 years) with a history of 5 years or less.

40

The suprarenal glands

Learning objective

✓ To know the physiology of the suprarenal glands and hormone-producing tumours that derive from the separate parts of the gland, and their management.

The suprarenal (adrenal) glands are paired glands situated above and medial to the upper pole of each kidney. The cortex derives from the mesoderm of the urogenital ridge, while the medulla derives from neural crest ectoderm. These different origins account for the different physiology of medulla and cortex, and the different pathology encountered surgically.

Physiology

Suprarenal cortex

The suprarenal cortex secretes three groups of steroids:

1 *glucocorticoids*, which regulate carbohydrate metabolism, protein breakdown and fat mobilization;
2 *androgenic corticoids*, which are virilizing;
3 *mineralocorticoids*, which regulate mineral and water metabolism. Aldosterone acts to retain sodium and water and to excrete potassium.

Glucocorticoids and androgens are under hypothalamic control via adrenocorticotrophic hormone (ACTH) secreted by the anterior pituitary gland; mineralocorticoids are under the control of the renin–angiotensin system (Chapter 11, p. 77). As the steroids share a similar biochemical structure, it is not surprising that there is some

Lecture Notes: General Surgery, 12th edition. © Harold Ellis, Sir Roy Y. Calne and Christopher J. E. Watson. Published 2011 by Blackwell Publishing Ltd.

overlap in actions; thus, hydrocortisone (cortisol), a glucocorticoid, also affects salt and water metabolism and has sex steroid effects (acne, hirsutism) if given in large amounts.

Suprarenal medulla

The suprarenal medulla is richly innervated with sympathetic preganglionic fibres, and produces the catecholamines adrenaline (epinephrine) and noradrenaline (norepinephrine) in response to autonomic stimulation.

Pathology

The main pathologies affecting the suprarenal gland are increased function, owing to tumour or hyperplasia; decreased function, owing to atrophy, infarction or removal; or abnormal function, owing to enzyme disorders.

Increased function

- *Glucocorticoids* (Cushing's syndrome): adrenocortical adenoma; ACTH-producing pituitary adenoma; ectopic ACTH production (paraneoplastic).
- *Androgenic corticoids*: virilism (the adrenogenital syndrome).
- *Mineralocorticoids*: primary hyperaldosteronism (Conn's syndrome).
- *Catecholamines*: phaeochromocytoma.

Decreased function

Hypoadrenalism is most commonly a sequel of a prolonged corticosteroid therapy, in which endogenous steroid production is suppressed, followed by abrupt steroid withdrawal. It may also be due to the following:

- *congenital* suprarenal hypoplasia;
- *autoimmune* destruction: Addison's disease;[1]
- *suprarenal infarction*: a rare consequence of stress or sepsis (notably meningococcal sepsis);
- *bilateral adrenalectomy*: intentionally (to treat Cushing's syndrome) or secondary to bilateral nephrectomy;
- *suprarenal infiltration* by secondary tumours from primaries in bronchus and breast;
- *bilateral tuberculosis* of the suprarenals.

Enzyme disorders

Congenital suprarenal hyperplasia, the collective description for the suprarenal hyperplasias resulting from increased ACTH secretion, may result from certain enzyme disorders. ACTH is produced in excess because glucocorticoids, the end point in the pathway of steroid hormone synthesis, are not produced as a result of one of many possible enzyme deficiencies. Instead, all the substrate synthesized is turned into an intermediate hormone, such as an androgen.

Cushing's syndrome

Cushing's syndrome[2] is produced by increased circulating corticosteroids. Excepting therapeutic exogenous steroid administration, the majority of cases result from a pituitary adenoma producing ACTH, resulting in hyperplasia of the suprarenal cortex (the disease that Cushing first described); about 10% are due to benign or malignant adrenocortical tumours or, rarely, ectopic ACTH production by a distant tumour, e.g. carcinoma of the bronchus.

[1]Thomas Addison (1773–1860), Physician, Guy's Hospital, London, UK.
[2]Harvey Cushing (1869–1939), Professor of Surgery, Harvard Medical School, Boston, MA, USA. He was one of the founders of neurosurgery.

Clinical features

The syndrome usually affects young adults (occasionally children), women more often than men. The appearance is characteristic: adiposity with central distribution, abdominal striae, a red moon face and diabetes. There may be osteoporosis, leading to vertebral collapse. Associated mineral and androgenic corticoid oversecretion produce varying degrees of hypertension, hirsutism and acne, with amenorrhoea in women or impotence in men.

Special investigations

These may be thought of as investigations to confirm the diagnosis, and investigations to identify the cause.

- *Urinary 24 hour cortisol level* is raised; but may also be raised in the obese and in patients under stress.
- *Plasma cortisol*: raised levels, and loss of the normal diurnal variation (low at night, up in the morning) is suggestive.
- *Dexamethasone suppression test*, in which the steroid dexamethasone is administered over a period of days and at different doses, and the plasma cortisol is measured: suppression of cortisol occurs with low-dose dexamethasone (1 mg) in normal subjects and high-dose (4 mg over 48 hours) dexamethasone in the presence of pituitary tumours; ectopic ACTH and suprarenal tumours do not suppress.
- *Plasma ACTH* is raised in the presence of ectopic or pituitary ACTH-driven disease; its secretion is suppressed by autonomous suprarenal tumours.
- *Computed tomography (CT) and magnetic resonance (MR)* are the best imaging modalities for localization of a tumour in the suprarenal gland.

Treatment

If it is due to bilateral hyperplasia, bilateral adrenalectomy is performed and the patient placed on a maintenance dose of hydrocortisone. Removal of the affected suprarenal gland is carried out in cases of adenoma or carcinoma.

Cases due to basophil adenoma of the pituitary respond to hypophysectomy, usually performed via a trans-sphenoidal approach.

Primary hyperaldosteronism (Conn's syndrome)

Conn's syndrome[3] is a rare syndrome produced by an aldosterone-secreting adenoma of the suprarenal cortex. Characteristically, there is a low serum potassium (which results in episodes of muscle weakness or paralysis), raised serum sodium and alkalosis together with hypertension. There may also be polyuria and polydipsia.

The condition is interesting because, although rare, it represents a curable cause of hypertension.

Special investigations

- *Serum electrolytes*: hypernatraemia and hypokalaemia.
- *Plasma aldosterone*: the diagnosis is confirmed by demonstration of excess aldosterone in the plasma.
- *Abdominal CT* may demonstrate the tumour, which is often small.
- *Selective angiography* and selective venous sampling from the suprarenal veins with aldosterone estimations may be needed to delineate the lesion.

Treatment

Laparoscopic adrenalectomy has become the standard procedure for unilateral lesions; it has the advantage of lower morbidity and a shorter hospital stay than the traditional open procedure.

The adrenogenital syndromes

These rare syndromes result from the hypersecretion of adrenocortical androgens, due either to a defect in the enzyme pathway of steroid production, commonly 21-hydroxylase deficiency (the congenital form), or to an autonomous tumour producing androgens (the acquired form).

[3]Jerome Conn (1907–1994), Physician, University of Michigan, Ann Arbor, MI, USA.

Congenital adrenogenital syndrome

Also known as congenital suprarenal hyperplasia, this is due to an inborn defect of normal steroid synthesis (especially hydrocortisone) by the suprarenal cortex. Excessive ACTH production by the pituitary then occurs with resulting hyperplasia of the cortex and hypersecretion of cortical androgens.

Acquired adrenogenital syndrome

In children it is always due to an adrenocortical tumour, which is usually malignant. In young adults, the condition may be caused either by a tumour or by cortical hyperplasia in cases of Cushing's syndrome, in which androgen production is excessive.

Clinical features

These are conveniently divided into three varieties depending on age of onset.

Infancy

In the congenital variety of the adrenogenital syndrome, the newborn female child has a large clitoris and is often mistaken for male (female pseudohermaphrodite). Growth is initially rapid, but the epiphyses fuse early so that the final result is a stunted child. There may be episodes of acute adrenocortical insufficiency, especially with stress or infection.

Childhood

Virilization occurs in the female child and precocious sexual development, particularly of the penis, in the male child. This can be well summarized as 'little girls become little boys and little boys become little men'.

Adults

Amenorrhoea, hirsutism and breast atrophy in women, often associated with other features of Cushing's syndrome. In men, feminization is seen, but this is extremely rare.

Differential diagnosis

The diagnosis is based on detecting the excessive amount of steroid precursors, such as 17αhydroxyprogesterone, which is raised in the most common congenital form, 21-hydroxylase deficiency.

Differentiation must be made from the masculinizing tumour of ovary, in which the 17-ketosteroid urinary excretion is normal, and also the common condition of simple hirsutism in women.

Treatment

Bilateral cortical hyperplasia in infancy is treated by suppressing the excess ACTH secretion with exogenous steroids (e.g. hydrocortisone); on this regimen the virilizing features clear, and growth progresses normally. In the acquired variety, when a tumour is present it can be removed by laparoscopic adrenalectomy, and hyperplasia can be treated by bilateral adrenalectomy with hydrocortisone maintenance treatment.

Non-functioning tumours of the suprarenal cortex

Small non-secreting adenomas of the suprarenal cortex are common postmortem findings which are of no significance, and which are increasingly detected by modern cross-sectional imaging techniques such as CT and MR. Lesions less than 3 cm in diameter which are proven to be non-secreting and which do not change on repeated imaging over a 6 month interval can be safely left *in situ*. Non-functioning carcinomas of the suprarenal cortex are rare; they resemble renal carcinoma in appearance (hence the original hypothesis that the hypernephroma was of suprarenal origin). They are highly malignant and frequently invade the subjacent kidney.

Adrenomedullary tumours

Classification

Primary

- Neuroblastoma.
- Phaeochromocytoma.
- Ganglioneuroma.

Secondary

A common site, especially from breast and bronchus.

Neuroblastoma

A highly malignant tumour of sympathetic cells occurring in children under the age of 5 years, and the most common malignant tumour in neonates and infants under 1 year old. It may be bilateral, and up to 80% are associated with chromosomal abnormalities.

Macroscopically, it varies from a small nodular tumour to a large retroperitoneal mass, containing areas of haemorrhage and necrosis. Microscopically, it arises from neuroblasts of the suprarenal medulla, or within any cells of neuroectodermal origin along the spine.

Capsular invasion occurs early with spread to adjacent tissues, the regional nodes and by the blood to bones and the liver.

Special investigations

- *CT, MR, ultrasound and bone scan* are all used to stage the disease.
- *Neurone-specific enolase* is a sensitive marker of disseminated disease, and can be used as a tumour marker following treatment.

Treatment

A combined approach with surgical removal of local disease together with chemotherapy and/or radiotherapy is necessary.

Prognosis

Early disease, localized to the area of origin and in the absence of distant or lymph node spread, carries a favourable prognosis, as do absence of chromosome abnormalities, and age under 1 year together with histologically well-differentiated tumour.

Phaeochromocytoma

A physiologically active tumour of chromaffin cells, which secretes adrenaline and noradrenaline in varying proportions. Ten per cent are malignant and 10% are multiple; 10% occur outside the suprarenal gland in the sympathetic chain or the organ of Zuckerkandl[4] near the aortic bifurcation; 10% are familial (the '10% tumour').

Any age may be affected, but the tumour is particularly found in young adults. The sexes are equally affected.

Clinical features

These are produced by excess circulating adrenaline and noradrenaline.

There is hypertension, which is paroxysmal or sustained, and which may be accompanied by palpitations, headache, blurred vision, fits, papilloedema and episodes of pallor and sweating. There may be hyperglycaemia with glycosuria. Attacks may be infrequent, or occur several times a day.

The diagnostic triad, with high specificity and sensitivity is as follows:

- *headache*, sudden in onset, and pounding;
- *tachycardia* and/or palpitations;
- sweating.

Occasionally, the tumour may coexist with neurofibromas and café-au-lait spots, medullary carcinoma of the thyroid or a parathyroid adenoma as part of a multiple endocrine neoplasia syndrome (Chapter 38, p. 324).

Special investigations

Identifying the presence of a phaeochromocytoma

- *Urinary catecholamines*, particularly vanillylmandelic acid collected over a 24 hour period, are usually raised, particularly during an acute hypertensive attack.
- *Fasting plasma catecholamine concentrations* are raised.

Locating a phaeochromocytoma

- *CT or MR* may demonstrate the site and size of the tumour.
- *[131]I-MIBG scan*: meta-iodobenzylguanidine (MIBG) is a structural analogue of

noradrenaline, which is taken up by chromaffin cells of the suprarenal medulla and concentrated in adrenergic granules; it is also taken up by phaeochromocytomas and is useful both in localizing occult primaries and in detecting secondary spread.
- *Selective venous sampling:* blood from the suprarenal veins is taken at angiography and catecholamine concentrations measured; a raised value in the blood obtained from the inferior vena cava at this level is useful confirmatory evidence of the presence of a tumour in the absence of abnormality on scanning.

Treatment

Surgical excision is performed. This is usually performed laparoscopically but larger tumours may require an open operation. Prior to surgery, the patient receives both alpha (e.g. phenoxybenzamine) and beta (e.g. propranolol) adrenergic blockade to negate the hypertensive effects of catecholamines which are released as a consequence of manipulation of the tumour during the operation.

The catecholamines produced by phaeochromocytomas cause marked vasoconstriction; hence, patients with phaeochromocytomas are relatively volume depleted. Immediately after removal of the tumour, the blood pressure may fall to very low levels; this is countered by volume replacement, although a noradrenaline infusion is sometimes required.

Ganglioneuroma

A benign, slow-growing tumour of sympathetic ganglion cells, which only becomes clinically manifest if it reaches a large size. Only about 15% arise in the suprarenal; the rest arise elsewhere along the sympathetic chain.

[4]Emil Zuckerkandl (1849–1910), Professor of Anatomy in Graz, and later Vienna, Austria.

41

The kidney and ureter

Learning objectives

✓ To understand the congenital renal anomalies and polycystic kidney disease. The reader should know the causes of haematuria and the appropriate investigation and management.

✓ To understand the causes, presentations and management of urinary tract infections.

✓ The causes of renal failure, its investigation and treatment should also be understood.

Congenital anomalies

Embryology (Figure 41.1)

The embryology of the kidney involves three separate stages. Initially, a pronephros develops in the posterior wall of the coelomic cavity. This is replaced by the mesonephric system, which comprises a long ridge of mesoderm, the mesonephros, with its duct, the mesonephric (Wolffian[1]) duct. The mesonephros itself then disappears except that, in men, some of its ducts become the efferent tubules of the testis. At the lower end of the mesonephric duct a diverticulum develops. This diverticulum becomes the ureteric bud, on top of which develops a cap of tissue, the metanephric mesenchyme. The metanephric mesenchyme gives rise to the glomeruli and the proximal part of the renal duct system. The ureteric bud forms the ureter, renal pelvis, calyces and distal ducts. The mesonephric duct atrophies in women, the remnant being called the epoöphron, and in men it gives rise to the epididymis and the vas deferens.

[1]Kaspar Friedrich Wolff (1733–1794), born in Berlin, Germany; Professor of Anatomy, St Petersburg, Russia.

Lecture Notes: General Surgery, 12th edition. © Harold Ellis, Sir Roy Y. Calne and Christopher J. E. Watson. Published 2011 by Blackwell Publishing Ltd.

The kidney originally develops in the pelvis of the embryo and then migrates cranially, acquiring a progressively more proximal arterial blood supply as it does so. This complex developmental process explains the high frequency with which congenital anomalies of the kidney, the ureter and the renal blood supply are found.

Common renal anomalies

- *Pelvic kidney*: owing to failure of cranial migration of the developing kidney. Occurs in 1 in 500–1000 subjects.
- *Horseshoe kidney*: produced by fusion of the two metanephric masses across the midline (see below). Occurs 1 in every 400 subjects.
- *Duplex system*: double ureters and/or kidneys owing to duplication of the metanephric bud.
- *Congenital absence* of one kidney (1 in every 2500 subjects). Congenital absence of a kidney is extremely rare, but should be borne in mind whenever the possibility of nephrectomy arises, for instance after kidney trauma.
- *Polycystic kidneys*: genetically determined tendency for abnormal cyst formation throughout both kidneys (see below). Occurs in 1 in 500–1000 subjects.

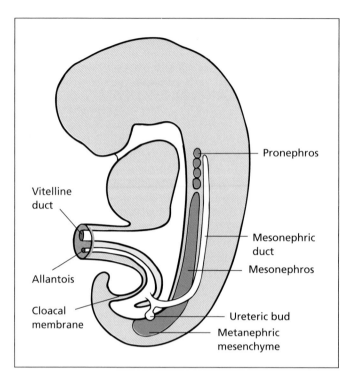

Figure 41.1 Development of the pro-, meso- and metanephric systems (after Langman).

- *Congenital hydronephrosis*: produced by neuromuscular incoordination at the pelviureteric junction.
- *Aberrant renal arteries*: one or more arteries supplying the upper or lower pole of the kidneys are very common; they represent the persistence of aortic branches that pass to the kidney in its lower embryonic position.

Polycystic disease, the various types of reduplication of the renal pelvis and the abnormal fusions are all associated with an increased incidence of infection when compared with kidneys that are anatomically normal.

Horseshoe kidney

During the kidneys' ascent from their pelvic position as the metanephros in the embryo, they may fuse. The commonest example is fusion of the lower poles across the midline, forming one large horseshoe-shaped kidney. The linked lower ends of the kidneys usually lie in front of the aorta in the region of the fourth or fifth lumbar vertebra and the ureters descend from the front of the fused kidneys.

Clinically, horseshoe kidneys may present as a firm mass in the pelvis, or with recurrent urinary tract infection. An intravenous urogram (IVU) will show rotation of the two renal pelvises with the ureters arising anteriorly close to the midline. Usually, the renal pelvises are directed laterally.

The main surgical importance of horseshoe kidneys is as the differential diagnosis of a lump in the pelvis, since the consequences of removing such renal tissue as an undiagnosed 'mass' are disastrous. Also, pelviureteric obstruction is more common, occurring in 10% of cases.

Duplex system

Instead of a single metanephric mass draining via a single ureter into the bladder, part of the system may be duplicated. Most common is separation of the renal pelvis into a double pelvis draining the upper and lower pole separately. This may extend distally as a bifid ureter, which unites to form a single ureter in its distal third, entering the bladder by a common ostium. Occasionally, a second diverticulum grows from the mesonephric duct, producing a double ureter. In this circumstance, the upper pole ureter always enters the bladder below and medial to the lower pole ureter, which enters the bladder in the normal position. Rarely, the upper pole ureter drains in an ectopic position directly into the urethra below the external sphincter in men, or into the vagina or perineum in women.

Duplex anomalies are usually asymptomatic, but may present as a cause of hydronephrosis (p. 340) or urinary tract infection. Ectopic ureters often present with infection owing to reflux up the abnormal ureteric orifice resulting in reflux nephropathy (chronic pyelonephritis) of the upper pole. Ectopic ureters opening into the urethra or onto the vagina or perineum are a cause of dribbling incontinence.

Polycystic disease

Pathology

The condition is characterized by multiple cysts throughout the renal substance, nearly always in both kidneys. These cysts are surrounded by attenuated renal tissue. The condition is inherited as an autosomal dominant form presenting in middle age; a more uncommon autosomal recessive form also exists, presenting in childhood with renal failure. Genetically, the dominant form may result from a number of different gene mutations, the most common being in the *PKD1* and *PKD2* genes; it is thought that a second, spontaneous somatic mutation is required for a cyst to form, accounting for the appearance of cysts in adulthood.

There may be associated multiple cysts in other viscera, particularly the liver (30%), lungs, spleen or pancreas (10%). In addition, there is a strong association with intracranial berry aneurysms and a history of subarachnoid haemorrhage. Diverticulosis coli is also more common in patients with polycystic kidneys.

Presentation of adult polycystic kidney disease

Polycystic kidney disease usually presents between 30 and 60 years of age with one of the following:

- *abdominal mass*: symptomless, bilateral, lobulated renal swellings found on routine examination;
- *haematuria*;

- *loin pain*, usually aching;
- *urinary tract infection*;
- *renal failure*: presenting with headache, lassitude, vomiting and a refractory anaemia;
- *hypertension*;
- *intracranial haemorrhage*, as a result of hypertension or 'berry' aneurysm.

On examination, the enlarged lobulated kidneys are usually readily palpable. There may be the clinical features of chronic uraemia, and the blood pressure is often raised.

Special investigations

- *Ultrasonography* is very accurate in detecting the multiple cysts in adults, but is less so in children because of the smaller size of the cysts.
- *Urea and creatinine* rise as renal function deteriorates.
- *IVU* demonstrates the typical elongated spidery calyces stretched out and indented by the cysts.

Treatment

Left untreated, many patients may survive in reasonable health well past middle age. Medical treatment is required in the management of the complicating hypertension and renal failure (dialysis and transplantation). Nephrectomy is performed for recurrent pain, infection and haematuria or, with very large kidneys, to provide enough room in the iliac fossae to accommodate a renal transplant; bilateral nephrectomy may be required to treat uncontrollable hypertension.

Renal cysts

Simple unilocular cysts of the kidney are quite common, the incidence increasing with age such that 50% of 50 year olds will be affected. A simple cyst may be small or may reach a very large size. Several cysts may be present and both kidneys may be affected. The cause is unknown, but may relate to two spontaneous somatic mutations in a tubular cell.

Clinical features

The cyst may be symptomless and may be found as a mass on routine clinical examination. If very large, it may present as an aching pain in the loin. Haematuria is absent, and this is an important point in differentiation from a renal carcinoma.

Special investigations

- *Urine* is clear, even on microscopic examination.
- *Ultrasonography* confirms a cystic mass.
- *IVU* demonstrates a round filling defect, which displaces but does not invade the calyces.
- *Computed tomography (CT)* shows one (or more) fluid-filled cysts, which do not enhance with intravenous contrast.

Ultrasound and CT are used to differentiate a simple cyst (thin wall, sharp and distinct border, homogeneous contents, non-enhancing) from a complex cyst that may be a renal cancer.

Treatment

No treatment is required for a simple cyst. Aspiration is performed if infection or malignancy is suspected. If cytology is unhelpful, then monitoring by serial CT or biopsy of the wall are performed to exclude malignancy.

Haematuria

Classification

Two useful rules are as follows:

1 when considering the causes of bleeding from any orifice in the body, always remember the general causes due to bleeding diatheses;
2 when considering any local cause of symptoms in the genitourinary tract, always think of the whole tract from the kidneys to the urethra.

Haematuria is an excellent example of these two general rules and the causes can be classified as follows (Figure 41.2).

General

- *Bleeding diatheses*, e.g. anticoagulant drugs, thrombocytopenic purpura. However, most patients with haematuria and a bleeding diathesis have underlying renal tract pathology.

Local

- *Kidney*: trauma, polycystic disease, glomerulonephritis, tuberculosis, infarction (from emboli in mitral stenosis or infective endocarditis), stone and tumour.
- *Ureter*: stone and tumour.
- *Bladder*: trauma, cystitis, stone, tumour and bilharzia.
- *Prostate*: prominent vessels in benign prostatic enlargement.
- *Urethra*: trauma, stone and tumour.

Management

Blood in the urine is an alarming symptom and usually brings the patient rapidly to the doctor. It should always be taken seriously and requires full history, examination and appropriate special investigations.

History

Haematuria accompanied by pain in one or the other loin suggests renal origin, and colicky pain indicates a stone in the renal pelvis or ureter, or partial ureteric obstruction by clot or necrotic papilla. Terminal bleeding with severe pain and frequency indicates bladder calculus. Prostatic bleeding is more likely to be initial or terminal and usually painless. Dribbling of blood from the urethra independent of micturition is typical of a urethral origin for the blood. Completely painless and otherwise symptomless, haematuria is suggestive of a tumour in the urinary tract.

A history of recent sore throat, especially in a child, would make a diagnosis of acute nephritis a possibility. Always check whether the patient is on anticoagulant therapy or if there is a history of bleeding tendencies; haematuria while on anticoagulation is still more commonly due to a renal pathology, which the anticoagulation has made symptomatic – full investigation is warranted.

Examination

One or the other kidney may be palpable; a carcinoma of the bladder may be felt on bimanual examination. An enlarged prostate, particularly if the patient is hypertensive, may suggest a prostatic source of bleeding, although other causes must be excluded before this diagnosis is finally made.

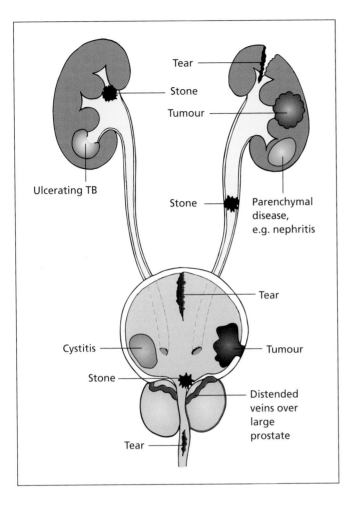

Figure 41.2 Some important causes of bleeding in the urinary tract.

Special investigations

- *Urine microscopy.* The presence of red cells will exclude haemoglobinuria and beeturia (following ingestion of beetroot). The presence of casts will indicate nephritis; pus cells and organisms suggest infection.
- *Urine cytology* is performed looking for evidence of malignancy; all but low-grade tumours should be detected.
- *IVU* may reveal a localized renal lesion or may show a filling defect in the ureter or bladder. Stones in the urinary tract will be displayed on this investigation; look for them carefully on the preliminary plain films, as they are obscured by contrast in the urogram. Upper tract (ureter and renal pelvis) urothelial tumours are usually demonstrated as filling defects in the contrast.

- *Ultrasonography* has replaced IVU as the investigation of choice, as it is able to detect parenchymal tumours, renal calculi and lesions in the collecting system and bladder. In cases of persistent haematuria, when ultrasonography is normal, further imaging by IVU or CT may be required.
- *Cystoscopy* will show any intravesical lesion in addition to bleeding from the prostate or blood emerging from one or the other ureter. Cystoscopy is best performed immediately after presentation with haematuria.

These are the minimum investigations required for anyone with haematuria. Other investigations such as CT and selective renal angiography may be required in some cases.

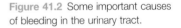

Injury to the kidney

The kidney may be injured by a direct blow in the loin or occasionally by a penetrating wound. The degree of damage varies from slight subcapsular bruising to complete rupture and fragmentation of the kidney or its avulsion from its vascular pedicle. Each kidney is contained within its own compartment of extraperitoneal fascia – the renal fascia. A closed rupture of the kidney is usually 'tamponaded' within this compartment; hence, most ruptures can be treated conservatively.

Clinical features

Clinically, there is usually local pain and tenderness and haematuria is a common finding. Retroperitoneal haematoma may cause abdominal distension due to ileus. There may be associated injury to other viscera, especially the spleen.

Special investigations

- *Urine*: macroscopic haematuria is usual.
- *IVU*: damage to the kidney may be shown by extravasation of contrast medium outside the renal outline or distortion or rupture of the renal calyces. Vascular pedicle disruption may manifest as delayed or non-enhancement of the renal parenchyma. IVU will also determine the presence of a normal kidney on the other side.
- *Ultrasound examination* may delineate a renal tear as well as indicating injury to other solid viscera, the liver and spleen. Views of other organs may be obscured if there is considerable intra-abdominal gas.
- *CT*: particularly useful in defining solid visceral injuries and is not affected by distended loops of bowel.

Imaging in renal trauma is indicated in anyone with penetrating trauma to the flank, back or abdomen, and in blunt trauma in patients with macroscopic haematuria, or microscopic haematuria and shock. The rapid data acquisition time and clarity of view of modern scanners make contrast-enhanced CT the investigation of choice.

Treatment

Associated injuries and shock will require appropriate treatment.

Penetrating injuries usually require surgical exploration after imaging. Blunt injuries can normally be managed conservatively, with bed rest, serial observations of the urine to determine whether or not the haematuria is clearing and careful clinical charting of blood pressure and pulse rate.

Nephrectomy is required in renal trauma in the following circumstances:

- *continued bleeding*, which threatens life;
- *severe hypertension* persisting after renal injury;
- *lack of function* in the affected kidney after several months, but only if symptomatic (e.g. recurrent infections, stone formation).

Hydronephrosis

Pathology

Hydronephrosis is a dilatation of the renal pelvis and calyces. The causes may be classified according to whether or not the hydronephrosis was consequent on obstruction of the renal tract, as follows.

1 *Hydronephrosis secondary to obstruction*:
  a within the lumen, e.g. ureteric calculus;
  b in the wall, e.g. transitional cell tumour, pelviureteric obstruction owing to neuromuscular incoordination;
  c outside the wall, e.g. retroperitoneal fibrosis, extrinsic tumour such as cervical cancer.
2 *Hydronephrosis without obstruction*: vesicoureteric reflux.

Obstruction may be unilateral (e.g. calculus stuck in one ureter) or bilateral (e.g. prostatic hypertrophy, urethral stricture, posterior urethral valve in newborn) with resultant bilateral hydronephrosis. It is important not to use the terms hydronephrosis and obstruction interchangeably.

Aberrant renal vessels were considered to be a common cause of hydronephrosis, because they frequently cross the dilated renal pelvis at its junction with the ureter. It is probably unusual for these aberrant vessels actually to initiate the hydronephrosis; more likely, they snare the congenitally dilated pelvis and merely act as a secondary constrictive factor.

Clinical features

An uncomplicated hydronephrosis on one side may be symptomless or may produce a dull, aching pain in the loin often mistaken for 'lumbago' or 'rheumatism'. Occasionally, there may be acute attacks of pain resembling ureteric colic, particularly after drinking large volumes of fluid (most notably beer).

Associated infection may present with fever, pyuria, rigors and severe loin pain. Bilateral hydronephrosis may present with the clinical features of uraemia. Very often, it is the underlying cause, e.g. the ureteric calculus, the enlarged prostate or the urethral stricture, that manifests itself clinically.

On examination, the enlarged kidney may be palpable. The size of this may vary according to the state of distension of the renal pelvis.

Complications

- *Infection*: resulting in pyonephrosis (p. 346).
- *Stone formation*: calculi readily deposit in the infected stagnant urine.
- *Hypertension*: secondary to renal ischaemia.
- *Renal failure*: where there is extensive bilateral destruction of renal tissue.
- *Traumatic rupture* of the hydronephrotic pelvis.

Special investigations

- *Ultrasound* shows a dilated collecting system (calyces and pelvis).
- *CT* may be required to determine the cause.
- *IVU* confirms the diagnosis, demonstrating an enlarged renal pelvis and swollen, dilated, club-like calyces. If renal function is severely impaired, the kidney may not secrete contrast.
- *Diuretic renography*, in which a furosemide injection is given at the time of, or 15 minutes before, MAG3 injection, will differentiate between an obstructed and non-obstructed dilated system, and will also provide information concerning the relative function of each kidney, which is important if nephrectomy is being considered.
- *Retrograde pyelogram*, via a catheter inserted into the ureter at cystoscopy, may be required to show the exact anatomy of the hydronephrosis and to demonstrate any obstructive cause in the ureter.

Treatment

Obstruction of a kidney may warrant percutaneous drainage or retrograde passage of a double pigtail ureteric stent. Obstruction with infection and obstruction in a solitary kidney are indications for emergency drainage.

Subsequent treatment is directed at removal of any underlying cause of the hydronephrosis. When the cause is a neuromuscular incoordination, an operation to widen the pelviureteric junction (pyeloplasty) may save the kidney from progressive damage.

A poorly functioning (particularly an infected) kidney is an indication for nephrectomy, provided that the other kidney has reasonable function.

Urinary tract calculi

Aetiology

Knowledge of stone formation within the urinary tract is still inadequate and many stones form without apparent explanation. Predisposing factors may be classified into four main groups:

1 inadequate drainage;
2 excess of normal constituents in the urine;
3 lack of inhibitors of stone formation
4 presence of abnormal constituents in the urine.

Inadequate drainage

Calculi may form whenever urine stagnates, e.g. within a hydronephrosis or in a diverticulum of the bladder.

Excess of normal constituents

Increased concentration of solutes in the urine, because of either a low urine volume or increased excretion, may result in precipitation from a supersaturated solution.

- *Inadequate urine volume*: renal stones are particularly common in people from temperate climates who go to live in the tropics, where dehydration produces extremely concentrated urine.
- *Increased excretion of calcium* (hypercalciuria) may be secondary to hypercalcaemia or, more commonly, idiopathic. Common causes of an

increase in serum calcium are hyperparathyroidism (Chapter 38, p. 324) and prolonged immobilization (e.g. an orthopaedic patient on traction or a paraplegic person confined to bed).

- *Increased serum uric acid* may be accompanied by uric acid stone formation. The most common cause is gout, but it may also occur following chemotherapy for leukaemia, lymphoma or polycythaemia.
- *Increased oxalate excretion* results from increased dietary intake, with strawberries, rhubarb, leafy vegetables and tea being among the culprits. Hyperoxaluria is also a complication of loss of the terminal ileum (e.g. in Crohn's disease or after surgical resection), which results in increased oxalate absorption by the colon.

Lack of inhibitors of stone formation

- Low levels of citrate and magnesium in the urine make calcium complexes less soluble, which promotes calcium oxalate and phosphate stone formation.

Presence of abnormal constituents

- *Urinary infection*, particularly in the presence of obstruction, e.g. hydronephrosis or chronic retention, produces epithelial sloughs upon which calculi may deposit. In addition, infection may alter the urine pH, favouring precipitation of certain solutes. A high pH, brought about by the presence of urea-splitting organisms such as *Proteus*, favours calcium phosphate stone formation, for example.
- *Foreign bodies*, such as non-absorbable sutures inserted at operation, ureteric stents, sloughed necrotic renal papilla or a fragment of broken urinary catheter, may act as a nidus for stone formation.
- *Vitamin A deficiency*, which may occur in primitive communities, results in hyperkeratosis of the urinary epithelium, which again provides the debris upon which stones may form.
- *Cystinuria*, caused by a mutation in one of two different genes responsible for amino acid transfer in the kidney, may result in cystine stone formation.

Composition of urinary calculi

The three common stones are oxalate, phosphate and urate.

- *Oxalate stones* (calcium oxalate) are the most common (60%). They are hard with a sharp, spiky surface, which traumatizes the urinary tract epithelium; the resultant bleeding usually colours the stone a dark brown or black.
- *Phosphate stones* (33%) are composed of a mixture of calcium, ammonium and magnesium phosphate ('triple phosphate stone'). They are hard, white and chalky. They are nearly always found in an infected urine and produce the large 'stag-horn' calculus deposited within a pyonephrosis.
- *Uric acid and urate stones* (5%) are moderately hard and brown in colour with a smooth surface. Pure uric acid stones are radiotranslucent but, fortunately for diagnosis, most contain enough calcium to render them opaque to X-rays.
- *Cystine stones* account for about 1% of urinary calculi.

Note that a stone found in the lower urinary tract may have arisen there primarily or it may have migrated there from a primary source within the kidney.

Clinical features (Figure 41.3)

Pain is the presenting feature of the great majority of kidney stones, but if the calculus is embedded within the solid substance of the kidney it may be entirely symptom free. Within the minor or major calyx system, the stone produces a dull loin pain. Impaction of the stone at the pelviureteric junction, or migration down the ureter itself, produces the dreadful agony of ureteric colic; the pain radiates from loin to groin, is of great severity and is accompanied by typical restlessness of the patient, who is quite unable to lie still in bed. Unlike the usual textbook description, the pain is not usually intermittent, but is continuous, although quite often with sharp exacerbations on a background of continued pain. There is often accompanying vomiting and sweating.

Haematuria, which may be microscopic or macroscopic, is frequently present so that detection of blood in the urine is an extremely helpful means of confirming the clinical diagnosis.

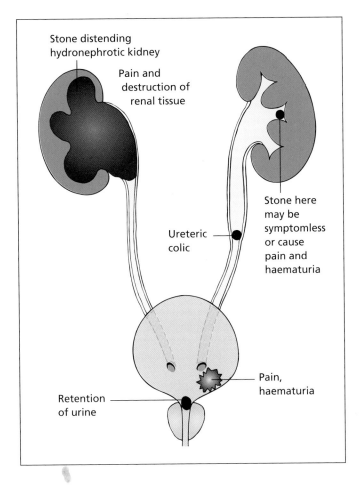

Stone distending
hydronephrotic kidney

Pain and
destruction of
renal tissue

Stone here
may be
symptomless
or cause
pain and
haematuria

Ureteric
colic

Pain,
haematuria

Retention
of urine

Figure 41.3 Diagram of the effects of urinary calculi.

Special investigations

These are usefully divided into investigations to confirm the diagnosis, and others to elucidate the aetiology of the stone.

Diagnostic investigations

- *Urine* is tested for the presence of blood.
- *Plain abdominal X-ray* specifically looking at kidneys, ureters and bladder (a 'KUB') will show the presence of stone in 90% of cases.
- *IVU* will demonstrate the exact anatomy of the renal system, e.g. the presence of associated hydronephrosis, although a completely obstructed kidney may show no function whatsoever.

    There is an important catch for the unwary; a small stone within the kidney may be completely obscured by the contrast of the pyelo-

gram. Never state that a kidney is free from stones without first carefully inspecting a plain X-ray of the renal area.
- *CT* is replacing IVU as the investigation of choice to confirm the diagnosis of renal colic since it is rapid, is more sensitive at detecting a stone than IVU, and can diagnose alternative pathologies if present (e.g. torted ovarian cyst, ruptured aortic aneurysm).
- *MAG3 renography* (mercapto-acetyl triglycine) may also be used to determine the presence of obstruction and impairment of function.

Investigation of the underlying cause

- *Urine microscopy and culture*: the urine is cultured for bacteria and examined microscopically for the presence of cystine crystals.

- *Analysis of the stone*, whether passed spontaneously or removed surgically, should be performed.
- *Uric acid* estimation. The serum uric acid is raised in gout with its associated uric acid stones.
- *Serum calcium* estimation is carried out. Hypercalcaemia (a value above 2.75 mmol/L) is suspicious of the presence of a parathyroid tumour, although the incidence of stones due to this cause is low.

Complications

- *Hydronephrosis*: see p. 340.
- *Infection*: pyelonephritis, pyonephrosis.
- *Anuria* due to either impaction of calculi in the ureter on each side, or blockage of the ureter in a remaining solitary kidney.

Treatment

Acute ureteric colic

Analgesia, either repeated injections of pethidine or rectal diclofenac, is given to relieve the severe pain. The great majority of small stones within the ureter (up to 5 mm) pass spontaneously. These ureteric stones tend to lodge at one of three places:

1 the pelviureteric junction;
2 the point at which the ureter crosses the pelvic brim;
3 the entrance of the ureter into the bladder.

The lower the stone, the more likely it is to pass spontaneously.

Ureteric calculi

If the stone remains in the ureter following an episode of acute colic and cannot or will not pass spontaneously, intervention is necessary. Extracorporeal shock wave lithotripsy (ESWL) is the first-line treatment. Other options include ureteroscopy with stone disintegration by holmium laser, electrohydraulic lithotripter, or extraction with the aid of a Dormia basket.[2] If non-invasive methods fail, the stone may have to be removed by open or laparoscopic operation (*ureterolithotomy*).

Renal calculi

A small calculus lodged in the solid substance of the kidney without symptoms can be left alone but kept under periodic survey. Larger renal stones require removal. Initially, ESWL is employed to shatter the stone without any open surgery. Ultrasonic shock waves are focused onto the calculus and cause it to shatter. The small fragments are passed spontaneously, often resulting in acute colic.

Stones that do not respond to ESWL may be removed percutaneously using a nephroscope (percutaneous nephrolithotomy).

Small symptomatic lower pole stones, which tend to be difficult to target with ESWL, may be treated by flexible nephroscopy and laser ablation.

Rarely is it necessary to perform open surgery simply to remove the stone, either through the kidney substance (*nephrolithotomy*) or, wherever possible, through its pelvis (*pyelolithotomy*). When the kidney is grossly and irreparably damaged, nephrectomy should be performed.

Acute calculous anuria

This may be due to blockage of both ureters by stones, or obstruction of a solitary kidney. It is best treated by percutaneous nephrostomy, although retrograde ureteric stenting is an alternative. If the patient is uraemic, haemo- or peritoneal dialysis may also be required. The stone is then removed as indicated above.

Treatment of the cause

In every case of renal stone, an attempt is made to determine the underlying cause and eliminate it. Thus, renal infection is dealt with and surgical correction of any obstructive lesion performed. A small percentage of recurrent and bilateral stones are found to be due to parathyroid tumour (Chapter 38, p. 324), removal of which will prevent further recurrences. In every case of renal calculus disease, the patient should be instructed to drink liberal quantities of fluid in order to encourage the production of a dilute urine.

Urinary tract infections

The urinary tract may be divided into the upper tract, comprising ureter and kidney, and the

[2]Enrico Dormia (1928-2009), Professor of Urology, Milan, Italy

lower tract, comprising bladder and urethra. Lower tract infections arise from ascending infection up the urethra. Upper tract infection may be due to either haematogenous infection of the kidney or an ascending infection from the lower urinary tract.

Cystitis

Cystitis is usually an ascending infection which, because of the short urethra, is more common in women, often following copulation. In men, it is commonly the consequence of urethral or prostatic obstruction. Urethral catheterization invariably results in bacterial colonization of the bladder.

The principal symptoms are of a stinging/burning pain on passing urine (dysuria), with increased frequency and urgency. Haematuria may be present, and examination confirms a low-grade pyrexia and suprapubic tenderness. Loin pain suggests ascending infection.

Special investigations

In women, recurrent infections are an indication for full investigation. In men and children, a single episode is unusual and merits investigation.

- *Urine microscopy and culture* to identify the causative organism (invariably bowel flora, usually *Escherichia coli*). The presence of pus cells with no growth is a feature of bladder cancer.
- *Ultrasound scan* of the bladder and kidneys may reveal dilatation of the upper tracts. A postmicturition ultrasound scan may demonstrate a large residual volume of urine within the bladder, suggesting obstruction or atony.
- *Plain abdominal X-ray* to exclude a bladder stone as a source of recurrent infection.
- *Cystoscopy*: bladder diverticula and other structural defects should be sought.

Treatment

Antibiotics are given according to sensitivity of the infecting organism. A high oral fluid intake is encouraged. Alkalinizing the urine with potassium citrate, and drinking cranberry juice, is helpful. Recurrent postcoital cystitis is an indication for prophylactic antibiotic therapy; an alternative is a self-start regimen of antibiotics in which the patient starts a course as soon as she becomes symptomatic. This latter approach is less likely to result in antibiotic resistance. Any underlying cause, e.g. calculus or prostatic obstruction, must be dealt with.

Reflux nephropathy

Reflux nephropathy, formerly termed chronic pyelonephritis, is the consequence of recurrent infections, resulting in shrunken, scarred kidneys. It is more common in childhood, as the growing kidney seems most susceptible, and reflux nephropathy accounts for almost 20% of chronic renal failure in adults. In childhood, it is due to a combination of two factors: vesicoureteric reflux and intrarenal reflux.

Vesicoureteric reflux

When the normal valve mechanism at the vesicoureteric junction is deficient, such as with an ectopic ureter in a duplex system, urine can pass back up the ureter during bladder contraction.

Intrarenal reflux

The collecting duct enters the calyx of the kidney, leaving the renal papilla. The ducts normally open obliquely, such that, as the pressure within the calyx increases, the ducts close, preventing urine from refluxing into the kidney (intrarenal reflux). If the ducts do not open obliquely, as is seen in compound papillae, intrarenal reflux may occur. If the urine is infected, the resultant inflammation leaves a permanent scar and loss of nephrons. Repeated episodes of infection result in major damage and loss of function.

Clinical features

While the typical features of urinary infection, namely dysuria, frequency and pyrexia, may be present, subclinical infection, often only signified by urinary incontinence at night, is common, particularly in children.

Special investigations

- *Micturating cystogram*: contrast is first introduced into the bladder, the patient voids, and reflux of urine during voiding can be recorded.

- *Indirect micturating cystogram*, an isotope (MAG3) study in which differential function of the kidneys can be assessed along with isotope reflux during micturition.
- *IVU* may show scarring, with a thin cortex overlying a distorted calyx, particularly at the upper and lower pole. The normal cupping of the calyces is reversed, and is termed clubbing.
- *DMSA (dimercaptosuccinic acid) scan*, which is used to demonstrate the degree of renal scarring as a result of reflux.

Treatment

The cause of the chronic pyelonephritis should be treated when identified. Long-term low-dose antibiotic prophylaxis is given to patients with asymptomatic or frequent infections.

Pyonephrosis

This is an infected hydronephrosis in which the kidney becomes no more than a bag of pus. If the ureter is obstructed, there may be little to find on examining the urine, although, more commonly, pyuria is a marked feature. Usually, the enlarged tender kidney is easily palpable.

Special investigations

- *Ultrasound* of the kidneys to confirm hydronephrosis.
- *IVU* shows little or no function and an enlarged renal shadow.
- *DMSA scan* will quantify the residual function in the kidney after treatment.
- *MAG3 renography* will indicate function and confirmation of obstruction.

Treatment

There should be urgent drainage by percutaneous nephrostomy, which will often identify the cause of the obstruction. If there is no residual renal function, nephrectomy is required.

Carbuncle of the kidney

This is better termed cortical abscess of the kidney and represents a haematogenous infection,

usually *Staphylococcus aureus*, coming from a primary focus such as a cutaneous boil.

Clinical features

There is pyrexia, toxaemia and pain and tenderness in the loin, and the kidney may be palpable.

Special investigations

- *Urine* is frequently sterile unless the abscess bursts into the calyceal system.
- *Full blood count*: there is a leucocytosis.
- *CT or ultrasonography* confirm the diagnosis.

Treatment

Percutaneous drainage together with antibiotics.

Perinephric abscess

Infection of the perinephric space is usually secondary to rupture of a carbuncle of the kidney. Rarely, it may complicate a pyonephrosis or infection of a traumatic perirenal haematoma.

Clinical features

There is the constitutional evidence of acute infection and in addition a diffuse tender bulge in the affected loin. This is particularly well seen when the back is carefully inspected with the patient lying prone.

Special investigations

- *Abdominal X-ray* showing kidneys, ureters and bladder (a 'KUB') may show loss of the psoas shadow owing to retroperitoneal oedema.
- *IVU* may be normal or may show the features of a renal cortical abscess or a pyonephrosis.
- *CT* will enable accurate localization of the abscess and its drainage.

Treatment

Surgical drainage is indicated only if CT-guided percutaneous drainage is unsuccessful.

Renal tuberculosis

Pathology

The kidney may be involved either as part of a generalized miliary spread of tuberculosis or more commonly as a focal lesion representing haematogenous spread from a distant site in the lungs (25% of patients have pulmonary tuberculosis), the bone or gut. The original focus may be quiescent at the time of active renal disease.

Early lesions are found near the junction of the cortex and medulla. These enlarge, caseate and then rupture into a calyx, eventually producing extensive destruction of renal substance. The ureter becomes infiltrated and thickened; its obstruction leads to tuberculous pyonephrosis. Rarely, a pyonephrosis becomes completely walled off as a symptomless, caseous and calcified mass ('autonephrectomy').

Spread of infected urine down the ureter frequently produces a tuberculous cystitis and may result in infection of the epididymis and seminal vesicles.

Untreated, the contralateral kidney often becomes involved, but this probably represents a separate haematogenous spread.

Clinical features

The patient is usually a young adult, often with a present or previous history of tuberculosis elsewhere. In the UK, the patient is likely to be an immigrant from a developing country. Symptoms in the early stages are mild and indeed may be entirely absent. There may be dysuria, frequency, pyuria or haematuria, which may be gross but is more usually slight or only microscopic. There may be loin pain on the affected side.

In more advanced cases, the dysuria and frequency become intense because of extensive involvement of the bladder, and then constitutional symptoms of tuberculosis, with fever, night sweats, loss of weight and anaemia, may be present. In some cases, a tuberculous epididymitis is the presenting feature (Chapter 46, p. 379).

Examination is usually negative, but the kidney may be tender and palpable. The epididymis and seminal vesicles may be enlarged and thickened if involved. The epididymis often feels craggy owing to calcification.

Special investigations

- *Urine* is commonly sterile to ordinary culture but contains pus cells and is acid in reaction ('sterile acid pyuria'); protein and usually red cells are also found. Acid-fast bacilli may be present on Ziehl–Neelson[3] staining of a spun deposit from an early morning specimen of urine. Three early morning specimens of urine are sent for culture, which takes 6 weeks.
- *IVU* may show failure of calyceal filling, irregularity of calyces and patchy calcification.
- *Chest X-ray* may show a primary lung focus.
- *Cystoscopy* may reveal a decreased capacity of the bladder, an oedematous mucosa on which tubercles may be seen, and perhaps a 'golf hole' ureteric orifice, the ureter being held rigidly open by surrounding fibrosis.

Treatment

Antituberculous therapy should not be commenced until the diagnosis has been confirmed as, once undertaken, treatment must be prolonged. Treatment usually involves isoniazid and rifampicin supplemented by pyrazinamide. Healing occurs with the production of fibrous tissue, which in early cases merely produces a small scar. In an advanced stage of the disease, this fibrous tissue may lead to stricture formation at the neck of a calyx or at the pelviureteric junction with a secondary hydronephrosis. Similar scarring of the heavily involved bladder may produce gross contraction on healing.

Surgery is indicated in only a minority of patients with advanced disease or when complications occur.

Renal failure

Acute renal failure

Acute renal failure is characterized by a reduced glomerular filtration rate (GFR), retention of nitrogenous waste (urea and creatinine rise),

[3]Franz Heinrich Paul Ziehl (1825–1898), Neurologist, Lübeck, Germany. Friedrich Karl Adolf Neelson (1854–1894), Professor of Pathology in Rostock, later Prosector in the State hospital, Dresden, Germany.

impaired acid–base balance (acidosis develops) and, usually, a reduced urine output.

An absence of urine production is termed *anuria*, whereas production of less than 400 mL/day in the adult is *oliguria*.

Aetiology

In the surgical context, acute renal failure may be a consequence of surgery or may be due to a surgically treatable lesion.

The causes of acute renal failure may be usefully divided into prerenal, renal and postrenal, in a similar way to the causes of jaundice relative to the liver. The presence of two kidneys means that the pathology must affect both kidneys in order to manifest, unless one kidney has previously failed or been removed.

Prerenal causes

Prerenal factors involve reduction in the blood flow to the kidney, resulting in a decreased GFR.

1 *Fluid loss*:
   a blood loss, e.g. haemorrhage;
   b plasma loss, e.g. burns, generalized peritonitis;
   c electrolyte loss, e.g. vomiting, diarrhoea, fistula, inadequate replacement.
2 *Impaired circulation*:
   a general factors, e.g. hypotension due to sepsis, cardiac failure;
   b local factors, e.g. aortic dissection in which the renal arteries are excluded from the circulation.

Renal perfusion is maintained in the presence of mild hypoperfusion by a number of regulatory mechanisms: vasoconstriction of splanchnic, muscular and cutaneous vascular beds, and alteration of afferent and efferent renal arteriolar tone. The GFR is normally maintained even if the mean arterial pressure falls to 60–80 mmHg. In hypertensive patients, the elderly and patients with pre-existing renal disease (e.g. diabetic nephropathy), autoregulation may be impaired and the GFR maintained only at higher mean pressures. Some drugs, particularly non-steroidal anti-inflammatory drugs (NSAIDs) and angiotensin-converting enzyme inhibitors, also impair the normal compensatory mechanisms and make the kidney more sensitive to hypovolaemia.

Renal causes

Renal causes of acute renal failure include factors directly acting upon the glomerular apparatus and tubules:

- acute tubular necrosis (ATN);
- acute cortical necrosis, due to severe ischaemia;
- myoglobin secondary to rhabdomyolysis, e.g. following a crush injury, or reperfusion of an ischaemic limb;
- drugs, e.g. antibiotics such as gentamicin, NSAIDs such as diclofenac;
- acute nephritis – interstitial nephritis or glomerulonephritis.

Postrenal (obstructive) causes

An obstruction lesion occurring at any level from the tubules to the urethra may cause renal impairment. Only in patients with a solitary kidney will an upper tract obstruction cause acute renal failure; otherwise, the obstruction is likely to be in the lower tracts and affect both kidneys.

Clinical features

The majority of cases of acute renal failure are prerenal in aetiology, which means that the kidneys will recover as soon as the circulation is restored. The diagnosis is usually clear: the patient has failed to pass urine and bladder catheterization reveals no urine or a mere trickle. The most common 'cause' of apparent oliguria while catheterized is a blocked catheter, and this should always be excluded.

Special investigations

Initial investigation should be rapidly performed, since rapid treatment may prevent life-threatening sequelae, and the shorter the period of failure, the more quickly renal function will be restored.

- *Serum electrolytes*: urea and creatinine are raised; potassium may be very high and demands immediate treatment (see below).
- *Renal tract Doppler ultrasound*: are there two kidneys, and are they perfused? Are they of normal size, or is one small, suggesting prior renal disease? Is there evidence of hydronephrosis/hydroureter? Is the bladder full, or empty? If obstruction is documented, it

should be rapidly relieved and this may require bladder catheterization or even nephrostomy.

- *Urine microscopy and stick test* for blood and protein. Some blood may be present as a consequence of urethral catheterization. Rhabdomyolysis is suggested by a positive stick test for blood without red cells on microscopy. Acute nephritis should be considered when blood and protein are present.

Management

Replenish the intravascular volume

Initial management requires a clinical assessment of the intravascular volume to determine the extent of volume depletion. The best signs are the following:

- *Jugular venous pressure* (JVP): is it visible and is it raised?
- *Postural hypotension*: is there a fall in blood pressure when the patient stands up? (If the patient cannot stand, the blood pressure should be measured lying and sitting up in bed.)

Depletion of intravascular volume is suggested by a postural fall in blood pressure and a low (not visible) JVP. Treatment requires rapid infusion of a fluid that remains in the intravascular compartment (blood, colloid or saline, but not dextrose). Infusion is continued until the JVP is visible and postural hypotension corrected. Potassium additives should not be given until a diuresis is established since patients are likely to be hyperkalaemic.

A *central venous catheter* may be inserted at this stage to measure accurately the central venous pressure; the target pressure is $10\,cmH_2O$ measured relative to the mid-axilla. In septic patients or those with cardiac disease, a pulmonary artery catheter (Swan–Ganz[4]) may be helpful, both for measurement of the pulmonary capillary wedge pressure and to determine systemic vascular resistance and so indicate the requirement for inotropes such as noradrenaline (norepinephrine).

[4]Harold J. C. Swan (1922–2005) and William Ganz (1919–2009), Cardiologists, Cedars of Lebanon Hospital, Los Angeles, CA, USA; Ganz later became Professor of Medicine, UCLA, Los Angeles.

Once volume repletion is achieved, the infusion is stopped until the urine output picks up. Further infusion would result in fluid overload, and would require dialysis to remove the excess fluid in the absence of renal function.

Dopamine and diuretics

If rehydration is unsuccessful in inducing a diuresis, a bolus of furosemide (100–500 mg over 30 min) should be given; a low-dose dopamine infusion (1 µg/kg/min) has been used in this setting but recent evidence questions its efficacy.

If these measures fail to induce a diuresis, it is likely that either ATN or, less commonly, acute cortical necrosis has occurred.

Hyperkalaemia

A potassium level of over 6.5 mmol/L should be treated immediately to avoid life-threatening ventricular arrhythmias. The electrocardiogram (ECG) changes with increasing potassium: first, the T waves become peaked (tenting); next, the P waves disappear; and, finally, the ECG becomes sinusoidal. Resolution of these appearances can be monitored with treatment.

Calcium gluconate (10 mL of 10% intravenously) should be given over a few minutes to stabilize the myocardium. Insulin and dextrose (15 units of soluble insulin in 50 mL of 50% dextrose) is given as an infusion over 10–20 minutes. This drives potassium into the cells, and lowers serum potassium by 1–2 mmol/L. Because these measures do not remove potassium from the body, a more definitive treatment is necessary before the potassium rises once more. This is best achieved by establishing a diuresis, but, if this fails, urgent dialysis is indicated. Potassium exchange resins (e.g. calcium resonium), taken by mouth or given by enema, may give good interim potassium control. However, they tend to cause constipation, so a laxative (e.g. lactulose 10–20 mL twice a day) should also be prescribed.

Acute tubular necrosis

Persistence of acute renal failure after correction of hypovolaemia is usually due to the development of ATN. This is characterized by a prolonged period of oliguria lasting anywhere from a few days to 3–6 weeks.

Pathology

The condition usually follows ischaemia to the kidneys. The blood supply to a nephron passes first to the glomerulus via afferent arterioles, and exits via the efferent arterioles to supply the tubules. In response to hypotension the efferent arterioles constrict to maintain blood flow to the glomerulus, but in so doing further reduce the blood flow to the tubules. Hence, although the glomerular apparatus is usually preserved, the tubules, especially the proximal tubules, suffer patchy ischaemic damage. The kidneys become enlarged and oedematous. As this damage recovers, renal function returns.

Clinical features

The features are of a persistent oliguria, unresponsive to replenishment of the intravascular circulating volume. The symptoms are those of acute renal failure described above.

Treatment

If ATN is established, the patient should be managed by regular dialysis until function returns. Recovery of function is characterized by a stepwise increase in urine output, although there may be a short polyuric phase during which maintenance of fluid balance can be difficult.

If function fails to return, it is more likely that acute cortical necrosis occurred with necrosis of glomeruli in addition to tubules.

Chronic renal failure

Chronic renal failure may be classified into three groups, like acute renal failure. Most causes are non-surgical, but some surgically correctable causes are given below.

1 *Prerenal*: renal artery stenosis.
2 *Postrenal (obstructive)*:
   a congenital posterior urethral valves;
   b prostatic hyperplasia/carcinoma, which causes chronic retention and upper tract dilatation;
   c urethral stricture;
   d cervical carcinoma, infiltrating the ureters;

   e urothelial tumour affecting bladder base or both ureters.

Symptoms are of malaise, weakness, confusion, hiccoughs with pallor, hypertension and fluid overload (e.g. pulmonary oedema, ankle oedema) on examination. The investigations are those of acute renal failure, and are directed at finding a treatable cause such as prostatic hypertrophy. In the absence of a treatable lesion, established renal failure is managed by renal replacement therapy with either peritoneal dialysis or haemodialysis, with a view to renal transplantation in the future.

Renal tumours

Tumours of the kidney are divided into those arising from the kidney substance itself and those originating from the renal pelvis.

Classification

Of the kidney itself

1 *Benign*:
   a adenoma (small and symptomless);
   b oncocytoma (uncommon tumour, characteristic 'scar' on CT);
   c angiomyolipoma (uncommon tumour, characteristic CT appearance);
   d haemangioma (a rare cause of haematuria).
2 *Malignant*.
   a Primary: nephroblastoma, adenocarcinoma.
   b Secondary: the kidney is an uncommon site for deposits of carcinoma although it may be involved in advanced cases of lymphoma and leukaemia, as well as tumours of breast and bronchus.

Of the renal pelvis

- Papilloma.
- Transitional carcinoma.
- Squamous carcinoma.

The two principal malignant tumours of the kidney are nephroblastoma in children and adenocarcinoma in adults.

Nephroblastoma (Wilms' tumour[5])

Pathology

This is an extremely anaplastic tumour, which usually arises in children under the age of 5 years, although it occasionally affects older children and adolescents. It probably originates from embryonic mesodermal tissue. Bilateral tumours are present in 5–10% of cases, and there is an association with congenital anomalies (aniridia, hemihypertrophy, macroglossia) in a few patients.

Macroscopically, the tumours are large and may be difficult to distinguish from neuroblastoma (Chapter 40, p. 333). They are pale on cut section, and contain areas of haemorrhage.

Microscopically, there is a mixture of mesenchymal and epithelial components, with spindle cells, epithelial tubules and smooth or striated muscle fibres.

The regional lymph nodes are soon invaded, and spread occurs by the bloodstream to the lungs and liver.

Clinical features

Rapid growth produces a large mass in the loin, although involvement of the renal pelvis is late and therefore haematuria relatively uncommon. Other features include weight loss and anorexia, fever and hypertension. Children may also present on account of metastases, which occasionally involve bone.

Special investigations

- *Ultrasonography* may distinguish the solid tumour from a cystic or hydronephrotic mass.
- *CT scan* is useful for staging and preoperative assessment, in particular to look at the contralateral kidney.

Treatment

When possible, nephrectomy is performed. In early disease, with no residual tumour following surgery, cytotoxic chemotherapy alone will give prolonged survival. For more extensive disease,

radiotherapy is given. When the tumour is unresectable, chemotherapy is given and nephrectomy performed once the tumour regresses.

This intensive therapy has improved the prognosis of a condition that previously could seldom be cured. Overall prognosis is 80% 5 year survival, with cure of early disease.

Adenocarcinoma (hypernephroma or Grawitz's tumour[6])

Pathology

This tumour accounts for 80% of all renal tumours. Men are affected twice as often as women. The patients are usually 40 years of age or over. It may be associated with familial conditions such as tuberose sclerosis and von Hippel–Lindau disease,[7] and can be bilateral.

Macroscopically, the tumour appears as a large, vascular, golden yellow mass, usually in one or the other pole of the kidney (hence its earlier name hypernephroma).

Microscopically, the tumour cells are typically large with an abundant foamy cytoplasm and a small central densely staining nucleus.

The tumour originates from the renal tubules and not from suprarenal rests, as was postulated by Grawitz.

Spread

- *Directly* throughout the renal substance with invasion of the perinephric tissues.
- *Via lymphatics* to the para-aortic lymph nodes.
- *Via bloodstream* with growth along the renal vein into the inferior vena cava (IVC), from which it may shower emboli. Metastases in the lung, bones and brain are common. Occlusion of the IVC results in a typical appearance with bilateral leg oedema.

The adenocarcinoma of the kidney is a tumour that may occasionally produce a solitary blood-borne deposit, so that removal of the primary

---

[5]Max Wilms (1867–1918), Professor of Surgery, first in Basle, Switzerland, and then in Heidelberg, Germany.

[6]Paul Otto Grawitz (1850–1932), Pathologist, Grefswald, Germany.
[7]Eugen von Hippel (1867–1939), Professor of Ophthalmology, Göttingen, Germany; Arvid Lindau (1892–1958), Pathologist, Lund, Sweden.

together with this deposit has been followed in some instances by prolonged survival.

Clinical features

The patient may present with symptoms either of local disease or of one of the paraneoplastic syndromes with which it may be associated.

Local disease

The classic triad of symptoms of a renal cell carcinoma, present in only 10% of cases, are as follows:

1 haematuria, present in half the cases – it may produce clot colic;
2 loin pain, aching, present in 40%;
3 loin mass, presenting in 25%.

Rarely, a left varicocele may occur (1%) as a consequence of tumour spread along the left renal vein occluding the confluence with the testicular vein on that side.

General features

In addition to local symptoms, the patient may present with the general features of malignancy, namely anaemia, loss of weight and occasionally a pyrexia of unknown origin, or as a consequence of secondary deposits, e.g. a pathological fracture.

Paraneoplastic syndromes

A number of hormones may be released from renal adenocarcinomas. Among the results are hypertension (renin production), polycythaemia (erythropoietin) and hypercalcaemia (ectopic parathormone production).

Incidental finding

Between 30% and 50% of cases are detected incidentally during imaging for symptoms unrelated to the renal tract.

On examination, the diseased kidney may be palpable.

Special investigations

- *Urine* nearly always contains either macroscopic or microscopic blood.
- *Ultrasonography* will differentiate cystic from solid mass.

- *CT* is the investigation of choice, providing accurate visualization of the tumour, indicating spread to lymph nodes and the chest and demonstrating caval invasion.
- *IVU* reveals distortion of the calyces by a polar tumour, which may occasionally show flecks of calcification.
- *Bone scan*, looking for metastatic disease, is indicated in the presence of a raised serum calcium or alkaline phosphatase.
- *Angiography* may be necessary if partial nephrectomy is considered.

Treatment

For small (<5 cm) polar tumours, partial nephrectomy is considered; central tumours and those over 5 cm in diameter are treated by radical nephrectomy. Cryoablation of small tumours may also be considered.

Postoperative immunotherapy with interleukin 2 reduces the incidence of recurrence. Two per cent of patients develop a second cancer in the contralateral kidney.

The five-year survival rate after successful resection is about 50%, but metastases may occur many years after nephrectomy. Poor prognostic factors include perinephric and lymphatic invasion.

Tumours of the renal pelvis

Transitional cell tumours of the renal pelvis vary in malignancy from benign papillomas to highly anaplastic transitional cell carcinomas.

A squamous carcinoma of the renal pelvis may occur when there has been squamous metaplasia of the epithelium; one-third of these cases are associated with renal calculus. Some may be associated with analgesic abuse and analgesic-associated nephropathy.

Clinical features

Patients present usually either with haematuria or with hydronephrosis due to ureteric obstruction. The tumour may seed down the ureter and even involve the bladder.

Treatment

Treatment is nephroureterectomy or, if feasible, local wide excision and plastic reconstruction.

42

The bladder

Learning objectives
- ✓ To know the causes, presentation and management of bladder cancer.
- ✓ To know about bladder stones and bladder diverticula, their causes and management.

Urachal anomalies

Urachal defects may result from anomalies of the primitive urachal connection. There are three principal anomalies.

1 *Urachal fistula*: a persistent urachal tract, resulting in a urinary discharge at the umbilicus.
2 *Urachal diverticulum*, an outpouching of the bladder, the urachal equivalent of a Meckel's diverticulum and the vitellointestinal duct.
3 *Urachal cyst*: where the urachus persists but is closed above and below. The cyst often becomes infected in later life, presenting with periumbilical pain and inflammation.

Treatment

In all cases treatment is excision.

Bladder exstrophy (ectopia vesicae)

Failure of fusion of the structures forming the anterior abdominal wall may cause a number of anomalies. Lower urinary tract changes include bladder exstrophy, where the ureters together with

Lecture Notes: General Surgery, 12th edition. © Harold Ellis, Sir Roy Y. Calne and Christopher J. E. Watson. Published 2011 by Blackwell Publishing Ltd.

the bladder trigone open directly onto the anterior abdominal wall below the umbilicus. This is usually associated with a failure of fusion of the pubic bones and, in men, there is an associated epispadias. Typically, there is a widened pelvis with a waddling gait.

The infant is completely incontinent of urine, with excoriation of the abdominal skin and a permanent unpleasant ammoniacal smell of infected urine. If the condition is untreated, the child may die of pyelonephritis, or else frequently develops a stratified squamous carcinoma of the bladder rudiment after initial metaplastic change.

Treatment

Traditional treatment is reimplantation of the ureters either into the colon or into an ileal loop (ureteroileostomy) combined with excision of the bladder itself as a prophylaxis against malignant change. Nowadays, complex reconstructive operations are performed soon after birth to fashion a new bladder.

Rupture of the bladder

The bladder may rupture either intraperitoneally or extraperitoneally.

Intraperitoneal rupture

This follows a penetrating wound (e.g. a bullet wound) or crush injury to the pelvis when the bladder is distended. Occasionally, it is consequent upon instrumentation of the bladder during transurethral resection of a tumour, and, rarely, the overdistended bladder of retention may rupture spontaneously.

Extraperitoneal rupture

More common; the bladder may be torn by a spicule of bone in a pelvic fracture or occasionally may be wounded during a hernia operation or repair of a cystocele.

Clinical features

Intraperitoneal rupture produces the typical picture of peritonitis with generalized abdominal pain, marked rigidity and a silent abdomen. *Extraperitoneal rupture* is associated with extraperitoneal extravasation of blood and urine producing a painful swelling that arises out of the pelvis. In this case, differentiation must be made from rupture of the membranous urethra (Chapter 44, p. 368), although this may not be possible until surgical exploration is carried out. Typically, however, a urethral tear is accompanied by anterior displacement of the prostate, which can be detected on rectal examination. In either circumstance, traumatic bladder rupture causes haematuria.

Special investigations

- *Computed tomography* demonstrates extravasation and any associated pelvic injury.
- *Cystography* will confirm rupture.
- *Urethrography* will demonstrate a urethral injury.

Treatment

Treatment is invariably surgical. The intraperitoneal rupture is sutured and the bladder drained by means of an indwelling urethral (Foley[1]) catheter. Small extraperitoneal ruptures are treated by urinary catheter drainage; larger leaks may necessitate exploration and repair, with drainage of the retropubic space and antibiotic therapy.

[1] Frederick Foley (1891–1966), Urologist, St. Paul, MN, USA.

Diverticulum of the bladder

The vast majority of diverticula of the bladder are secondary to bladder outflow obstruction, although a small number are congenital in origin. As it is usually the male bladder which becomes obstructed, 95% of diverticula occur in men. Congenital diverticula have all the layers of the bladder wall; acquired diverticula contain only the mucosa.

Pathology

The muscle of the bladder wall hypertrophies as a result of obstruction, and becomes trabeculated. Outpouches of mucosa occur between the bands of muscle fibres. One or more of these sacs may increase in size to form a fully developed diverticulum which, because it is devoid of practically all muscle in its wall, is unable to empty and undergoes progressive distension.

Complications

- *Urinary infection* because of urinary stagnation.
- *Calculus formation* because of a combination of infection and stasis.
- *Malignant change* may occur in its wall, as commonly as elsewhere in the bladder mucosa. Such tumours are more difficult to treat, and may have a worse prognosis owing to the absent muscle wall.
- *Hydronephrosis* may rarely occur owing to pressure of the diverticulum against the adjacent ureter.

Clinical features

The majority of diverticula remain silent unless they undergo one of the complications listed above. Some are found incidentally during investigation of the underlying obstructive lesion, e.g. a prostatic hyperplasia or urethral stricture. Occasionally, a large, uninfected diverticulum gives the strange symptom of double micturition ('*pis en deux*'). In this circumstance, the patient empties his bladder but a substantial amount of the urine passes into the distensible diverticulum. No sooner does micturition end than the diverticulum passively empties again into the bladder, giving the surprised patient the desire once again to empty his bladder.

Special investigations

- *Intravenous urogram (IVU)*: contrast medium enters the diverticulum.
- *Cystoscopy*: the mouth of the diverticulum can be visualized.

Treatment

Intervention is indicated for the complications of a diverticulum, but most are managed conservatively; the treatment of outflow obstruction usually suffices.

Bladder stone

The varieties of bladder calculi are the same as renal stones, namely phosphate, oxalate, urate and rarely cystine.

Aetiology

Bladder stones either originate in the kidney and pass down the ureter into the bladder, where they remain and grow, or originate *de novo* in the bladder. Stones that arise in the bladder are due to the following:

- *Stasis and infection*: bladder stones commonly arise as a consequence of outflow obstruction (e.g. urethral stricture or prostatic enlargement). They may be secondary to an atonic bladder in a paraplegic person, and may have arisen first within a bladder diverticulum.
- *Foreign body*: a calculus will deposit on a long-term indwelling catheter or on any foreign body inserted into the bladder.

Clinical features

The typical triad of symptoms of bladder stone are frequency, pain and haematuria. In addition, patients sometimes complain of intermittent stopping of the urinary flow as the stone blocks the internal urinary meatus like a ball valve, and occasionally actual retention of urine may occur if the stone impacts in the urethra.

- *Frequency* is more troublesome during the day than at night, probably because, in the upright position, the stone lies over, and irritates, the bladder trigone.
- *Pain* is felt in the suprapubic region, in the perineum and the tip of the penis; it particularly occurs at the end of micturition, when the bladder contracts down upon the calculus.
- *Haematuria* tends to occur as the last few drops of urine are passed.

Special investigations

- *Plain abdominal X-ray* (specifically a 'KUB' to show kidneys, ureters and bladder): the majority of bladder stones are radio-opaque and are readily visible.
- *Cystoscopy* allows stones to be seen as well as to be fragmented and retrieved.

Treatment

Unless the stone is very small, when there is a possibility that it will pass spontaneously, it should be removed either by crushing with an endoscopic lithotrite under direct vision or by disintegration with extracorporeal shock wave lithotripsy.

Bladder tumours

Pathology

Bladder tumours may be classified as follows, together with their relative incidence.

Benign

- Transitional cell papilloma (<1%).

Malignant

1 *Primary*:
   a transitional cell carcinoma (90%);
   b squamous carcinoma arising in an area of metaplasia (7%);
   c adenocarcinoma (uncommon, but may occur in urachal remnants) (2%);
   d sarcomas (rare).
2 *Secondary*: direct invasion from adjacent tumours, i.e. colonic, renal, ovarian, uterine, prostatic tumours.

Transitional cell papilloma

Transitional cell papillomas, more properly called inverted papillomas on account of their inward growth into the bladder wall, grade imperceptibly into malignant tumours. Many pathologists regard them as low-grade carcinomas, especially because they have a tendency to recur after treatment, to seed elsewhere in the bladder and to undergo frank malignant change.

Most benign papillomas can be controlled by fulguration or resection via an operating cystoscope. Because of the high risk of further lesions occurring, once the patient has developed a papilloma, he or she should undergo regular cystoscopic surveillance.

Transitional cell carcinoma (TCC)

These are commonly found in middle-aged and elderly patients. Men are far more frequently affected than women.

Aetiology

Risk factors include cigarette smoking (twofold increase in incidence), and workers in the aniline dye and rubber industry because of the excretion of carcinogens such as β-naphthyl amine in the urine. The manufacture of many of the more dangerous dyes and chemicals has been abolished in this country. There is a high incidence of malignant change in the exposed bladder mucosa of ectopia vesicae (p. 353), in the bladder infected with schistosomiasis and in association with the long-term catheterization in paraplegic patients; in these cases, characterized by chronic inflammation and mucosal metaplasia, squamous carcinoma is common.

Pathology

Although any part of the bladder may be involved, growths are particularly common at the base, trigone and around the ureteric orifices. They are often multiple, signifying a field change throughout the transitional urothelium with the tendency for tumours to develop anywhere from the renal pelvis to the urethra.

Macroscopic appearance

The well-differentiated TCCs form fine fronds, which resemble seaweed floating in the urine. The more malignant tumours are sessile, solid growths, which infiltrate the bladder wall, then ulcerate, often with marked surrounding cystitis. Carcinoma *in situ* may produce a suspicious red area of bladder mucosa.

Microscopic appearance

The TCCs have a connective tissue core and no involvement of the stem. The carcinomas may be well- or poorly differentiated transitional cell tumours but, rarely, keratinizing squamous cell tumours or adenocarcinomas may be seen.

Spread

- *Local* with infiltration of the bladder wall, the prostate, urethra, sigmoid colon and rectum or, in women, the pelvic viscera. The ureteric orifices may be occluded, producing hydronephrosis and ultimately renal failure. The pelvic skeleton may be directly invaded.
- *Lymphatic*, to the iliac and para-aortic lymph nodes.
- *Blood-borne* spread occurs late to the liver, lungs and bones.
- *Implantation* may take place into the scar if open operation is performed.

Clinical features

Bladder tumours usually present with painless haematuria (macroscopic or microscopic). Malignant tumours may also cause dysuria, frequency and urgency of micturition. Occasionally, the patient may present with hydronephrosis caused by ureteric obstruction or with retention of urine caused either by clot or by growth involving the urethra. In late cases, there may be severe pain from pelvic invasion or uraemia from bilateral ureteric obstruction.

Examination is usually negative, but tumours invading muscle may be palpable bimanually at the time of cystoscopy.

Special investigations

- *Urine examination* usually reveals blood, either to the naked eye or microscopically.
- *Urine cytology* is usually positive in high-grade (G3 and carcinoma *in situ*) carcinomas; a positive urine test always indicates TCC in the urinary tract, but a negative cytology does not exclude it.

- *IVU* may demonstrate a filling defect and perhaps ureteric obstruction or hydronephrosis. At the same time, the presence of pelvic bony secondaries may be revealed.
- *Flexible cystoscopy* under local anaesthesia in the clinic is the most valuable investigation, permitting diagnosis and biopsy.

Treatment

Initial assessment of all tumours involves bimanual examination and transurethral resection under general anaesthesia; further treatment of TCC depends on the grade and stage of the tumour.

Staging

Staging is generally according to the TNM system (Chapter 7, p. 39). The local staging (T) involves both bimanual palpation and histological examination to ascertain the depth of invasion through the bladder wall, and the grade of the tumour (G1, well differentiated, to G3, poorly differentiated). Carcinoma *in situ* (CiS) is a high-grade tumour confined to the epithelium.

Low-risk superficial cancers

Well-differentiated (G1 and G2) tumours that do not invade the bladder wall (pTa) or invade only the lamina propria (pT1) are treated by endo-scopic resection followed by intravesical chemotherapy (mitomycin) to prevent recurrence. Follow-up cystoscopy is required to detect and treat recurrence. This severity of disease has a low chance (10–15%) of progression to muscle-invasive disease.

High-risk superficial cancers

High-risk superficial disease (G3pT1 and CiS) has a much greater chance of progression to muscle invasion (30–60%). Treatment comprises intravesical bacille Calmette–Guérin (BCG) therapy,[2] radiotherapy or early cystectomy.

Muscle-invasive cancers

Muscle-invasive cancers (pT2 and greater) have a poor prognosis, with approximately 50% 5 year survival. Treatment can be primary cystectomy or radiotherapy with cystoscopic follow-up (and cystectomy if recurrence is diagnosed, so-called 'salvage cystectomy'), or deep transurethral resection with or without systemic chemotherapy.

At cystectomy, the bladder and distal ureters are removed, along with the prostate or gynaecological organs, with implantation of the ureters into a tube of ileum brought out as a stoma (an ileal conduit).

Chemotherapy may be used for metastatic disease but is relatively ineffective.

[2] Léon Calmette (1863–1933), Director of Pasteur Institute, Paris, France. Camille Guérin (1872–1961), Veterinary Surgeon, Lille, France.

43

The prostate

Learning objectives
- ✓ To know the causes and treatment of both benign and malignant prostatic enlargement.
- ✓ To know about the presentation of urinary retention and its treatment.

There are two common conditions of the prostate that require consideration: benign enlargement and carcinoma.

Benign enlargement

Pathology

Some degree of enlargement of the prostate is extremely common from the age of 45 onwards, but this enlargement often produces either no or only minor symptoms. Seventy per cent of men have benign hyperplasia by the age of 70.

The prostate, like the breast and thyroid, is composed of glandular tissue and stroma, which have periods of activity and involution throughout life under the influences of a changing milieu of hormones. Associated with these periods, the gland may become enlarged, with excessive proliferation of both fibrous and epithelial tissue.

Enlargement of the lateral lobes of the prostate results in encroachment on the prostatic urethra. The median lobe may also enlarge as a rounded swelling overlying the posterior aspect of the internal urinary meatus. The three lobes may then obstruct the urethral lumen, impeding the passage of urine. Occasionally, only the median lobe is enlarged.

Lecture Notes: General Surgery, 12th edition. © Harold Ellis, Sir Roy Y. Calne and Christopher J. E. Watson. Published 2011 by Blackwell Publishing Ltd.

Pathological consequences of outflow obstruction

- *Trabeculation of the bladder*: as a result of the obstruction, the bladder hypertrophies and the thickened muscle bands produce trabeculation.
- *Bladder diverticula* form from saccules between muscle bands.
- *Bladder stones* form as a consequence of urinary stasis, particularly in diverticula.
- *Urinary infection* may occur (especially after catheterization).
- *Hydronephrosis* results from back pressure on the ureters, which may result in renal failure.
- *Renal failure*, due to progressive hydronephrosis, resulting in anaemia and uraemia. It is commonly referred to as obstructive nephropathy.

Clinical features

There are three types of symptoms that result from prostatic hyperplasia.

- *Obstructive symptoms* consequent upon bladder outflow impedance.
- *Irritative symptoms* due to the muscular instability of the bladder (detrusor instability).
- *Symptoms of the sequelae*, such as infection or renal failure.

It is important to realize that lower urinary tract symptoms are not always due to prostatic hyperplasia and bladder outflow obstruction. They may be due to the ageing process of the bladder since they may also occur with age in women.

Obstructive symptoms

The narrowing of the prostatic urethra by the lateral lobes on each side and the possible median lobe enlargement cause the patient difficulty in passing urine, with a poor and intermittent stream. There may be difficulty starting (hesitancy), and dribbling at the end of micturition (terminal dribbling).

Associated with the prostatic enlargement, there may be partial obstruction and congestion of the prostatic plexus of veins, which may produce haematuria, which usually occurs at the end of micturition when the bladder contracts around the enlarged intravesical part of the prostate. As a cause of haematuria, bleeding from distended veins should only be diagnosed after exclusion of intravesical and upper tract tumours.

Eventually, the bladder is likely to fail to overcome the obstruction and this results in retention of urine. This may be acute, with sudden onset and severe pain, or chronic, in which the bladder gradually becomes distended and the patient develops dribbling overflow incontinence, with little or no pain. It is in the latter group that uraemia is likely to occur. In some instances, a complete obstruction then supervenes ('acute on chronic obstruction').

Symptoms of detrusor instability

Involuntary contractions of the distended bladder result in frequency, urgency and nocturia. Urinary tract infection may exacerbate the symptoms, or precipitate acute retention (see below).

Symptoms of renal failure

The obstruction to the outflow of the bladder may result in renal failure, with drowsiness, headache and impairment of intellect owing to uraemia. It is therefore always wise to examine the bladder for enlargement and to determine the blood urea in an elderly man with inexplicable behavioural changes.

Examination

The patient with an enlarged prostate, if uraemic, is likely to be pale and wasted, with a dry, furred tongue; he may be mentally confused. Examination of the abdomen may reveal a large bladder, which may reach to the umbilicus or even above. The swelling has the typical globular shape of the bladder arising from the pelvis, and is dull to percussion. If there is acute obstruction, the bladder will be tender to palpation.

On rectal examination, the prostate will be enlarged. Typically, in benign enlargement the lateral lobes are enlarged and a sulcus is palpable between them in the midline posteriorly. This is in contrast to carcinoma, which usually involves the posterior part of the gland and obliterates the sulcus with a craggy, hard mass. The size of the prostate may appear to be larger than it really is if the bladder is grossly enlarged and pushes the prostate down towards the examining finger. The gland should therefore be palpated again after catheterization and before operation. Occasionally, only the middle lobe is enlarged. In such cases, the prostate appears normal in size on rectal examination, in spite of marked symptoms or even retention of urine. The diagnosis is established at cystoscopic examination.

Special investigations

- *24 hour frequency/volume chart.* The patient records when he passes urine, and how much he passes in a 24 hour period.
- *Serum urea and creatinine* to identify renal failure.
- *Haemoglobin* is estimated, since uraemia inhibits the bone marrow and leads to anaemia.
- *Prostate-specific antigen* (PSA) is a sensitive indicator of prostatic carcinoma, and has superseded measurement of serum acid phosphatase. A PSA concentration below 4.0 ng/mL is normal. Refinements in PSA include measurement of the free/total PSA ratio, which is over 0.15 in normal men.
- *Urinalysis* for the presence of leucocytes. *Culture* is performed if urinalysis is positive: an infected renal tract severely complicates prostatic disease. Most patients with prostatic disease do not have infected urine until the bladder and urethra have been instrumented.
- *Urine flow rate assessment.* A void volume of at least 200 mL is required for meaningful assessment of maximum flow rate. A maximum flow rate of less than 10 mL/s indicates obstructed flow or weak bladder contractility. A flow rate over 15 mL/s is

unlikely to be obstructed. Urodynamics (pressure flow assessment) can be used to distinguish outflow obstruction from poor detrusor contraction, which will not improve following prostate surgery.

- *Ultrasound scan* may demonstrate bladder enlargement, hydronephrosis and hydroureter. Following voiding, it can be used to estimate the amount of residual urine in the bladder. Normally, there is none; however, in the presence of bladder outflow obstruction the bladder cannot be completely emptied. Ultrasound has replaced the intravenous urogram (IVU) in the routine investigation of patients with outflow obstruction.

Complications of prostatic hyperplasia

These are classified as follows:

1 *Prostatic complications*:
  a acute retention;
  b chronic retention;
  c haemorrhage.
2 *Bladder complications*:
  a diverticula;
  b urinary infection;
  c stone formation.
3 *Renal complications*:
  a hydronephrosis.
  b uraemia.

Treatment

This depends on whether the patient is an elective case, with troublesome prostatic symptoms, especially marked nocturnal frequency, or whether he presents urgently with retention (see p. 364).

Conservative management

If the patient has few lower urinary tract symptoms, he is encouraged to perform simple bladder training. This simply means getting the patient to hold his urine for approximately 10 minutes after he would ordinarily want to void. One-sixth improve; one-third remain stable; and the rest develop worsening symptoms.

Medical therapy

This is indicated for moderately or severely symptomatic patients.

1 *Selective α_1-adrenergic antagonists* (e.g. tamsulosin) are the mainstay of treatment for symptoms due to bladder neck obstruction. They act by causing relaxation of the smooth muscle of the bladder neck, improving symptoms and urinary flow rate.
2 *5α-reductase inhibition* (e.g. finasteride) blocks the conversion of testosterone to its active metabolite, dihydrotestosterone, in the prostate. The beneficial effect may take up to 6 months to appear.

Surgery is indicated for symptomatic patients in whom medical therapy has failed and who have bladder outflow obstruction on flow rate and pressure/flow assessment. Surgery is also indicated for the complications of bladder outflow obstruction.

Surgical therapy

Surgery is indicated for symptomatic patients in whom medical therapy has failed and who have bladder outflow obstruction on flow rate and pressure/flow assessment. Surgery is also indicated for the complications of bladder outflow obstruction.

Transurethral prostatectomy

The prostate can be removed endoscopically by means of an operating cystoscope, using a diathermy cutting loop or laser fibre. This is useful in dealing with fibrotic and malignant prostatic obstruction but it is also used routinely for benign enlargement. The mortality and morbidity in skilled hands are very low, and this technique is now the treatment of choice in all but very enlarged prostates. Removal of too much gland may damage the urethral sphincter mechanism.

Open prostatectomy

If the prostate is very large or if there is some coexistent intravesical pathology, such as a large diverticulum or tumour that requires removal at the same time, an open operation may be necessary. This is performed either by the transvesical route or by the retropubic approach.

Complications of prostatectomy

Transurethral prostatectomy has a low morbidity and mortality, particularly in view of the elderly population in which it is usually performed.

- *Haemorrhage*: primary haemorrhage is more common with malignant glands, with large resections, and in patients on aspirin or clopidogrel, which should therefore be stopped preoperatively. Postoperative irrigation and warming the patient are important in stopping fibrinolysis.
- *Transurethral resection (TUR) syndrome*: absorption of large volumes of the irrigating fluid through the open prostatic veins may result in hyponatraemia and confusion.
- *Infection* is particularly common in patients who are catheterized before surgery; prophylactic antibiotics are given.
- *Retrograde ejaculation* is almost certain after TUR.
- *Impotence* occurs in 5–15% of patients, depending on the level of potency preoperatively.
- *Bladder neck stenosis*, due to stricturing of the bladder neck following resection, may occur and presents with outflow obstruction.
- *Urinary incontinence* is uncommon but may occur if the resection is extended below the verumontanum with damage to the urethral sphincter.
- *Recurrent lower urinary tract symptoms*: late recurrence may be due to either regrowth of an adenoma or malignant change.

Carcinoma

Pathology

Carcinoma of the prostate is the most common cancer in men in the UK, but is rare below the age of 50. Above this age the incidence increases markedly, and it is estimated to affect 80% of men aged 80, though only 4% of men will die from it; it is more common to die with the disease than from it. Many prostates with apparent benign hyperplasia have a malignant focus on careful histological examination of the resected gland or of autopsy material.

Macroscopic appearance

The tumour is usually situated in the posterior part of the prostate beneath its capsule and appears as an infiltrating, hard, pale area.

Microscopic appearance

An adenocarcinoma, usually moderately differentiated but occasionally anaplastic. The degree of differentiation is quoted in terms of the Gleason grade[1] from 2 to 10.

Spread

- *Local*: there is invasion of the periprostatic tissues and adjacent organs (i.e. the bladder, urethra, seminal vesicles) and, rarely, invasion around and ulceration into the rectum.
- *Lymphatic*: to the iliac and para-aortic nodes.
- *Blood-borne*: especially to the pelvis, spine and skull, usually as osteosclerotic lesions. Secondaries may also be found in the liver and lung.

Clinical features

Prostate cancer may be asymptomatically detected on PSA screening or present with symptoms that are identical to those of benign enlargement. In addition, the patient may present with symptoms from secondary deposits, particularly with pain in the back from involvement of the vertebrae; occasionally, surgery is required for the relief of spinal cord compression. As with cancer anywhere, the patient's general condition is likely to be poor, with weight loss and anaemia.

Bimanual examination of the prostate may reveal four different stages (the Tumour assessment of the TNM staging; Figure 43.1):

T1 The prostate feels benign, with no palpable tumour.

T2 A hard nodule in one lobe of the prostate or abolishing the normal sulcus between the two lateral lobes. The tumour is confined to the prostate.

T3 A hard mass in the prostate together with infiltration of the tissues on either side of the prostate or into the seminal vesicles.

T4 A hard mass in the prostate which is fixed to the pelvic side wall or is invading the bladder.

Special investigations

The same initial investigations are performed as for benign enlargement.

[1] Donald Gleason (1920–2008), Pathologist, Minneapolis, MN, USA.

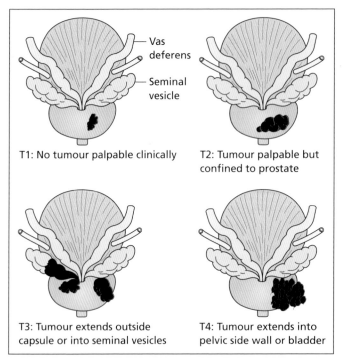

Figure 43.1 The clinical staging of prostatic carcinoma.

- *PSA concentration* in the blood is usually raised in the presence of prostate carcinoma. A PSA over 20 ng/mL suggests disseminated disease. PSA is also useful as a tumour marker to follow the response to treatment.
- *Transrectal ultrasound* gives good definition of the prostate. It can detect small tumours and can assess extracapsular spread. It is also used to guide needle core biopsies, which are performed systematically through the gland, obtaining 10–15 cores.
- *Transrectal prostatic biopsy, or prostatic chippings* retrieved at transurethral resection, will confirm the diagnosis and grade of tumour.
- *Bone scan* is indicated if the PSA is greater than 20 ng/mL, or if there is bone pain. It will show the presence and extent of bony metastases.
- *Magnetic resonance (MR) imaging* is indicated in patients with higher grade tumours and those undergoing radical surgery to identify lymphadenopathy.

Treatment

Treatment is based on the likelihood of tumour confinement to the gland, derived from the Gleason grade score, serum PSA and clinical stage, a prediction of the extent of spread of the tumour.

Localized disease

Small well-differentiated tumours in elderly men may be treated by 'watchful waiting', particularly if their anticipated life expectancy is poor (less than 10 years).

- *Radical prostatectomy*, removing the prostate, seminal vesicles and pelvic lymph nodes with anastomosis of the bladder neck to the urethra just distal to the prostate, is the treatment of choice in young patients with a high chance of localized disease. The side-effects include impotence in half the patients, and urinary incontinence in a few.
- *Radical radiotherapy* with or without hormone treatment has a lower impotence rate and virtually no chance of incontinence, but may leave proctitis or bladder irritation.

The long-term efficacy of each technique is yet to be subjected to a full randomized clinical trial, partly because the slow rate of growth of prostate cancer necessitates long follow-up.

Metastatic disease

Carcinoma of the prostate is more usually discovered at a stage when it has already spread beyond its capsule and may well have involved other organs, particularly the pelvic cellular tissues, bladder base and bone. The mainstay of treatment of this disease is androgen suppression or the use of specific androgen antagonists, which will produce symptomatic relief in disseminated prostatic cancer in about 75% of patients.

- *Gonadotrophin-releasing hormone agonists*, e.g. buserilin and goserilin, are the mainstay of treatment. They inhibit the release of luteinizing hormone from the anterior pituitary, with consequent reduction of testicular production of testosterone. Initiation of therapy may cause a flare of testosterone production, and hence a flare of disease, so a short 3 week course of androgen therapy is given.
- *Cyproterone acetate*: a steroid androgen antagonist.
- *Castration* of patients with prostatic carcinoma often relieves their symptoms and sometimes produces dramatic remissions in the course of the disease.
- *Oestrogen administration*, e.g. stilboestrol (with aspirin to prevent thromboembolic disease), may be used when the disease becomes hormone refractory. Stilboestrol may produce gynaecomastia, nipple and scrotal pigmentation and testicular atrophy. More importantly, it may result in fluid retention and precipitate congestive cardiac failure.

Palliation produced by hormonal treatment of prostatic cancer suppresses PSA to normal levels for an average of 2 years, after which it slowly rises, with symptoms returning a few months later. When the cancer is refractory to hormone therapy, the average life expectancy is 6 months.

Radiotherapy may relieve the pain of bony deposits and can also be used for local control to supplement hormonal therapy.

Urinary obstruction due to the prostatic carcinoma may resolve on hormonal therapy; if not, an endoscopic prostatectomy is indicated.

Prostatitis

Once commonly due to tuberculosis, bacterial infection of the prostate is now more often due to faecal organisms, particularly *Escherichia coli* and *Streptococcus faecalis*. Non-bacterial prostatitis does not have an identifiable cause, although an autoimmune process after prior sensitization, possibly by an infection, may be responsible. Not uncommonly, patients may present with the symptoms of prostatitis in the absence of any inflammation (prostatodynia). These two forms, non-bacterial prostatitis and prostatodynia, have been reclassified as chronic pelvic pain syndrome.

Clinical features

In addition to asymptomatic prostatitis seen histologically in prostatic chippings at the time of resection, the following three forms of prostatitis are recognized.

Acute bacterial prostatitis

The patient presents with fever, rigors, perineal pain and difficulty voiding, together with symptoms of a urinary tract infection; he may present with acute retention. In addition, pain on ejaculation and blood in the semen (haematospermia) may be present. Rectal examination reveals an enlarged exquisitely tender prostate, and occasionally an abscess may be palpable. Epididymitis is a common accompaniment, owing to infection passing along the vas deferens.

Treatment is a 6 week course of antibiotics with good prostatic penetration (e.g. ciprofloxacin or trimethoprim).

Chronic bacterial prostatitis

This presents as recurrent urinary tract infections. The prostate feels much firmer, and may resemble a carcinoma. Diagnosis is made by urine samples before and after prostatic massage, and appropriate antibiotic therapy started.

Chronic pelvic pain syndrome

This is a common insidious problem affecting up to 9% of adult men. Characteristically, the patient experiences pain in the perineum, scrotum, tip of penis or bladder, along with pain on ejaculation or micturition. Symptoms of urinary frequency and a feeling of incomplete emptying are common.

The aetiology of the syndrome is unclear; cryptic infection, an autoimmune process and pelvic muscle abnormality have all been suggested.

Treatment options include pelvic floor relaxation, doughnut seat cushions, α-blockers, non-steroidal anti-inflammatory drugs, antibiotics and repetitive prostatic massage.

Bladder neck obstruction

Bladder neck obstruction may be due to congenital valves in the region of the prostatic urethra and internal meatus, or fibrosis of the prostate.

Posterior urethral valves

Congenital valves, which usually produce hydronephrosis and retention of urine in childhood. They are usually diagnosed on antenatal ultrasound, and the diagnosis confirmed by micturating cystourethrogram. Early treatment by surgical incision of the valves before renal failure occurs is important.

Bladder neck fibrosis

Bladder neck fibrosis produces the symptoms of prostatic hyperplasia but without enlargement of the prostate. It is usually a consequence of scarring following instrumentation or prostatic resection.

Treatment

Endoscopic incision of the bladder neck is performed.

Urinary retention

Urinary retention may be acute, chronic or acute on chronic.

- *Acute retention* presents with inability to pass urine, suprapubic pain and a suprapubic mass. The differential diagnosis that must always be considered is a ruptured abdominal aortic aneurysm, in which the mass may be pulsatile, the pain radiates into the back and the patient is shocked (causing anuria).
- *Chronic urinary retention* is a more insidious process with gradual enlargement of the bladder, dribbling incontinence and little or no pain.

The definitive treatment of urinary retention can only be decided upon after three essential steps have been carried out. These are as follows:

1 diagnosis of the cause;
2 assessment of renal damage caused by the back pressure;
3 assessment of the general condition of the patient – is the patient fit for any surgical procedure that may be necessary?

Diagnosis of the cause

The diagnosis can be classified into the following:

1 *General causes* (no organic obstruction to urinary flow):
  a postoperative;
  b central nervous system (CNS) disease, e.g. tabes, multiple sclerosis, spinal tumour;
  c drugs, e.g. anticholinergics, tricyclic antidepressants.
2 *Local causes*:
  a in the lumen of the urethra, e.g. stone or blood clot;
  b in the wall, e.g. stricture;
  c outside the wall, e.g. prostatic enlargement (benign or malignant), faecal impaction, pelvic tumour, pregnant uterus.

General causes of retention of urine must always be borne in mind. The most common cause of acute retention is indeed seen postoperatively. The patient is not used to passing urine lying in bed, is weak and often in pain. Usually, the condition can be overcome by giving an injection of opiate and sitting the patient with his legs over the side of the bed within earshot of a running tap; if this does not succeed, catheterization may be required. The catheter can either be removed once the bladder has been emptied or, more commonly, left *in situ* until the following morning. Sometimes a patient with an enlarged prostate is precipitated into retention of urine following some other surgical procedure and it may then be necessary to proceed to prostatectomy.

In every case, the CNS must be carefully examined, as retention of urine may be due to interruption of the sacral nervous pathway. There is a tendency to think of retention of urine in an elderly man as being invariably due to prostatic disease, but every now and then one of these patients will be found to have a spinal tumour, tabes dorsalis or some other neurological condition such as the autonomic neuropathy of diabetes.

The diagnosis of the cause of retention is made by the usual three steps.

History

This may reveal the typical progressive symptoms of prostatism, a story of urethral infection suggesting stricture, a preceding episode of ureteric colic suggesting stone, etc.

Examination

This includes a rectal examination to determine the size and nature of the prostate, palpation of the urethra for stone or stricture, inspection of the urethral meatus and examination of the CNS.

Special investigations

- *X-ray of the pelvis* may reveal a calculus at the bladder base or bony secondaries from prostatic carcinoma.
- *PSA* should be measured, but not until 6 weeks have passed following the episode of retention since this can elevate the PSA. A raised value is suggestive of carcinoma.

Assessment of the degree of renal damage

The patient with retention of urine may have damaged his kidneys by back pressure; obviously, this is far more likely to occur in long-standing cases of chronic retention, but the possibility must be considered in every case. This assessment again is made under the three following headings.

History

Renal failure is suggested by headaches, anorexia, vomiting and mental disturbance.

Examination

Is the patient pale and drowsy with the dry, coated tongue of uraemia?

Special investigations

- Urea and cr*eatinine* are estimated: a blood urea over 7 mmol/L and/or creatinine over 135 μmol/L suggest at least some degree of renal impairment.

Assessment of the general condition of the patient

The average patient with retention of urine admitted to hospital is an elderly man. Before proceeding to major surgery, his general condition must obviously be carefully investigated, again under the three headings.

History

Exercise tolerance, the presence of cough and sputum and a history of previous coronary episodes are enquired into.

Examination

Chest, cardiovascular system and blood pressure.

Special investigations

- *Chest X-ray and electrocardiogram* are performed if necessary.
- *The haemoglobin* level is checked.

Scheme of management of acute urinary retention

The three common causes for an emergency surgical admission of a man with acute urinary retention are benign prostatic hyperplasia, malignant disease of the prostate and urethral stricture. The scheme shown in Figure 43.2 outlines the management of such cases. An attempt is made to catheterize the patient under full aseptic precautions.

Benign prostatic enlargement

Proceed to prostatectomy as soon as convenient if the renal function and general condition of the patient are satisfactory. If renal damage or general poor condition preclude operation, drainage by urethral catheter is continued until these can be improved. If the patient is in such poor health that operation is inappropriate, for example a bedridden patient, then he is best managed by permanent urethral drainage, the catheter being changed regularly and urinary antiseptics used if necessary, should urinary infection occur. A self-retaining Foley catheter[2] is far kinder to the patient than a leaky and smelly permanent suprapubic cystostomy tube.

---

[2] Frederick Foley (1891–1966), Urologist, Boston, MA, then St. Paul, MN, USA.

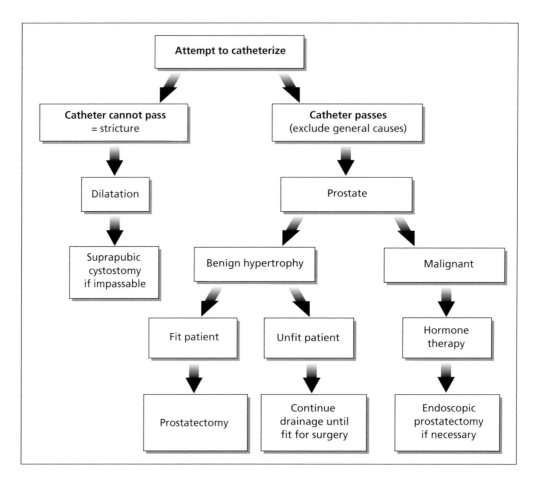

Figure 43.2 Treatment of acute retention.

Malignant disease of the prostate

In the presence of metastatic spread, hormone therapy is commenced. Endoscopic prostatectomy is required for localized tumours, or large tumours if symptoms persist on hormonal therapy.

Urethral stricture (Chapter 44, p. 368)

The catheter will not pass and the urethra must be gently dilated with bougies under local or general anaesthetic. Following this, it is possible to catheterize the patient and to continue with regular urethral dilatations or, preferably, to divide the stricture endoscopically with an optical urethrotome. Rarely, the stricture is impassable and the patient requires a temporary suprapubic cystotomy prior to urethrotomy. Occasionally, a

plastic operation on the stricture is indicated, but only rarely is permanent suprapubic drainage required.

Chronic urinary retention

If there is evidence of renal impairment, the patient is catheterized, and the catheter left in for a period to allow the renal function, and the general condition, to improve. Following relief of the hydronephrosis that accompanies chronic obstruction, there is a polyuric phase, and intravenous fluid replacement may be required to keep up with the fluid losses. Bleeding is common following decompression of a chronically distended bladder; there is no advantage in the intermittent catheter clamping that was once advocated when draining such bladders.

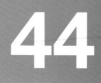

The male urethra

Learning objectives
✓ To know the congenital anomalies of the male urethra.
✓ To know the different types of urethral injury and their management. The reader should also know the causes, investigation and treatment of urethral stricture.

Congenital anomalies

Hypospadias

The male urethra is formed by the inrolling of the genital folds, which themselves form the corpus spongiosum. If the genital folds fail to develop or fuse completely, the tube is either short or absent. The urethra thus opens onto the ventral surface of the penis anywhere from the perineum up to the glans. Hypospadias is associated with an abnormal prepuce that is deficient ventrally, and so appears hooded. Proximal hypospadias is associated with a downward curvature of the penis on erection, termed *chordee*. Treatment involves plastic procedures utilizing the prepuce as a skin flap; circumcision before correction of the abnormality is therefore contraindicated.

Epispadias

The urethra opens dorsally on the penis. It is associated with other anterior abdominal wall defects including exstrophy of the bladder.

Posterior urethral valves (see also Chapter 43, p. 364)

A valve-like membrane at the level of the verumontanum. This can obstruct the flow of urine,

Lecture Notes: General Surgery, 12th edition. © Harold Ellis, Sir Roy Y. Calne and Christopher J. E. Watson. Published 2011 by Blackwell Publishing Ltd.

resulting in chronic retention of urine and uraemia in infants.

Injury to the urethra

This may be classified into rupture of the bulbous urethra and rupture of the membranous urethra.

The bulbous urethra

This may be damaged by a direct blow, e.g. a fall astride a bar (such as a bicycle cross-bar) or a kick in the perineum, or during forcible dilatation or cystoscopy. The patient will complain of severe pain in the perineum and usually bright-red blood will be seen dripping from the external meatus. There will be marked bruising in the region of the injury.

The membranous urethra

This is injured in pelvic fractures, especially those involving dislocation of a portion of the pelvis; it is torn at its junction with the prostatic urethra. As with extraperitoneal rupture of the bladder (Chapter 42, p. 354), blood and urine are extravasated in the extraperitoneal space and produce a swelling dull to percussion above the pubis. If the urethra is torn from the bladder, the prostate is displaced and there will be a feeling of emptiness on rectal examination.

The attempted passage of a catheter in a patient with a pelvic fracture can be both misleading and dangerous: misleading in that the catheter may pass along a partially ruptured posterior urethra into the bladder so that the diagnosis is missed, and dangerous in that the catheter may complete the tear in a partially ruptured urethra or produce a false passage.

Management

Satisfactory management depends on a high index of suspicion leading to early diagnosis, as extravasation of urine is liable to lead to secondary infection, which will greatly complicate the condition. The presence of bleeding from the meatus, or a fracture of the pelvis, combined with urinary retention, should alert to the possibility.

Initial management

- *Rectal examination* is performed to determine whether the prostate is palpable and in the normal position. An absent or high prostate implies a complete rupture of the membranous urethra, and urgent exploration is indicated.
- *A urethrogram* using water-soluble contrast medium will identify extravasation or loss of continuity, and localize the site of injury.
- *Contrast-enhanced computed tomography* is usually required to evaluate pelvic injuries fully.
- *The ABC of resuscitation* should not be forgotten, since many of these injuries occur in conjunction with a pelvic fracture.

Membranous urethral injuries

- *Complete rupture*, in which rectal examination confirms that the prostate (and therefore bladder) is floating out of the pelvis. Initial management is the passage of a suprapubic catheter. Subsequent management depends on the associated injuries, for example whether the pelvis is to be fixed by internal fixation. Surgery is either performed early, around the time of the pelvic fixation, or after an interval of around 6 weeks.

  Primary anastomosis is rarely possible. Instead, the base of the bladder and the urethra are approximated. The retropubic space is explored and the haematoma evacuated. A urethral catheter is passed and railroaded into the bladder. The bladder is approximated to the ruptured urethra by means of sutures in the anterior prostatic capsule. The urethral catheter will remain *in situ* for 2 weeks.

- *Incomplete rupture*. If there is little extravasation, and continuity is preserved, a well-lubricated urethral catheter should be passed carefully, and left in place for 10 days.

Bulbous urethral injuries

- *Complete rupture*. A complete laceration is an indication for urgent open repair, with suture of the tear and diversion of the urinary stream by suprapubic drainage.
- *Incomplete rupture*. If there is little extravasation, and continuity is preserved, a well-lubricated urethral catheter may be passed carefully, and left in place for 10 days. Alternatively, a suprapubic catheter can be inserted.

Complications

- *Stricture formation* often occurs following injuries to the urethra because of scarring; subsequent repair may be necessary.
- *Impotence* occurs in half the patients, as a consequence of either a pelvic injury involving the terminal branches of the internal iliac arteries or injury to the nerves supplying the penis.

Urethral stricture

Aetiology

Congenital

- Meatal stenosis in hypospadias.

Acquired

1 *Trauma*:
   a urethral instrumentation including catheterization;
   b rupture of the urethra;
   c previous urethral or prostatic surgery.
2 *Postinfection*:
   a gonococcal;
   b non-specific urethritis, e.g. *Chlamydia*.
3 *Carcinoma of the urethra* (extremely rare).

Clinical features

The patient with a urethral stricture complains of difficulty in passing urine with a poor stream and states that only by straining can he empty his bladder. He is usually younger than 50 years (in contrast to prostatic disease), and may suffer urinary infection and acute retention as a consequence of the stricture.

Special investigations

- *Urethrogram* will demonstrate the location and length of the stricture.
- *Urethral ultrasound* will define the stricture and assess the presence of corporal fibrosis, which is of prognostic value in determining the chance of recurrence.
- *Urinary flow rate*: the stricture limits the flow of urine, and measurement of the flow rate shows a flat plateau.
- *Urethroscopy* will visualize the stricture and facilitate treatment.

Treatment

Optical urethrotomy is the first-line treatment. Urethral strictures have a high chance of recurrence depending on the length of the stricture and the degree of corporal fibrosis. About 50% of strictures recur after optical urethrotomy, although this rate can be reduced to 20% by getting the patient to use intermittent self-catheterization with disposable catheters.

Recurrent strictures can be treated by further optical urethrotomy or urethroplasty, with either simple resection of the stricture with end-to-end anastomosis of the ends, or interposition of a tube of buccal mucosa.

The management of acute retention due to urethral stricture is outlined on Chapter 43, p. 366.

45

The penis

Learning objectives
✓ To understand phimosis and paraphimosis and their treatment.
✓ To know about carcinoma of the penis, its presentations and treatment.
✓ To know the causes of impotence and its treatment.

Phimosis

Phimosis is gross narrowing of the preputial orifice. It occurs rarely as a congenital lesion, but may result from scarring following the trauma of forcible retraction of the prepuce (see below) or as a result of chronic balanitis.

Clinical features

On micturition, the prepuce is seen to balloon and the urinary stream is reduced to a dribble.

Treatment

Circumcision is performed. In some cases of chronic balanitis with considerable inflammation of the prepuce, a dorsal slit is an efficient, but less aesthetic, method of cure.

Paraphimosis

Paraphimosis results from pulling a tight foreskin proximally over the glans. The foreskin acts as a constricting band, interfering with venous return from the glans, which therefore swells painfully.

Lecture Notes: General Surgery, 12th edition. © Harold Ellis, Sir Roy Y. Calne and Christopher J. E. Watson. Published 2011 by Blackwell Publishing Ltd.

Once swelling starts, it becomes more difficult to replace the foreskin.

Paraphimosis commonly occurs after an erection. It may also occur following urethral catheterization, when the foreskin is forcibly retracted over the glans to expose the meatus. Once the catheter is inserted, the thickened scarred prepuce constricts the venous return, producing a paraphimosis. Hence it is important to ensure always that the patient's prepuce is pulled forward again after the insertion of an indwelling catheter – if not, paraphimosis may follow.

Treatment

Once a paraphimosis has become established, it is difficult to reduce. There are two commonly used courses of action. Under a penile local anaesthetic block, the glans is squeezed for a few minutes to reduce the oedema, and enable the foreskin to be reduced. If squeezing fails, the foreskin may be slit dorsally to release the constricting band.

Having once had a paraphimosis, the patient should be considered for a formal circumcision to prevent recurrence.

Non-retractile prepuce

Many male infants are presented to the doctor or nurse because the parents notice that the prepuce cannot be retracted. In fact, the foreskin is normally firmly adherent to the glans until 3 years of age. Over the next 3 years, the congenital adhesions between the glans and the foreskin lyse, progressively separating from the glans.

Forcible attempts to retract the foreskin traumatize the tissues, and the resultant scarring may lead to a true phimosis. Inability to retract the foreskin in the infant is not an indication in itself for circumcision; indeed, in the 'nappy' stage the prepuce protects the delicate glans and the urethral orifice from the excoriation of ammoniacal dermatitis.

Circumcision

Circumcision is the resection of the foreskin, leaving the glans exposed. Indications for circumcision include the following:

- phimosis;
- paraphimosis;
- religious custom;
- non-retractile prepuce over 6 years of age.

Having the prepuce removed reduces the risk of carcinoma of the penis, probably because it prevents the accumulation of smegma, which is carcinogenic.

Ammoniacal dermatitis

This is a common cause of inflammation of the penis in children and is due to the presence of ammonia liberated by urea-splitting organisms. This is especially liable to occur if the child's nappies are infrequently changed and he is allowed to remain wet. The ammonia causes a painful, red, oedematous rash on the perineum, penis and foreskin.

Treatment

Treatment is to change the child's nappies frequently, wash the area with warm water and to cover the skin with a protective barrier cream such as zinc oxide. Secondary bacterial or candidal infections may occur and require appropriate antimicrobials.

Circumcision should be avoided in the presence of ammoniacal dermatitis, as a meatal ulcer is likely to result.

Balanitis

Balanitis is an acute inflammation of the foreskin and glans and is usually due to the common pyogenic organisms, for instance coliform bacilli, staphylococci and streptococci. It may result in phimosis from scarring.

It is important to test the urine for sugar to exclude diabetes, which may predispose to the inflammation, in which case *Candida* may be the infecting organism.

Treatment

Treatment consists of administering the appropriate antibiotic after the organism has been cultured and its sensitivity has been determined. Local toilet with weak disinfectant solutions may give relief symptomatically.

Carcinoma

Pathology

This tumour usually affects elderly subjects. It is uncommon in the UK, although relatively frequently seen in Africa and the East. It is almost invariably associated with the presence of retained smegma and is virtually unknown among Jews, who are circumcised soon after birth.

The most frequent site of the tumour is in the sulcus between the glans and the prepuce.

Macroscopic appearance

The premalignant stage is a persistent red patch on the penis progressing to either a papillary growth on the glans or an infiltrating ulcer; the latter is more common.

Microscopic appearance

The lesions are squamous carcinomas, which are usually well differentiated.

Spread

- *Local*: the tumour may fungate through the prepuce to present as an ulcerating lesion on the penile skin. Proximal spread along the shaft may destroy the substance of the penis.

- *Lymphatic*: the inguinal lymph nodes are frequently involved, often bilaterally.
- *Blood-borne* spread occurs late and is unusual.

Clinical features

The patient may present with an ulcer on the glans or because of a purulent or blood-stained discharge from below the non-retractile prepuce. He may wait until the tumour has ulcerated through the prepuce or until most of his penis has been destroyed by growth. Surprisingly enough, carcinoma of the penis never seems to occlude the urethra sufficiently to produce retention of urine.

Treatment

Diagnosis is achieved by biopsy, which often necessitates excision of the foreskin.

Early growths can be treated adequately by local radiotherapy using iridium wires, or by partial amputation of the penis if the urethra is encroached upon. Survival from early disease is good (near 100% at 5 years).

When the regional lymph nodes are involved, which is the case in 50% of patients at presentation, treatment is more difficult. Radical surgery may effect a cure, and consists of total amputation of the penis and bilateral block dissections of the inguinal lymph nodes, usually with some form of plastic surgical reconstruction. This operation, although mutilating, does not interfere with micturition because both the internal and external sphincters are preserved. After a total amputation of the penis, the patient will need to micturate sitting down.

Inoperably fixed lymph nodes are treated by palliative irradiation.

In summary,

- *urethra intact*: radiotherapy;
- *urethra involved*: amputation;
- *lymph nodes involved*: block dissection if operable, radiotherapy as a palliative measure if matted together and fixed.

Impotence

Impotence is the inability to achieve, or sustain, an erection satisfactory to permit penetration for sexual intercourse.

Aetiology

Impotence most commonly occurs as a consequence of ageing, such that 70% of 70 year olds have some difficulty with obtaining an erection (although 70% of 70 year olds also have sexual intercourse once a month). Aside from ageing, the other causes of erectile impotence are as follows.

Neurogenic

Erection is mediated via efferent parasympathetic fibres from S2, S3, S4. Reflex erection requires afferent signals via the pudendal nerve, while psychogenic erection requires outflow from the brain via the spinal cord. Causes of neurogenic impotence include the following:

- *congenital*: spina bifida;
- *spinal causes*: spinal cord injury, spinal cord tumour;
- *central causes*: hypothalamic injury, cerebral infarction/tumour;
- *postsurgical causes*: e.g. pelvic surgery such as anterior resection, abdominoperineal resection and radical prostatectomy.

Vascular

Erection requires increased arterial flow into the erectile tissue of the penis, together with some degree of venous outflow inhibition. Arterial disease affecting flow in the internal iliac arteries, as may result from aortoiliac disease, can cause impotence and buttock claudication (Leriche's syndrome[1]).

Hormonal

- *Diabetes mellitus*, the most common hormonal cause, but probably acting via a diabetic neuropathy.
- *Pituitary failure*, primary testicular failure, hypothyroidism, and most other endocrine diseases may contribute to impotence.

Pharmacological

Some drugs, in particular antihypertensive agents, tranquillizers and oestrogens, may cause impotence. Alcohol is also a common cause.

---

[1] René Leriche (1879–1955), Professor of Surgery successively in Strasbourg, Lyon and Paris, France.

Psychogenic

Psychogenic impotence is usually of sudden onset, and the patient continues to have nocturnal erections and erections following masturbation, suggesting there is not a physical cause.

Special investigations

A full history and examination are conducted to determine the cause. Other investigations include the following:

- *urine dipstick* to detect diabetes;
- *hormone screen*: abnormalities in the blood levels of testosterone, follicle-stimulating hormone, luteinizing hormone, prolactin and thyroxine should be excluded.

Treatment

Treatable medical causes are excluded, and hormonal disturbances are corrected when possible. Other treatments include the following:

- *Sildenafil*, a phosphodiesterase type 5 inhibitor, is taken 1 hour before intercourse. It causes vasodilatation of the corporus cavernosum, but is contraindicated in patients on nitrate therapy, e.g. for ischaemic heart disease, since this combination can result in severe hypotension.
- *Sublingual apomorphine* has a faster action than sildenafil, but is associated with nausea.
- *Alprostadil* (prostaglandin E1), given by intrapenile injection or by direct intraurethral application, is also effective.
- A *vacuum condom*, or an *intrapenile inflatable prosthesis* may be required.

46

The testis and scrotum

Learning objectives

✓ To know the different causes of testicular maldescent and their treatment.

✓ To have knowledge of testicular torsion, how it presents, its differential diagnosis and treatment.

✓ To know the different causes of scrotal lumps, their differing clinical features and treatment, including the diagnosis and management of testicular tumours.

Abnormalities of testicular descent

Embryology

The testis arises from the mesodermal germinal ridge in the posterior wall of the abdominal cavity. It links up with the epididymis and vas deferens, which develop from the mesonephric duct. As the testis enlarges, it undergoes caudal migration. By the third month of fetal life it is in the iliac fossa; by the seventh month it reaches the inguinal canal; by the eighth month it has reached the external inguinal ring; and by the ninth month, at birth, it has descended into the scrotum. During this descent, a prolongation of peritoneum, called the processus vaginalis, projects into the fetal scrotum; the testis slides behind this and is thus covered in its front and sides by peritoneum. The processus vaginalis becomes obliterated at about the time of birth, leaving the testis covered by the tunica vaginalis. As expected from the embryology, abnormalities of descent are more common in premature infants (20% incidence) than in full-term infants (2%).

Lecture Notes: General Surgery, 12th edition. © Harold Ellis, Sir Roy Y. Calne and Christopher J. E. Watson. Published 2011 by Blackwell Publishing Ltd.

Classification of maldescent

Testicular maldescent can be subdivided according to whether or not the testis followed the normal course of descent.

Ectopic testis (uncommon)

A testis that has strayed from the normal line of descent is termed ectopic. The commonest position is in the superficial inguinal pouch, which lies anterior to the external oblique aponeurosis. The testis reaches this site after migrating through the external inguinal ring and then leaves the normal track of descent to pass laterally. Other situations are the groin, the perineum, the root of the penis and the femoral triangle.

Undescended testis (common)

A testis that has followed the normal course of descent but has stopped short of the scrotum is termed an undescended or, more properly, an incompletely descended testis. It may lie anywhere from the abdominal cavity, along the inguinal canal, to the top of the scrotum. The vast majority are due to a local defect in development. The affected testis is always small and it is probable that this imperfect development impairs descent rather than that the imperfect descent impairs development. The incompletely descended testis is usually accompanied by persistent patency of the processus vaginalis, presenting as a congenital inguinal hernia. Unilateral undescended testes are four times as common as bilateral. The condition of bilateral undescended impalpable testes is termed *cryptorchidism*.

Most, if not all, testes that are going to descend do so within the first few months of life. If the testis is not in its normal scrotal position in early childhood, it is very unlikely that it will be capable of spermatogenesis. However, the interstitial cells are functional, so that secondary sex characteristics develop normally.

Differential diagnosis: the retractile testis

The most common mistake in diagnosis is to fail to differentiate a true maldescent from a retractile testis. The retractile testis is a normal testis with an excessively active cremasteric reflex, resulting in the testis being drawn up to the external inguinal ring. It is a common condition and often the parents think that the testes have failed to descend; indeed, when the scrotum is palpated the testes may not be felt. However, careful examination will probably reveal the testis at the external inguinal ring or at the root of the scrotum and the testis can, by downward stroking or by gentle traction, be coaxed into the scrotum. A useful trick is to place the child in the squatting position for the examination; this often encourages a retractile testis to descend into the scrotum. It is also worthwhile asking the parents to examine the child when he is relaxed in a warm bath; again, the retractile testis may then slip into its normal position.

If the testis is easily palpable in the groin and remains easy to feel when the child tenses his abdominal wall muscles, it is lying in the ectopic position and not in the inguinal canal – where it is usually impalpable or, at the most, in a thin boy, detected as a vague, tender bulge.

Treatment

The child with retractile testes is normal; reassurance of the parents is all that is required.

The ectopic or undescended testis must be placed in the scrotum if it is to function as a sperm-producing organ. The optimum age for surgery has been revised in recent times, and current recommendations are for surgery around the age of 2. After that age, definite changes in the testis can be seen on microscopy, which may lead to impaired spermatogenesis. The operation, termed orchidopexy, consists of mobilizing the testis and its cord, removing the coexisting hernial sac and fixing the testis in the scrotum without tension.

Complications of maldescent

- Defective spermatogenesis, sterility if bilateral.
- Increased risk of torsion.
- Increased risk of trauma.
- Increased risk of malignant disease, even if surgical correction is carried out.
- Inguinal hernia – persistence of the processus vaginalis.

Scrotal swellings

Examination

When considering any swelling in the scrotum, the following three questions should be considered in turn (Figure 46.1).

1 *Can the examiner's fingers meet above the swelling?* If this is not possible, the swelling arises from the abdomen and is an inguinoscrotal hernia.
2 *If it is possible to palpate clearly the upper edge of the swelling, is the swelling cystic?* If it is cystic on transillumination and the testis is palpable separate from the swelling, the swelling is a cyst of the epididymis. However, if the testis is not palpable because it lies within the cyst, it is a hydrocele.
3 *If the swelling is solid, the following must be considered:*
   a the swelling is an abnormal testis, e.g. a tumour or (rarely) a gumma;
   b the epididymis is involved – this is usually an inflammatory condition, either acute or chronic.

   The latter is either tuberculous or the residual chronic thickening that may persist for many months after an acute pyogenic infection that has been treated with an antibiotic.

Special investigation

Ultrasound of the swelling is valuable in determining whether there is an underlying solid mass in

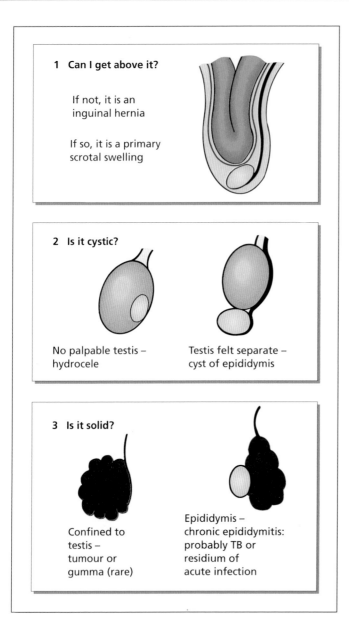

1 Can I get above it?

If not, it is an inguinal hernia

If so, it is a primary scrotal swelling

2 Is it cystic?

No palpable testis – hydrocele

Testis felt separate – cyst of epididymis

3 Is it solid?

Confined to testis – tumour or gumma (rare)

Epididymis – chronic epididymitis: probably TB or residium of acute infection

Figure 46.1 The differential diagnosis of a scrotal swelling.

relation to the presence of a scrotal cystic swelling, and may indicate its nature.

Cysts of the epididymis

Epididymal cysts arise as cystic degeneration of one of the epididymal or para-epididymal structures, and so are common in middle-aged and elderly men. They are often multiple, may be bilat-eral, and produce a fluctuant and usually highly translucent swelling in the scrotum. As they arise from the epididymis, the testis is palpable sepa-rately from, and in front of, the cyst. This is the main differentiating point from a hydrocele. The contained fluid may be water-clear or may be milky and contain sperm; hence, the old term spermatocele. Clinically, there is no way of differ-entiating between a cyst of the epididymis and a spermatocele, and the latter term is best abandoned.

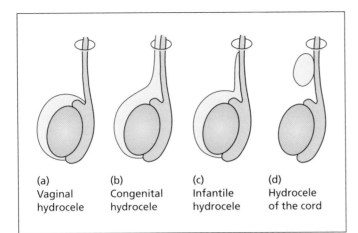

(a)
Vaginal
hydrocele

(b)
Congenital
hydrocele

(c)
Infantile
hydrocele

(d)
Hydrocele
of the cord

Figure 46.2 (a–d) The anatomical classification of hydroceles (the ring at the upper end of each diagram represents the internal inguinal ring).

Large cysts of the epididymis may trouble the patient by getting in the way of his clothes and chafing his legs. If producing symptoms, cysts of the epididymis should be removed surgically. Aspiration is usually unsuccessful because of recurrence.

Hydrocele

A hydrocele is an excessive collection of serous fluid in the processus vaginalis, usually the tunica. Hydroceles may be classified as follows.

Primary or idiopathic hydrocele (Figure 46.2)

This is usually large and tense. There is no disease of the underlying testis. Primary hydroceles may be subdivided into the following:

- *Vaginal hydrocele.* The vaginal hydrocele is the usual type of hydrocele surrounding the testis and separated from the peritoneal cavity. The patient presents with a cystic transilluminable swelling in the scrotum. On examination, the testis is difficult to feel and lies at the back of the swelling which, owing to the anatomy of the tunica, encompasses the anterior and lateral portions of the organ.
- *Congenital hydrocele.* Congenital hydrocele is associated with a hernial sac, the still patent processus vaginalis. It opens into the peritoneal cavity through a narrow orifice. When elevated it gradually empties.

- *Infantile hydrocele.* Infantile hydrocele extends from the testis to the internal inguinal ring but does not pass into the peritoneal cavity.
- *Hydrocele of the cord.* Hydrocele of the cord is rare. It lies in, or just distal to, the inguinal canal, separate from the testis and the peritoneum, and represents a length of patent processus vaginalis in which the upper and lower parts have closed. Diagnosis is confirmed by the simple test of downward traction on the testis, which pulls the hydrocele of the cord down with it. The equivalent in the female is a hydrocele of the round ligament within the inguinal canal, termed a *hydrocele of the canal of Nuck*.[1]

Secondary hydrocele

A secondary hydrocele is usually smaller and lax and the testis is diseased. It is due to the serosal sac surrounding the testis becoming filled with an exudate secondary to tumour or inflammation of the underlying testis or epididymis.

Treatment

Infants

Hydroceles in infants should be left alone because most disappear spontaneously. If the hydrocele persists after the first year, operative treatment is

---

[1]Anton Nuck (1650–1692), Professor of Anatomy and Medicine, Leiden, The Netherlands.

advisable. The sac is identified and excised, care being taken not to damage any other structures in the cord.

Adults

In young adults, the possibility of tumour should be borne in mind. Ultrasound examination will usually differentiate a normal from an abnormal testis in this situation.

The hydrocele can be treated by aspiration, the resultant fluid being straw-coloured with flecks of cholesterol in it. Operative treatment is the treatment of choice in all but the very elderly, as hydroceles recur after aspiration.

Secondary hydroceles require treatment for the underlying condition.

Acute infections of the testis and epididymis

Acute infections usually arise as an ascending infection via the vas deferens, spreading first to the epididymis and thence to the testis; occasionally, infection may be blood-borne.

Blood-borne infection

The commonest blood-borne agent to infect the testis is the *mumps virus*, the testicular manifestation of which usually follows within a week of the onset of parotid enlargement. Occasionally, it may occur in the absence of other manifestations. Diagnosis is confirmed clinically and by the rising level of mumps antibodies in the serum. Young adults are particularly likely to be affected; there may be residual damage to the testis and, if both sides are involved, fertility may be impaired.

Ascending infection

Ascending infection is usually a consequence of a preceding urinary tract infection (e.g. with *Escherichia coli*) or a urethritis or prostatitis from a sexually transmitted organism such as gonorrhoea or *Chlamydia*, which result in epididymitis. Epididymitis may also follow urethral stricture in which straining causes reflux of urine up the vas, or instrumentation of the urethra such as during prostatectomy.

Clinical features

The patient will have a very painful swelling of the epididymis, often with a secondary hydrocele and constitutional effects (pyrexia, headache and leucocytosis). There may be a history of dysuria, suggesting a urinary tract infection, or urethral discharge, suggesting a sexually transmitted organism. Examination of the urine may reveal the presence of organisms and pus cells, but the urine need not be abnormal. Rectal examination of the prostate may reveal coexistent prostatitis.

Treatment

Treatment is bed rest and the appropriate antibiotic given over a prolonged course (6 weeks); ciprofloxacin is a typical first-line agent with good specificity for the organisms most often encountered. If frank abscesses have formed (verified by ultrasound), drainage is required. However, with early adequate treatment, resolution is more likely. The patient will often have residual swelling of the epididymis, which may be rather firm, and differentiation from the tuberculous epididymitis may be difficult unless the history of the previous acute attack is obtained. When epididymitis arises as a consequence of *Chlamydia* or other sexually transmitted disease, it is important that the sexual partner is also treated; doxycycline is the antibiotic of choice.

Differential diagnosis

As with all acutely painful conditions of the testis, torsion must be excluded. If the patient is in his teens, torsion is more likely; if he is in his twenties and sexually active, epididymitis is more likely. However, if doubt exists, urgent exploration is mandatory.

Chronic infections of the testis

Gumma

Although once common, syphilis of the testis is now a rarity. The testis is enlarged and is clinically difficult to distinguish from a carcinoma. On penicillin therapy, gummas of the testis melt away.

Tuberculosis

This may occur in association with tuberculosis in other parts of the genitourinary tract by ascending infection, but more commonly is a consequence of haematogenous spread.

Clinical features

The patient usually presents with swelling of the epididymis. The vas deferens may be thickened and feel nodular. A cold abscess may develop in relation to the epididymis and rupture through the scrotum, usually posteriorly, resulting in a chronic sinus. The seminal vesicles may be enlarged and palpable on rectal examination.

Diagnosis depends on isolating tubercle bacilli from the urine or biopsy material, and/or evidence of tuberculosis elsewhere.

Treatment

This is the same as for tuberculosis in other situations. If a chronic sinus has developed, unilateral orchidectomy is probably the best form of treatment, as the testis is unlikely to be functional, is a continued source of infection and may lead to spread of the disease elsewhere.

Torsion of the testis

Aetiology

Usually this is a torsion of the spermatic cord in a congenitally abnormal testis, often maldescended or hanging like a bell clapper within a completely investing tunica vaginalis. Occasionally, true torsion of the testis occurs without involving the cord, when there is an extensive mesorchium between the testis and epididymis. It is probably impossible for torsion to occur in an anatomically completely normal testis. Untreated, the testis undergoes irreversible infarction within a few hours and there is a typical transudation of blood-stained fluid into the tunica vaginalis. Torsion is more common in undescended and ectopic testes.

Clinical features

Torsion of the testis is a surgical emergency, which usually occurs in children or adolescents. There may be a history of mild trauma to the testis or of previous attacks of pain in the testis due to partial torsion and spontaneous untwisting. Cycling, straining, lifting and coitus are typical precipitants.

The history is of a sudden onset of severe pain in the groin and lower abdomen, often accompanied by vomiting. The abdominal pain occurs because the nerve supply of the testis is mainly from the T10 sympathetic pathway. Rarely, the pain is limited to the abdomen. Patients with torsion of the right testis have been mistakenly operated on for acute appendicitis because the testis has not been examined with care, or more often not at all.

Examination of the scrotum reveals a swollen testis, painful to touch and lying high in the scrotum.

Differential diagnosis

The differential diagnosis is from acute epididymitis and torsion of a testicular appendage; epididymitis does not come on suddenly.

1 *Epididymitis.* The testis does not lie so high in the scrotum, there is a systemic reaction with pyrexia and leucocytosis and there is usually a history of urinary infection with pus cells and organisms in the urine. A useful factor in differential diagnosis is the age of the patient, as torsion of the testis is unusual after the age of 20 years, whereas epididymitis is rare before that age.
2 *Torsion of a testicular appendage.* Two embryological remnants exist around the testis, the appendix testis and the appendix epididymis, which may themselves twist. They present in a similar fashion to testicular torsion, but on examination the testis does not lie high in the scrotum, and a dark blue pea-like swelling may be visible through the scrotal skin.
3 *Strangulated inguinal hernia.* Torsion may also mimic a strangulated inguinal hernia.

Colour Doppler ultrasound of the testis may be helpful in diagnosis, provided it can be carried out rapidly by an experienced operator, and without delaying surgical exploration.

Treatment

If there is *any* doubt as to the diagnosis, it is best to explore the testis as soon after admission as possible, because every hour increases the likelihood of irreversible damage to the testis. If still viable, the testis is untwisted and sutured to the tunica vaginalis. If infarcted, it is removed. In every case, fixation of the other testis should be performed at the same time, since any congenital anomaly is likely to be bilateral and torsion of the opposite testis may therefore occur.

Varicocele

This is a condition of varicosities of the pampiniform plexus of veins. It usually occurs on the left, and manifests first in adolescence. It is present in nearly 10% of men, the proportion increasing with age and being higher in infertile men.

Its origin is said to be due to the drainage of the left testicular vein at right angles into the left renal vein, unlike the right testicular vein, which drains obliquely into the inferior vena cava. Patients with varicocele have absent or incompetent valves at the junction with the left renal vein.

Occasionally, a varicocele can be secondary to a tumour or other pathological process blocking the testicular vein. The best known example of this is a tumour of the left kidney involving the renal vein and obstructing the drainage of the left testicular vein.

Clinical features

A varicocele may cause a dragging sensation in the scrotum. It is also associated with defective spermatogenesis, and patients with varicocele are often subfertile. On examination *in the standing position*, the varicose veins within the scrotum feel like a 'bag of worms', but there may be little to feel when the patient lies down.

Treatment

Usually, the varicocele requires no treatment apart from reassurance that the condition is not likely to give rise to any dangerous complications. If the weight of the varicocele and testis causes an ache, close-fitting underpants may help. If the patient demands treatment, the varicocele can be cured radiologically by embolizing the left testicular vein; it may also be treated surgically by ligating and dividing all the testicular veins as they traverse the inguinal canal. There is *no* evidence that treatment of a varicocele has any effect on male infertility.

Disorders of the scrotal skin

Idiopathic scrotal oedema

Characteristically affecting prepubescent boys, this inflammatory condition is characterized by an erythematous, oedematous swelling of the scrotal skin. It may involve both sides of the scrotum, and can extend into the groins. Unlike torsion, it is painless, and the testicular apparatus is normal on examination. Spontaneous resolution within a few days is usual.

Fournier's gangrene

Fournier's gangrene,[2] or synergistic gangrene of the scrotum, is a result of synergistic infection with several species of bacteria, both aerobic and anaerobic; haemolytic streptococci, staphylococci and *E. coli* are common isolates.

The patient is often diabetic and catheterized; there may be a history of minor trauma, perianal abscess or surgery, although there is no obvious precipitating factor in half the cases. The patient develops sudden pain in the scrotum, and rapidly becomes profoundly toxic.

This is a surgical emergency. Treatment involves high-dose broad-spectrum antibiotics and wide debridement of affected skin, often twice daily.

Carcinoma of the scrotum

Rare nowadays, this tumour is noteworthy as the first described industrial malignant disease. Percival Pott[3] (1779) noted an association with chimney sweeps, in whom chimney soot acted as a carcinogen when ingrained into the scrotal skin. Later, it was described in workers with mineral oils whose trousers were soaked by the carcinogenic oils.

Presenting as an ulcerating growth, it is usually a squamous carcinoma and is treated by wide excision with block dissection of affected inguinal nodes.

---

[2]Jean Alfred Fournier (1832–1914), 'Professeur des maladies cutanées et syphilitiques', Hôpital St. Louis, Paris, France.
[3]Percival Pott (1714–1788), Surgeon, St Bartholomew's Hospital, London, UK.

Tumours of the testis

Testicular tumours are the most common solid malignancy in young adult men, although they are relatively uncommon, representing around 2% of malignancies in men.

Aetiology

Testicular tumours are associated with undescended and ectopic testis (sevenfold risk). There is also an increased incidence in patients who are infertile, and those who have had a previous contralateral testicular malignancy.

Pathology

There are two main forms of malignant tumours of the testis – seminoma and non-seminomatous germ cell tumours (NSGCTs), of which teratoma is the main type. Rare tumours include lymphoma, which affects an older age group.

Seminoma

The seminoma (60%) arises from cells of the seminiferous tubules, usually occurs between 30 and 40 years of age and is relatively slow growing. Macroscopically, the tumour is solid, appearing rather like a cut potato on section. Microscopically, cells vary from well-differentiated spermatocytes to undifferentiated round cells with clear cytoplasm. Some 10% arise in undescended testes.

Teratoma

Teratoma (40%) occurs in a younger age group, the peak incidence being 20–30 years. It is thought to arise from primitive totipotential germ cells. Macroscopically, it has a markedly cystic appearance and used to be called fibrocystic disease. The cut surface may appear like a colloid goitre, and areas of haemorrhage and infarction are common. Microscopically, the cells are very variable and the tumour may contain cartilage, bone, muscle, fat and other tissues.

Spread

- *Local*: the testis is progressively destroyed by the tumour. Spread through the capsule is unusual, but occasionally in an advanced case there may be ulceration of the scrotum.
- *Lymphatic*: to the para-aortic nodes via lymphatics accompanying the testicular vein. In advanced cases, there may be enlargement of the supraclavicular nodes especially on the left side.
- *Blood-borne*: spread from the teratoma occurs relatively early to the lungs and liver. In the seminoma this tends to be late in the disease.

Clinical presentations

- As a lump in the testis.
- As a hydrocele.
- Rarely as a painful rapidly enlarging swelling, which may be mistaken for orchitis.
- As secondaries, usually metastatic growths in the lung (presenting as breathlessness), as a mass in the abdomen due to involved abdominal lymph nodes or as a cervical lymphadenopathy.

Tumours of the testis usually present as a painless, swollen testicle, or a lump on a testicle that is hard and may be associated with an overlying secondary hydrocele, which sometimes contains blood-stained fluid. There is often a misleading history of recent trauma, and rarely it may present having undergone torsion.

Occasionally, gynaecomastia may be a presenting feature, owing to the production of paraneoplastic hormones.

Special investigations

- *Scrotal ultrasound* may reveal a solid tumour in a hydrocele; the value of a negative ultrasound in the exclusion of malignancy depends on the skill of the ultrasonographer.
- *Tumour markers*: NSGCTs (e.g. teratomas) usually produce α-fetoprotein and many produce β-human chorionic gonadotrophin (β-HCG); some pure seminomas also produce β-HCG. These are useful not only in making a diagnosis but also in subsequent follow-up.
- *Chest X-ray and abdominal CT* to seek secondary spread and so stage the disease.

Treatment

If it is suspected that the testicular swelling is due to a tumour, early exploration is mandatory. The spermatic cord is exposed through an inguinal incision, occluded by an atraumatic clamp and the testis delivered. The clamp prevents vascular dissemination of tumour cells. If the diagnosis is now obvious, immediate orchidectomy is performed. If the diagnosis is in doubt, a biopsy is taken and submitted to frozen section examination. Orchidectomy is performed if the malignancy is confirmed. Inguinal, rather than scrotal, exploration is performed to avoid exposure to the scrotal lymphatics, which drain to the inguinal nodes, unlike the spermatic cord, which drains to the internal iliac nodes.

Seminomas are highly radiosensitive so that, following orchidectomy, radiotherapy is given to the ipsilateral iliac and para-aortic lymph nodes. For extensive disease, cytotoxic chemotherapy may also be given.

Teratomas are not as radiosensitive and are best treated by combination cytotoxic chemotherapy. Retroperitoneal lymph node dissection also has a role, particularly in the treatment of residual tumour after chemotherapy. As cytotoxic chemotherapy is likely to render the patient infertile, prior sperm banking is now offered.

Prognosis

Node-negative cases have an extremely good prognosis of nearly 100% 5 year survival. Even with early abdominal lymph node spread, there is still a 95% 5 year survival and, with disseminated disease, long-term survivals are often achieved with chemotherapy.

Male infertility

The majority of couples who are trying for a pregnancy will be rewarded within 2 years. However, one in 10 couples suffer infertility, with the problem distributed evenly between each partner, with one-third of cases due to factors in both the man and the woman.

Aetiology

Congenital disorder

- *Chromosome abnormality*, e.g. Klinefelter's syndrome (XXY).[4]
- *Developmental anomaly*, e.g. testicular maldescent, absent vas deferens.

[4]Harry Fitch Klinefelter (1912–1990), Associate Professor of Medicine, Johns Hopkins Hospital, Baltimore, MD, USA.

Physical problems

- *Post-infection*, e.g. following mumps orchitis or epididymitis.
- *Trauma*, with subsequent atrophy.
- *Neurological*, e.g. spinal injury, producing erectile and ejaculatory dysfunction.
- *Temperature*, e.g. varicocele, tight-fitting underpants.
- *Iatrogenic*, e.g. vasectomy, damage during orchidopexy or hernia repair.

Hormonal

- *Pituitary insufficiency*, e.g. from a pituitary tumour or craniopharyngioma.
- *Liver failure*, causing increased circulating oestrogens.

Drugs

- *Chemotherapy and radiotherapy* for cancer, usually teratoma or seminoma – patients are offered sperm-bank facilities prior to treatment.

Clinical features

A full history and thorough examination are required to exclude obvious contributory pathology. Previous surgery or infection of the testicular apparatus is particularly important, especially as a child. Coexisting diabetes or renal or hepatic failure may contribute to infertility, as can smoking.

Examination should include assessment of hair distribution and general build for evidence of testicular failure (female distribution). Examination of the penis and scrotal contents is particularly important, verifying the course of the vas deferens on each side, the size of the testis and the presence of a varicocele (with the patient standing). The presence of hypospadias (Chapter 44, p. 367) should be noted as this may affect where the sperm are deposited.

Special investigations

Before embarking on investigation, it should be ascertained that coitus is occurring regularly. Invasive tests are withheld until the infertile partner is identified.

- *Semen analysis*. Ideally, this is produced following a period of abstinence of 3 days and is examined within 4 hours. A semen volume over 2 mL, with over 20 million sperm per millilitre, of which 50% are motile at 4 hours, and at least 14% of normal morphology, is acceptable.

- *Hormone assays* in patients with no sperm (azoospermia), or few sperm. Raised prolactin is suggestive of a pituitary tumour. Raised follicle-stimulating hormone levels, with small testes, suggests primary testicular failure.
- *Seminal fructose levels*. Fructose is produced by the seminal vesicles, and is absent in disease of the seminal vesicles and in congenital absence of the vasa deferentia.
- *Transrectal ultrasound* is performed where a low-volume ejaculate is produced to detect obstruction.

Treatment

Non-specific measures

Non-specific measures, if no cause is found, include wearing loose-fitting underpants, avoiding hot baths and cessation of smoking and excess alcohol intake. Regular intercourse throughout the menstrual cycle is encouraged.

Surgical

Any underlying disease is treated.

- *Vasectomy reversal* is attempted.
- *An epididymal blockage* is corrected.
- *Testicular biopsy* is performed with sperm retrieval only where facilities for sperm storage exist.

The role of varicocele ligation in the treatment of male infertility is not supported by evidence.

Assisted conception

In vitro fertilization (IVF), in which fertilization of the ovum takes place outside the body, has revolutionized the treatment of infertility.

Complementary techniques include intracytoplasmic sperm injection (ICSI), microsurgical epididymal sperm aspiration, percutaneous epididymal sperm aspiration, percutaneous testicular sperm aspiration and open testicular sperm extraction. Nowadays ICSI, with sperm procurement through one of the above methods, or IVF are the treatments of choice, with birth rates per cycle of treatment of 15–20%.

Since the advent of contraceptive medication, there has been an increase in the age of planned conception with the result that more and more couples are having difficulty in conception, with fewer children available for adoption.

47

Transplantation surgery

Learning objectives

✓ To know about organ donation.

✓ To know the principles behind organ matching and immunosuppression, together with the different types of transplant and their complications.

Historical background

Early attempts at organ transplantation were fraught with failure owing to a lack of appreciation of the immune response that resulted in rapid destruction of the transplanted organ. It was not until 1954 that successful replacement of a diseased organ with a transplanted organ occurred, when the immune response was bypassed by performing kidney transplants between identical twins. In 1960, the first immunosuppressive drugs were used with which the immune response could be partly controlled, permitting longer useful function of organs from unrelated donors. In the subsequent decade, regular haemodialysis, and later peritoneal dialysis, became increasingly available, able to support patients with kidney failure while awaiting transplantation. In the 1980s, the more powerful immunosuppressant ciclosporin permitted transplantation of the liver, heart, lungs and pancreas, and afforded better results following kidney transplantation. With the advances in immunosuppression, better techniques of organ preservation and improved anaesthetic and intensive care management, organ transplantation to replace diseased organs is now an accepted treatment offering transplant recipients the possibility of long-term survival.

Lecture Notes: General Surgery, 12th edition. © Harold Ellis, Sir Roy Y. Calne and Christopher J. E. Watson. Published 2011 by Blackwell Publishing Ltd.

Classification of grafts

- *Autograft*: transplant from one part of the body to another, e.g. skin graft.
- *Allograft*: between members of the same species, e.g. human to human.
- *Isograft*: between identical twins.
- *Xenograft*: between members of different species, e.g. pig to human.
- *Structural grafts*: act as a non-living scaffold. Can be of biological origin (e.g. arterial and heart valve grafts) or synthetic (e.g. Dacron vascular prosthesis).

In addition to classifying a graft according to its source, organ grafts are also classified according to where they are implanted relative to the native organ.

- *Orthotopic*: the diseased organ is removed and replaced by the transplanted organ lying in the normal anatomical position, e.g. heart, lung and liver transplants are usually orthotopic.
- *Heterotopic*: the transplanted organ is placed in a different position from the normal anatomical position, e.g. kidney and pancreas transplants. The diseased organ is not usually removed.

This chapter will discuss organ allografts for the functional replacement of diseased organs such as kidney, liver, heart, lungs and pancreas.

Organ donors

There are two potential sources of donor organs.

Living donors

Living donation is possible when removal of either a paired organ (e.g. the kidney) or part of an unpaired organ (e.g. the liver or lung) leaves the donor with sufficient residual organ function, and provides an organ or part of an organ for a recipient. Live donation is most common in kidney transplantation, in which the donor can maintain adequate renal function with only one kidney and donate the other to a relative, partner or, less commonly, a friend. As with any operation, there are risks to the donor, especially of postoperative events such as chest and wound infection, deep vein thrombosis and pulmonary embolism; the risk of death following kidney donation is estimated to be between 1 in 1600 and 1 in 3200. In the UK, there are now more living kidney donors than deceased kidney donors. Donation of a portion of the liver, either to a child or to another adult, involves a major operation and runs the risk of leaving the donor with borderline liver function from the remaining liver lobe; the risk of death following donation of a liver lobe is estimated at between 1 in 100 and 1 in 200. Live donation of a lung lobe is also possible, the recipients usually being children.

Deceased donors

There are two types of organ donation from deceased donors:

Donation after brain stem death

Most organs for transplantation come from donors who have sustained a lethal brain injury following a head injury, intracranial haemorrhage or primary brain tumour, and who have been certified dead by 'brain stem' criteria (Chapter 15, p. 125). The organs are removed from the donor in the operating theatre after isolating their vascular pedicles and while the heart is still beating; when circulation ceases the organs are rapidly cooled by perfusion *in situ* with an ice-cold organ-preservation solution.

Donation after cardiac death (non-heart-beating donation)

When patients have sustained a catastrophic brain injury, but do not fulfil the criteria for the diagnosis of death by brain stem criteria, the supervising doctors may nevertheless decide that future treatment is futile. In such circumstances life-supporting treatment is withdrawn and the patient dies, death being certified by the absence of a circulation. Following cardiac arrest the donor is transferred to the operating theatre, where the organs are rapidly cooled, perfused with preservation solution and removed. Unlike organs from brain dead donors, organs removed from donors after cardiac death suffer a period of warm ischaemia prior to cooling. During this period, the organs switch from aerobic to anaerobic metabolism, which depletes intracellular energy stores and causes the accumulation of lactic acid. Unchecked, this process rapidly results in cell death. Organs vary in their tolerance of warm ischaemia, with kidneys remaining viable for about 60 minutes whereas the liver tolerates less than 30 minutes. In such cases, the initial function of the organs is inferior to those removed following brain stem death, but the ultimate function is satisfactory.

Exclusions to organ donation

There are three main reasons why a potential donor may be unsuitable.

1 *Potential transmission of infection.* The transplanted organ could carry with it viral infections such as hepatitis B and C and human immunodeficiency virus, and any bacterial infection that was disseminated in the donor. Likewise, donors in whom there is a risk of prion infection such as new variant Creutzfeldt–Jakob disease are unsuitable.
2 *Malignancy.* Malignant disease in the donor can be transplanted into the recipient, where it may become established in the immunosuppressed environment. Therefore, with the exception of low-grade primary brain tumours (which do not spread outside the central nervous system) and superficial non-melanoma skin tumours, active

malignancy is a contraindication to organ donation.

3 *Impaired function of donor organ.* If the function of the organ is impaired in the donor, it is unsuitable for transplantation. For example, a heart with severe coronary artery disease is unsuitable, while a donor with polycystic kidneys is an unsuitable kidney donor but may be a suitable heart donor.

Organ preservation

Once removed from the donor, the organs must be maintained in their optimum state prior to transfusion. This is achieved by a combination of (1) cooling the organ to approximately 4°C to reduce metabolic activity and (2) perfusing it with, and storing it in, a preservation solution that contains a pH buffer to counter the lactic acid accumulation and a compound to prevent cell swelling by osmosis. One such solution is the University of Wisconsin (UW) solution. In this solution, a kidney can be preserved for 36–40 hours, and a liver for up to 20 hours, although in both cases the shortest possible preservation period, or *cold ischaemia time* (the time between cessation of circulation in the donor and implantation in the recipient), is desirable. No comparable preservation solution exists for the heart and lungs, and implantation must occur within 4–6 hours, to ensure immediate life-sustaining function of these organs. An alternative for kidney preservation is to place the organ on a machine that continuously pumps ice-cold preservation fluid through it.

Organ recipients

Patients are considered for transplantation when they are in chronic organ failure without hope of recovery, but still fit enough to withstand the operative procedure. For kidney transplantation, potential transplant recipients should be on or about to start dialysis. Patients with chronic liver disease are placed on the transplant waiting list when their liver disease warrants, such that their risk of death without a transplant is greater than the risk of death following transplantation. For example, in patients with primary biliary cirrhosis,

an elevation of serum bilirubin concentration over 100 μmol/L is an indication for transplantation. In acute liver failure, transplantation is indicated if the synthetic function of the liver is severely impaired, as best reflected by the degree of elevation of prothrombin time.

The immunology of organ transplantation

The major histocompatibility complex

When an organ is transplanted, it is recognized as foreign by the host's immune system and the rejection response is initiated. The recognition is mediated by an interaction between host T lymphocytes (T cells) and histocompatibility antigens on the surface of the allograft (the foreign organ). The major histocompatibility complex (MHC) is a group of genes that encode molecules (antigens) expressed on the surface of cells. The MHC molecules are of two principal sorts. MHC class I antigens are present on all nucleated cells. MHC class II antigens are present on certain cells (e.g. macrophages, monocytes and dendritic cells), and can be induced to appear on others by the presence of cytokines such as interferon γ (IFN-γ).

The human leucocyte antigen system

The human leucocyte antigen (HLA) system describes the locus on chromosome 6 containing the genes encoding the MHC antigens in the human. HLA-A, -B and -C loci encode class I molecules, whereas class II molecules are encoded by HLA-DP, -DQ and -DR loci. The extensive polymorphism at the loci, in particular the A and B loci, results in differences in the MHC antigens on allografts recognized by the host lymphocytes.

Organ matching

There are three levels of organ matching that can be performed, of which ABO matching is required for all transplants. Lymphocytotoxic cross-matching is required in recipients who have previously been exposed to other HLA antigens following previous blood transfusions or transplants or in childbirth. MHC matching is at present restricted to kidneys, where the availability of dialysis enables recipients to wait for an optimally matched kidney, and the better tolerance of cold ischaemia provides the necessary time required to tissue type the donor organ and move it between centres to the best-matched recipient. This system requires central coordination of a large pool of recipients and donors which, in the UK, is based in Bristol.

ABO matching

Just like blood transfusions, the existence of preformed ABO antibodies means that the transplanted organs must be ABO compatible. Thus, while a group A recipient can have an organ from either a group A or group O donor, a group O recipient can have only a group O organ because of the presence of preformed antibodies to group A (and B) antigens. Crossing the ABO barrier results in hyperacute rejection except in the case of the liver, which is relatively resistant to this process. Nevertheless, abiding by the ABO rules is also advisable in liver transplantation since the long-term outcome is better.

Crossing the ABO barrier is possible without hyperacute rejection in certain circumstances. In children, the development of anti-A and anti-B antibodies does not occur until after the first year. It is thus possible to perform ABO-mismatched heart transplants in very young children with excellent results. Some adults have low titres of ABO antibody, which can be removed immediately prior to an ABO-mismatched kidney transplant from a live donor.

Lymphocytotoxic cross-match

To detect circulating antibodies in the recipient against donor HLA antigens, a direct lymphocytotoxic cross-match is performed. This involves mixing donor cells (lymphocytes) from peripheral blood, lymph node or spleen with the recipient's serum in the presence of rabbit complement and observing for cytolysis. Alternatively, the presence of anti-donor antibodies can be detected using flow cytometry. Presence of such antibodies in the cross-match test is associated with hyperacute rejection; hence, a positive cross-match is a contraindication to transplantation of all organs (except the liver).

MHC matching

In order to minimize the immune response to an organ allograft, the recipient's MHC antigens can be matched to the donor. The best matching, in fact perfect matching, comes from an identical twin. The inheritance of MHC antigens follows Mendelian genetics,[1] and the antigens are codominantly expressed with a degree of linkage. Therefore, within a family, there is a one in four chance that two siblings will share the same MHC antigens; a one in two chance of them differing by one haplotype; and a one in four chance of them inheriting a completely different set of HLA antigens. One in four living related sibling donors will thus offer a significant immunological advantage by complete HLA identity.

Unrelated donor–recipient pairs are also matched with a view to minimizing differences between MHC antigens. Three HLA loci, A, B and DR, are specifically considered. The object of organ matching is to reduce the number of mismatched antigens out of the six possible MHC antigens encoded by the three loci. This strategy has been shown to be beneficial for renal transplantation. Retrospective analysis has also shown a benefit of matching for the survival of heart transplants, but the short preservation time prevents prospective matching.

Rejection

Hyperacute rejection

Patients may develop antibodies to foreign HLA molecules following exposure to them during childbirth, blood transfusion or a previous transplant. When the recipient has preformed antibodies to HLA or ABO blood group antigens on the donor, the recipient antibody (HLA or ABO) binds to the donor cells, triggering graft destruction in minutes or hours.

Acute rejection

Acute rejection occurs when the initial dose of immunosuppression is inadequate to prevent the recipient's immune system attacking the graft. Clinically, acute rejection is characterized by a

[1]Gregor Mendel (1882–1884), Augustinian Priest and Scientist, St Thomas's Abbey, Brno, Czech Republic.

pyrexia, enlargement and tenderness over the transplanted organ, and biochemical dysfunction (a rise in creatinine in a kidney transplant, elevated liver enzymes in a liver transplant). It is confirmed by biopsy of the organ. The most common time for acute rejection is between 5 and 28 days after transplantation, and it usually responds to an increase in immunosuppression.

Chronic rejection

Chronic rejection, more properly termed chronic allograft damage, is an insidious process of graft attrition, which generally results in graft loss. It is characterized by a progressive vasculopathy in the graft, the aetiology of which is related to tissue compatibility between donor and recipient, to the immunosuppression, to damage to the graft during the transplant, to hypertension and possibly also to infection of the graft by cytomegalovirus. Although the vascular lesions are broadly similar in different organs, the time-course is not. In liver transplantation, chronic rejection may occur as early as the first month, whereas in kidney and heart transplantation it usually occurs after the first year.

Principles of immunosuppressive therapy

Immunosuppressive therapy following organ transplantation is a balance between giving enough drug to prevent rejection, but not too much to make the patient susceptible to opportunist infection. In addition, individual drugs have their own undesirable side-effects, which may be reduced by combining drugs with different modes of action and with different side-effect profiles, rather as is done with cancer chemotherapy regimens. A common protocol would be to combine a steroid (e.g. prednisolone) with an anti-nucleotide such as azathioprine or mycophenolate and an inhibitor of T-cell activation such as ciclosporin or tacrolimus, the so-called 'triple therapy'.

There are two other factors that influence immunosuppressive therapy. Some organs, such as intestine and lung, have an increased susceptibility to rejection, so higher doses of immunosuppression are required. Second, with most organs,

after the initial few months the incidence of rejection is much less as the graft undergoes a degree of acceptance, so the total amount of immunosuppression may be reduced. This may be achieved either by reducing the dosage of the agents used or by discontinuing one or more of the initial immunosuppressive agents.

Complications of transplantation

Following transplantation, the complications can be divided into early (those occurring in hospital) and late.

Early complications

Early complications may be related to the four components of the transplant procedure.

1 *The surgical operation*, such as wound infection, anastomotic breakdown and vascular anastomotic thrombosis.
2 *The quality of the organ*, dependent both on the donor organ and on the quality of the preservation, in particular the age of the donor and the duration of ischaemia. A donor organ with a long cold ischaemic time would be expected to perform less well initially.
3 *The immunological response* of the recipient to the donor (acute rejection).
4 *The effects of immunosuppression*. Initially, high doses of immunosuppression are used, and it is in the early stages that the infective complications of immunosuppression are seen, in particular wound and chest infections; viral infections such as herpes simplex (cold sores) are also common early after transplant.

Late complications

The late complications of transplantation are either immunological, related to the immunosuppression, or the result of recurrent disease.

1 *Immunological complications* include acute and chronic rejection.
2 *Immunosuppressive complications* reflect the difficulty in achieving immunosuppression sufficient to stop rejection, but low enough to stop adverse effects. Such complications include the following:

a drug side-effects, e.g. nephrotoxicity of ciclosporin and tacrolimus;

b infection occurs more commonly, particularly opportunist infections such as *Pneumocystis jiroveci* (formerly *P. carinii*) and cytomegalovirus;

c malignancy, which is more common after transplantation, particularly virus-related tumours such as Epstein–Barr[2] virus-related lymphomas and squamous carcinomas of the skin (in which human papilloma virus DNA can often be isolated).

3 *Recurrent disease.* In some cases, the original disease may recur in the transplanted organ. For example, glomerulonephropathies such as immunoglobulin A nephropathy and focal segmental glomerulosclerosis recur in the transplanted kidney; hepatitis B and C viruses reinfect the transplanted liver.

Results in clinical organ transplantation

Kidney transplantation

Kidney transplantation has been a routine treatment for over 30 years, and there are several survivors with transplants functioning for that period. In the UK, 2500 kidney transplants are performed annually, with over 7000 people on dialysis awaiting transplantation. The shortfall in supply is reflected worldwide.

The kidney is transplanted heterotopically into the iliac fossa, with the donor renal vessels anastomosed to the external iliac vessels of the recipient, and the donor ureter anastomosed to the bladder directly to produce a new ureteric orifice. Unless the recipient's own kidneys are a danger to the recipient (e.g. a source of infection) they are left *in situ*.

As with other organ transplants, results are usually quoted in terms of 1 year and 5 year graft survival, in which the losses in the first 12 months are higher and reflect the early complications, whereas the 5 year figures reflect the rate of chronic losses from recurrent disease or chronic rejection. One year graft survival following renal

transplantation is between 90% and 95%, and is over 99% when the kidney resulted from an HLA-identical sibling donation. Thereafter, there is a gradual loss of around 3% per annum, giving a 5 year survival of 70–80% (better still for related grafts).

Pancreas transplantation

It is likely that transplantation for the treatment of diabetes will eventually involve β-cells or islets, possibly with the help of genetic engineering, but, although several hundred islet grafts have so far been attempted in humans, long-term results have been poor until recently. Better short-term and long-term results follow transplantation of the vascularized pancreas. However, pancreatic transplantation involves a large operation, the principal complications of which include graft pancreatitis and consequent peritonitis as well as graft thrombosis. The favoured technique is to place the pancreas in the iliac fossa vascularized from the iliac vessels, with the exocrine drainage into a loop of small intestine.

Diabetic nephropathy is the main indication for pancreas grafting and is usually combined with a kidney transplant from the same donor. Approximately 70% of grafts are functioning after 3 years. There is accumulating evidence that combined kidney and pancreas transplantation prolongs life in patients with type 1 diabetes and renal failure compared with kidney transplantation alone, in addition to reducing the number of cardiovascular events and improving other diabetic complications such as autonomic neuropathy.

Liver transplantation

Liver transplantation is the treatment of choice for many forms of fatal liver disease. Patients are offered the operation before they become too sick for what is the most formidable of surgical assaults. The three main indications for liver transplantation are:

1 *complications of cirrhosis*: hepatocellular carcinoma, recurrent variceal haemorrhage, intractable ascites and poor synthetic function;

2 *acute hepatic necrosis*, e.g. paracetamol poisoning;

3 *metabolic disease*, e.g. oxalosis (in which kidney grafting may also be required).

---

[2]Michael Anthony Epstein (b. 1921), Professor of Pathology, University of Bristol, Bristol, UK. Yvonne Barr (b. 1932), Epstein's assistant, Middlesex Hospital, London, UK.

Around 85–90% of liver transplant recipients survive for 1 year, and the 5 year figure is around 70%, with a lower annual loss than kidney transplants after the first year.

Heart, lung and combined heart–lung transplantation

Heart transplantation is a relatively straightforward operative procedure in a unit where open heart surgery is performed. The main indications are atherosclerotic coronary artery disease and cardiomyopathy. Solitary lung transplantation without the heart is more common than combined heart–lung transplantation in which both lungs are transplanted *en bloc* with the heart; in the latter case, only three anastomoses are required, namely aortic, tracheal and right atrial. The most common indications for lung transplantation are primary pulmonary hypertension, chronic obstructive airways disease and cystic fibrosis. The survival of recipients of both heart and combined heart and lung grafts is approximately 70% at 3 years.

Index

Lecture Notes: General Surgery, 12th edition. © Harold Ellis,
Sir Roy Y. Calne and Christopher J. E. Watson. Published 2011 by
Blackwell Publishing Ltd.